Bipolar II Disorder

Modelling, Measuring and Managing

Bipolar Disorder is now more commonly viewed as a spectrum of conditions rather than a single disease entity. Bipolar II Disorder exists on this spectrum as a condition where the depressive episodes are as severe as in Bipolar I Disorder, but where the mood elevation states are not as extreme, often leading to failure to detect a condition thought to affect up to 6% of the population.

This book reviews, for the first time, our knowledge of this debilitating disorder, covering its history, classification and neurobiology. In a unique section, fourteen internationally recognised experts debate management strategies, building to some consensus, and resulting in treatment guidelines where no such advice currently exists. It should be read by all health professionals managing mood disorders and will also be informative to those with Bipolar II who wish to learn more about the condition.

Gordon Parker is Scientia Professor at the School of Psychiatry, University of New South Wales and Executive Director of the Black Dog Institute.

Bipolar II Disorder

Modelling, Measuring and Managing

Edited by

Gordon Parker

Scientia Professor, School of Psychiatry, University of New South Wales;
Executive Director, Black Dog Institute, Sydney, Australia

With the editorial assistance of

Kerrie Eyers

Publications Consultant, Black Dog Institute, Sydney, Australia

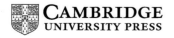

CAMBRIDGE
UNIVERSITY PRESS

CAMBRIDGE UNIVERSITY PRESS
Cambridge, New York, Melbourne, Madrid, Cape Town, Singapore, São Paulo,
Delhi, Dubai, Tokyo

Cambridge University Press
The Edinburgh Building, Cambridge CB2 8RU, UK

Published in the United States of America by Cambridge University Press, New York

www.cambridge.org
For information on this title: www.cambridge.org/9780521123587

© Cambridge University Press 2008

First published 2008
First paperback edition 2009

Printed in the United Kingdom at the University Press, Cambridge

A catalogue record for this publication is available from the British Library

ISBN 978-0-521-87314-7 hardback
ISBN 978-0-521-12358-7 paperback

Contents

List of contributors   *page* viii
Preface
Gordon Parker   xi

Introduction
Gordon Parker   1

1   Bipolar disorder in historical perspective
Edward Shorter   5

2   The bipolar spectrum
James Phelps   15

3   Defining and measuring Bipolar II Disorder
Gordon Parker   46

4   Bipolar II Disorder in context: epidemiology, disability and economic burden
George Hadjipavlou and Lakshmi N. Yatham   61

5   Is Bipolar II Disorder increasing in prevalence?
Gordon Parker and Kathryn Fletcher   75

6   The neurobiology of Bipolar II Disorder
Gin S. Malhi   83

7   The role of antidepressants in managing Bipolar II Disorder
Joseph F. Goldberg   94

8   The use of SSRIs as mood stabilisers for Bipolar II Disorder
Gordon Parker   107

9   Mood stabilisers in the treatment of Bipolar II Disorder
George Hadjipavlou and Lakshmi N. Yatham   120

10   The use of atypical antipsychotic drugs in Bipolar II Disorder
David Fresno and Eduard Vieta   133

11   The role of fish oil in managing Bipolar II Disorder
Anne-Marie Rees and Gordon Parker   141

12   The role of psychological interventions in managing Bipolar II Disorder
Vijaya Manicavasagar   151

13   The role of wellbeing plans in managing Bipolar II Disorder
Margo Orum   177

14   Survival strategies for managing and prospering with Bipolar II Disorder
Meg Smith   195

15   A clinical model for managing Bipolar II Disorder
Gordon Parker   204

16   Management commentary
Terence A. Ketter and Po W. Wang   217

17   Management commentary
Franco Benazzi   232

18   Management commentary
Michael Berk   237

19   Management commentary
Eduard Vieta   240

20   Management commentary
Philip B. Mitchell   244

21   Management commentary
Joseph F. Goldberg   247

22   Management commentary
Robert M. Post   252

23   Management commentary
Allan H. Young   259

24 Management commentary
Guy M. Goodwin 262

25 Management commentary
Sophia Frangou 265

26 Management commentary: What would Hippocrates do?
S. Nassir Ghaemi 269

27 Management commentary
Michael E. Thase 278

28 Rounding up and tying down
Gordon Parker 282

Appendix 1: Black Dog Institute Self-test for Bipolar Disorder:
The Mood Swings Questionnaire 296
Index 298

Contributors

Franco Benazzi
Hecker Psychiatry Research Center,
Forli, Italy

Michael Berk
Barwon Health and The Geelong Clinic,
University of Melbourne,
Victoria, Australia; Orygen Youth Health;
Mental Health Research Institute,
Melbourne, Australia

Kathryn Fletcher
School of Psychiatry, University of
New South Wales;
Black Dog Institute, Sydney, Australia

Sophia Frangou
Section of Neurobiology of Psychosis,
Institute of Psychiatry,
London, UK

David Fresno
Bipolar Disorders Programme,
University of Barcelona Hospital Clinic,
Barcelona, Spain

S. Nassir Ghaemi
Emory University,
Atlanta, USA

Joe Goldberg
Mount Sinai School of Medicine,
New York; Affective Disorders Program,
Silver Hill Hospital,
New Canaan, USA

Guy M. Goodwin
Department of Psychiatry,
University of Oxford,
Warneford Hospital,
Oxford, UK

George Hadjipavlou
Department of Psychiatry,
University of British Columbia,
Vancouver, Canada

Terence A. Ketter
Bipolar Disorders Clinic,
Stanford University School of Medicine,
Stanford, USA

Gin S. Malhi
CADE Clinic,
Department of Psychiatry,
Northern Clinical School,
University of Sydney;
Black Dog Institute,
Sydney, Australia

Vijaya Manicavasagar
School of Psychiatry,
University of New South Wales;
Psychological Services,
Black Dog Institute,
Sydney, Australia

Philip B. Mitchell
School of Psychiatry,
University of New South Wales;
Black Dog Institute,
Sydney, Australia

Margo Orum
Black Dog Institute,
Sydney, Australia

Gordon Parker
School of Psychiatry,
University of New South Wales;
Black Dog Institute,
Sydney, Australia

James Phelps
PsychEducation.org; Co-Psych.com

Robert M. Post
Department of Psychiatry,
Penn State College of Medicine,
Hershey;
Bipolar Collaborative Network, USA

Anne-Marie Rees
School of Psychiatry,
University of New South Wales;
Black Dog Institute,
Sydney, Australia

Edward Shorter
Department of Psychiatry,
Faculty of Medicine,
University of Toronto,
Ontario, Canada

Meg Smith
University of Western Sydney,
Penrith South;
Black Dog Institute,
Sydney, Australia

Michael Thase
Department of Psychiatry,
University of Pennsylvania School of
Medicine and University of Pittsburgh
Medical Center,
Philadelphia, USA

Eduard Vieta
Bipolar Disorders Programme,
University of Barcelona Hospital Clinic,
Barcelona, Spain

Po W. Wang
Department of Psychiatry and Behavioral
Sciences, and Bipolar Disorders Clinic,
Stanford University School of Medicine,
California, USA

Lakshmi N. Yatham
Mood Disorders Centre,
University of British Columbia,
Vancouver, Canada

Allan H. Young
Department of Psychiatry,
University of British Columbia,
Vancouver, Canada

Preface

Gordon Parker

This is, we believe, the first monograph focusing on Bipolar II Disorder by itself. 'By itself' raising an obvious question. If Bipolar II is a true mood disorder, is distinctly more common than Bipolar I (or manic depressive illness) but has comparable disability, sequelae and suicide rates, why has it not invited any previous definitive overview? The answer will be quickly apparent to readers.

Firstly, Bipolar II is a relatively 'new' condition, in the sense of it being defined and detailed only over the last few decades. Secondly, its status as a 'condition' is challenged by many. Thirdly, its detection by professionals is low and delayed. Fourthly, it is commonly viewed as a mild condition (e.g. 'bipolar lite'), and as therefore of little consequence in terms of its differentiation from unipolar depression. Fifthly, there are no treatment guidelines for its management, with clinical management – if conceding such a diagnosis – generally extrapolating strategies from the management of Bipolar I Disorder.

Most psychiatric monographs are written when there is a bank of knowledge. Not on this occasion. Here, author after author, all with expertise in the bipolar disorders, note the lack of a clear knowledge base and of any formalised clinical guidelines. This book was designed, however, to detail both what is currently known or debated, and what needs to be clarified. We aim to provide an advance on current clinical management, which has had to operate largely within a vacuum over the last decade – despite rapidly increasing interest in Bipolar II Disorder.

This book proceeds in two broad ways. To begin with, individual chapters review specific issues of relevance. All are informative but there is a predictable lack of integration as each writer addresses their specialist domain. Next, an unusual strategy, a set of international researchers turn from simply interpreting research studies, to considering the clinical nuances that *they* have observed. We learn what they actually do on a day-to-day basis, and their management recommendations. Personal views iterate with thoughtful interpretations of the literature. The tone is consequently quite different to most clinical overviews. Rather than reference, rely on and often reify previously published treatment guidelines, here the writers bring freshness to their clinical observations – providing new knowledge rather than overviewing old information. Despite some disparate individual views, it is possible to observe integration emerging, but without the collective tone of a 'consensus conference' – which often reflects the majority lining up with the views articulated by the most dominant and charismatic members.

The two sections – respectively prioritising literature overviews and clinical observation – combine to provide management strategies that should assist clinicians. Such strategies are not 'black and white', nor beyond debate and challenge, and are not necessarily easy to assimilate – but it is rich material that provides as many hypotheses for clinicians as for researchers. Most importantly, most of the multiple treatment options considered and questioned by clinicians are examined – so that this monograph should prove of practical use to clinicians and many who suffer from this condition.

A brief overview of the book. We start with an introduction – a young man's essay captures the day-to-day oscillations experienced by those with Bipolar II Disorder. Of greater salience is the tone of the writing. The reader can detect the exuberant chords and cadences of an individual communicating during a 'high' – a quality which is sometimes palpable in patients during their first visit and which may alert the clinician to the possibility of a bipolar mood disorder. This personal story sets a scene in many ways.

The first six chapters overview historical, definitional, classification and measurement issues, consider epidemiological nuances, and identify the limited research examining neurobiological underpinnings to Bipolar II Disorder. The status of Bipolar II Disorder is considered, from its 'non-existence', to it being a discrete categorical type, or its lying within a spectrum, and that it may even exist in the absence of any elevated mood states. Such thoughtful considerations of its status (most evident in Chapter 2) help explain why Bipolar II Disorder has long resisted encapsulation. The chapters following on from these six provide contemporary overviews of a number of possible management strategies, including psychotropic drugs (i.e. antidepressants in general, SSRIs, mood stabilisers, and antipsychotics), fish oil, and psychological interventions, and two chapters consider wellbeing plans and survival strategies.

In Chapter 15, one model for managing Bipolar II Disorder is presented – as a template for consideration and debate by a number of international experts – with their astute independent observations allowing some integration. By close, I suggest that we can no longer view ourselves as having little understanding of the condition. Consensus may not have been achieved, but that is rarely truly achievable in psychiatry. Agreement on many issues is clearly evident. While ambiguities remain, many have now been defined and their parameters are marked out for resolution by researchers and sharp clinical observations. The hope then is that this book will not only be helpful to clinicians in their daily practice but also to the research community in highlighting key questions that remain to be answered.

I would like to express my appreciation to a number of people. My particular thanks to the many authors who willingly responded to the demands involved in preparing this book, and who provided thoughtful, comprehensive and informative chapters. Then to Kerrie Eyers, who, as in-house editor, has rigorously and precisely edited the volume; and to my secretary Yvonne Foy, who has addressed the multiple administrative demands responsively and smoothly. Many thanks to Black Dog Institute colleagues (Kathryn Fletcher, Dusan Hadzi-Pavlovic, Gin Malhi, Vijaya Manicavasagar, Philip Mitchell, Amanda Olley, Anne-Marie Rees, Meg Smith, Lucy Tully) who contributed to the research underpinning my chapters and to independent chapters. My gratitude to the editors and publishers of the *American Journal of Psychiatry* and *Journal of Affective Disorders* for permission to republish from papers published in their journal, and to Allen & Unwin publishers for permission to republish the 'D club' essay. Sincere appreciation to Richard Marley, Alison Evans and Lesley Bennun of Cambridge University Press for their professional excellence at every stage of this production. Finally, I salute my wife Heather, for her support and graciousness in allowing me the time to write.

Introduction

Gordon Parker

In 2005, the Black Dog Institute held an essay competition, inviting those who had experienced the 'black dog' to describe how they lived with and mastered their depression. Most individuals portrayed depressive episodes with classic melancholic features – with a number of these individuals also depicting 'highs' indicative of bipolar disorder. One such essay is published here. There are several reasons for its reproduction in this forum. Firstly, it is delightfully written. Secondly, its writ large tone is informative. Its author bursts into print with the energy, exuberance and creativity of a 'high', followed shortly by a sombre description of the anergia and enervating blackness of depression. In essence, the essay's structure depicts the roller coaster ride experienced by so many with bipolar disorder. Thirdly, while the author was aware of his depression – his membership of the 'D Club' – he was not aware (raised in subsequent discussion) of the possibility of having bipolar disorder. As detailed through this book, many individuals experience Bipolar II Disorder for decades before receiving an accurate diagnosis – while many others never receive such a diagnosis. It is the depression (the big 'D') that perturbs their lives and drives them to present for treatment of the lows. But bipolar disorder missed is bipolar disorder mis-managed. Fourthly, this essay is beautifully multi-layered. The author captures the enormity of depression but, in being quintessentially upbeat, he demonstrates true resilience, and is touchingly devoid of self-pity.

While this essay captures the factual day-to-day existence of the Bipolar II world, the tone provides the signature chord heard in the conversational style of many who experience Bipolar II Disorder. My gratitude to this Australian writer for allowing his essay to be published anonymously below.

The 'D' Club

I'm the perfect party guest. Put me anywhere and I'll energise. Sit me next to the nerd and we'll be digitising computers and code, saddle me up to an artist and it'll

Bipolar II Disorder. Modelling, Measuring and Managing, ed. Gordon Parker. Published by Cambridge University Press. © Cambridge University Press 2008.

be all art house and film noir, introduce me to a mum and we'll be gushing over the newborn. Well, until baby needs a nappy change. Yep, I'm an energetic kind of guy. I'm into things. All things. Passion is my mantra. Be passionate – be proud. T'is cool. T'is sexy. What's more, people respond. I ask questions. They give me answers. It's like I have a truth serum aura or something. My intuition is strong, it is real, it is Instinct . . . it is David Beckham.

Well now that you have my RSVP profile and we're on intimate terms, I can tell you a little secret. A kind of friend for life, confidant, I trust you a whole lot, secret – I'm not always the bundle of kilowatts you see before you. I'm not always the interested, interesting persona that invigorates and epitomises the successful young professional – the man about town who's hip, happening, sporty and fashionable.

Yep, while I sit here typing this on my new ultra-portable, carbon-coated, wireless notebook, because looks are important, I am reminded of my darkest hours. 'My achey breaky heart' hours. And I hated that song from Billy Ray Cyrus and his mullet. Only a few months ago I finished Series 5 of 'Desperate Individuals'. It's my own spin-off from 'Desperate Housewives', except with a limited budget there were no major co-stars or Wysteria Lane . . . just a cast of two, with my sofa taking the supporting role.

Truth be known, my sofa deserves a Logie. A Logie for the best supporting furniture in a clinically depressed episode. Oh Logie schmogie. My sofa does what it always does when I'm alone in my depressive mindlessness. Cradles me, protects me and warms me. We've become quite acquainted over the years since my late teens. We hide from the phone together, cry together and starve together. Ain't that a shit! I have a relationship with a couple of cushions. At least they cushion me from a world I can no longer face, expectations I can no longer live up to, productivity that has left me behind. It makes for good television. Because my life as a depressive is today's cable. It's 100% reality. It's repetitive. It's boring. It's cheap. It's a mockumentary to everyone but the participant. My sofa doesn't eat, you can tell that from the crumbs under the cushions, and with clinical depression, I'm not hungry either so we're a perfect match. Food? My tongue is numb and I can't taste anything so why bother.

Looking back, it's hard to see when each period of depression started. That's because most depressive episodes end up being a blur; a juvenile alcoholic stupor forgetting the hours between midnight and 4 am, except in my mental state it's a whopping six months that are hazy and foreign. Seconds don't exist in my world of depressive dryness. Seconds have become hours. Hours are now days. Months are lost in a timeless void of nothingness. No sleep, no interest, no energy. And it is here that life becomes its most challenging. Don't get me wrong, I'm all for the comfortable picture theatre vicarious experience with stadium seating and pop-corn. I just wish depression was a two-hour affair on a cold Sunday afternoon instead of the rigor-mortic torture that makes it too painful to stay in bed, but even more painful to get up.

Depression is incoherence – the death of wellbeing, direction and life. Everything aches. Everything! Your head. Your eyes. Your heart. Your soul. Your skin aches. Can you smell it? Oh yeah, ache smells and I've reeked of it. My grandmother ached. She told me just before she died of cancer. From then on I saw the ache in her eyes. Sometimes in the middle of a depressive episode, I see it in mine. To look in the mirror and see your own total despair is . . . horrendous.

Now all of this is sounding downright pessimistic and I mustn't dwell on the pain of the past. After all, I'm here to tell my story when many others are not. For I write this not to recapitulate history but to shed a little light on an illness that will affect so many at some time in their life.

For those of you who have been or are currently clinically depressed, welcome to the club – the members-only D Club. Here's your card and welcome letter, and don't forget that we have a loyalty programme. You get points for seeking help, points for talking to friends and family, and points for looking after yourself.

Now news headlines would count the economic cost of depression, which is in the billions, but from a human perspective, it's simply a hell of a lot of agony.

The good news is that public perceptions, which not long ago relegated mental illness to that of social taboo, are slowly being broken. Courage, dignity and honesty can be used to describe former Western Australian Premier Dr Geoff Gallop's address detailing his depression at the start of 2006. Here's a small excerpt:

'It is my difficult duty to inform you today that I am currently being treated for depression. Living with depression is a very debilitating experience, which affects different people in different ways. It has certainly affected many aspects of my life. So much so, that I sought expert help last week. My doctors advised me that with treatment, time and rest this illness is very curable. However, I cannot be certain how long I will need. So in the interests of my health and my family I have decided to rethink my career. I now need that time to restore my health and wellbeing. Therefore I am announcing today my intention to resign as Premier of Western Australia.'

Stories like Dr Gallop's allow more of us to talk about how depression can affect our health, jobs, families, partners and friends. It's not a sign of weakness to express our inability to function mentally. It is in fact a sign of courage, openness, sincerity and trust. It is not unusual for those of us who have or are suffering from depression to feel guilty as if we have somehow brought this illness on ourselves, that we are weak, it's all in our head, or that we're somehow protecting those around us by hiding our mental paralysis. Truth be known, so many of us are lost in today's frenetic lifestyle that we don't see the signs of unhappiness and helplessness in our loved ones. Sometimes it takes a meltdown to even see it in ourselves. But it is only through acknowledging mental illness that we can get treatment and start to finally feel better. Who would've thought that asking for help would be so hard? For someone suffering from clinical depression, just to talk can be exhausting. During my last episode, I had repeating visions of falling asleep on my grandmother's lap because there I could forget the worries of my world. Memories of her gentle hand caressing the back of my neck are safe and warm. A simple gesture can mean so much.

Today, instead of my grandmother, I have dear friends who offer to cook, clean, wash and care for me. They fight my fierce independence and depression-induced silence with frequent visits and constant dialogue. Their lives haven't stopped, they don't feel burdened and they haven't moved in. They are now simply aware that I have a mental illness, and we are closer because of it. I too have taken responsibility to seek assistance from qualified medical practitioners. Don't get me wrong, taking the first, second and third steps to get help from a doctor can be traumatic. It's not easy admitting that you're not coping with life. And finding a physician who you feel comfortable with and antidepressants that work can take time. But I am testimony that you've got to stick with it.

And so as I sit here and start to daydream as I look out of the window, I am reminded of a recent time when I lost my ability to sing, to share in laughter, to swim, to eat, to talk, to enjoy; when waking up was just as difficult as going to bed. It's a frightful place that sends shivers up my spine. However it's a fleeting memory, because Mr Passion, that energetic kind of guy is back, and he doesn't have time to dwell on the past. This D Club member is in remission and it's time to party.

Acknowledgement

The 'D' club' essay was originally published in *Journeys with the Black Dog: Inspirational Stories of Bringing Depression to Heel*, edited by Tessa Wigney, Kerrie Eyers and Gordon Parker. Allen & Unwin, 2007.

REFERENCE

Dr Geoff Gallop (2006). Press release. Statement from the Premier of Western Australia. Content authorised by the Government Media Office, Department of the Premier and Cabinet, 16 January.

Bipolar disorder in historical perspective

Edward Shorter

Psychiatric disorders are like children laughing and playing gaily at the park, while behind a screen other children, dimly seen, cry out to us for help. We want to come to their aid but their shapes are like shadows. Nor can we locate them.

Bipolar disorder is like one of these children. We have it before us in the pharmaceutical advertising, the woman going up and down on the merry-go-round and helped with 'mood stabilizers'. Meanwhile, behind the screen there are other forms. Maybe a historical analysis will help us to see them more clearly.

Physicians have always known the alternation of melancholia and mania. The consistency of description across the ages gives the diagnosis a certain face validity, and it would be as idle to ask who was the first to describe their alternation as to ask who first described mumps. Aretaeus of Cappadocia, around 150 years after the birth of Christ, wrote of the succession of the two illnesses. It is clear from the context (Jackson, 1986, pp. 39–41) that he was using the two terms to describe what we today would consider mania and melancholia. Yet Aretaeus did not consider the alternation of mania and melancholia to be a separate disease.

For these remote centuries I use 'bipolar disorder' to mean the succession of melancholia and mania. A word of clarification: in the twentieth century, after the writings of Kleist and Leonhard, 'bipolar disorder' implies that there is a separate unipolar depressive disease. By contrast, the term 'manic-depression' suggests that there is only one depression, whether linked to mania or not. But the term manic-depression itself did not surface until 1899. To describe mania, melancholia and their alternation in previous centuries, I shall simply call it bipolar disorder and crave the reader's indulgence.

So the big question is not who first described bipolar disorder, but rather is it one disease or two? The decades and centuries of clinical experience that lie behind us constitute a mountain of evidence of some weight. And in this tremendous accumulation of practical learning, has bipolar disorder been considered one disease? Or two: the alternation of two separate diseases, mania and melancholia?

A third possibility: is bipolar disorder an alternation of several different kinds of mood disorder that includes episodes of catatonia, melancholia, psychotic

Bipolar II Disorder. Modelling, Measuring and Managing, ed. Gordon Parker. Published by Cambridge University Press. © Cambridge University Press 2008.

depression, mania and hypomania – with each an independent illness entity in its own right? Conrad Swartz has suggested that, in this kind of alternation, the term 'multipolar disorder' might be more appropriate than 'bipolar disorder' (Swartz, personal communication, 24 Oct., 2006). When we find these syndromes occurring over the years in the same patient, is it one illness or several?

For psychiatrists of the past, it was quite consistent to see melancholia cede to mania. Vincenzo Chiarugi, psychiatrist at the Bonifazio mental hospital in Florence, Italy, at the end of the eighteenth century, described a female patient, aged 35, who switched from deep melancholia to mania. Chiarugi thought this a case of 'true melancholy' and by no means out of the ordinary. The clinicians of the day often used such terms as mania and melancholia in a sense quite different from ours, yet, on the basis of the case report (Chiarugi, 1794, pp. 95–96), Chiarugi was dealing with manic-depression.

In the world of patients as well, alternating mania and melancholia have been known since time immemorial. As Thomas Penrose, the curate of Newbury in Berkshire, England, penned (Penrose 1775, p. 19) in the 1780s of a young woman disappointed in love:

Dim haggard looks, and clouded o'er with care,
Point out to Pity's tears, the poor distracted fair.
Dead to the world – her fondest wishes crossed
She mourns herself thus early lost.

Now, sadly gay, of sorrows past she sings,
Now, pensive, ruminates unutterable things.
She starts – she flies – who dares so rude
On her sequester'd steps intrude?

In the Voitsberg district of Austria early in the nineteenth century, such alternations of melancholia and mania were regarded by the valley dwellers as quite typical, and one of the features that distinguished them from the hill dwellers. Said a Dr Irschitzky in 1838, 'We know from experience, that among the valley folk now and then melancholia occurs, mostly for religious reasons, and frequently acute insanity (mania). These mental illnesses follow in a quite natural manner from the constitution and the character of these people . . . whereby frequently mania serves as an interlude' (Irschitzky, 1838, p. 243).

Among the first observers to see this alternation of mania and melancholia as parts of the same disease was Carl Friedrich Flemming, director of the Sachsenberg mental hospital in Germany, who in 1844 described '*Dysthymia mutabilis*', the kind of mood disorder that arises when *Dysthymia atra* (black depression) and *Dysthymia candida* (low-level mania) alternate. 'Between both of them (atra and candida) there is a not infrequent connection, *Dysthymia mutabilis*, which sometimes shows the character of one, sometimes the character of the other.' Flemming saw other kinds of depression too, such as *melancholia attonita*, or retarded melancholia (Flemming, 1844, pp. 114, 129).

Flemming's proposed coinage, appearing in a then obscure German-language journal, was soon forgotten in an era when Paris was the centre of the enlightened world. And it was in Paris that bipolar disorder as a separate entity was famously announced a few years later. In 1850, Jean-Pierre Falret, a staff psychiatrist of the Salpêtrière Hospice in Paris gave a lecture to the Psychiatric Society in which he briefly mentioned 'circular insanity' (*la folie circulaire*), thus giving the alternation of mania and melancholia a separate name. (This was Falret senior, as opposed to his son Jules Falret, also noted for the coinage of new illness entities in psychiatry.) Falret said it was different from 'melancholia and mania as such'. The paper was published the following year in the Gazette des Hôpitaux, but little was made of it (Shorter, 2005, p. 166). Three years later, in 1854, Falret's rival at the Salpêtrière, Jules Baillarger, covered the same ground again, but this time calling the alternation of mania and melancholia a separate disease in and of itself, different from what he said Falret had described, the switching back and forth of two separate disease entities. As noted above, Falret had indeed claimed the alternation of the symptoms as different in character from mania and melancholia alone, but only in one sentence (Baillarger, 1854a). Shortly thereafter, Falret shot back that it was in fact he who had the priority and not Baillarger (Falret, 1854), and Baillarger responded furiously at the same meeting of the Academy of Medicine (Baillarger, 1854b). In retrospect it is unclear who of the two squabbling academicians deserves the priority, though Falret did touch on the subject in 1850 (and neither knew of Flemming's earlier work). But it would be fair to say that, in Paris in the early 1850s, bipolar disorder was born for an international audience, yet without the careful apparatus of psychopathology and nosology that came later.

The baton now passed to the Germans, and for the next hundred years the principal contributions to bipolar disorder would be made by German professors. In 1878, Ludwig Kirn, a psychiatry resident who had trained at the Illenau asylum, published a postdoctoral thesis on 'the periodic psychoses' in which he gave a detailed psychopathological account of bipolar disorder, something the French clinicians had omitted in favour of grand generalisations (Kirn, 1878). German nationalists, with their dislike of the French, considered this the first description of the disorder *tout court*, but it in fact was not (Kirchhoff, 1924, p. 167).

In these years, many German psychiatrists – including Wilhelm Griesinger and Heinrich Neumann – described bipolar disorder in one form or another. For most, the usual course was switching from melancholia into mania, and then into terminal dementia, more or less as Falret had first described. But in 1882, Karl

Kahlbaum, one of the great names in the history of German psychiatry – because of his insistence on using the 'clinical method' to study psychopathology – proposed the term 'cyclothymia' for recoverable alternations of melancholia and mania, but – in not tipping into dementia (as in Heinrich Neumann's 'typical insanity') – instead the patients got better. Another such cyclical episode might then occur, and so forth. Also, the 'mania' that Kahlbaum described was not a full-blast onslaught affecting all mental functions but a kind of exaggerated elation without psychosis (Kahlbaum, 1882). It corresponded roughly to what Berlin psychiatrist Emanuel Ernst Mendel had called a year previously 'hypomania' (Mendel, 1881), and – in essence – the ancestor of 'Bipolar II Disorder'.

Then came the great earthquake in German nosology: Emil Kraepelin and his historic classification of psychiatric illnesses, the basic outlines of which have endured more or less intact until the present. The classification, based on course and outcome, became the first real conceptualisation of manic-depressive illness, a disease having an undulating course rather than an irreversible downhill slide as in chronic psychosis (which Kraepelin called '*dementia praecox*'). Kraepelin therefore is the first investigator to have conceptualised mania and melancholia in the context of a nosological organising principle, namely clinical course. Thomas Ban once observed: 'Many people described what was to become manic-depressive illness but it was Emil Kraepelin who conceptualised it as a class of illness because of his adoption of temporality as an organising principle of psychiatric nosology' (Ban, personal communication, 9 November, 2006).

In 1899, in the sixth edition of his textbook, Kraepelin lumped together all depression (except that beginning in middle age) and all mania under the category manic-depression (Kraepelin, 1899). For Kraepelin, it was the sole mood disorder – there was no 'unipolar' depression. Kraepelin thought it a matter of indifference whether the illnesses recurred periodically, or whether mania and melancholia were linked together or not. Thus, with Kraepelin's work what we most emphatically call 'bipolar disorder' ceased to be a separate disease. The concept of alternating mania and melancholia as a disease of its own became lost sight of because Kraepelin considered *all* mood disorders to be part of 'manic-depressive illness'. Although we commonly say that bipolar disorder is the successor of Kraepelin's manic-depressive insanity (*das manisch-depressive Irresein*), this is erroneous: Kraepelin put all cases of depression and mania, alternating or not, into manic-depression. Our use of the term 'bipolar disorder' alternately implies that there is a separate class of unipolar depression.

Two further comments about Kraepelin's manic-depressive illness should be made. Firstly, in later editions, he popularised Wilhelm Weygandt's concept of the existence of 'mixed psychoses', that is, manic and depressive symptoms appearing simultaneously. Weygandt had ventured the notion in a post-doctoral thesis, which was not an automatic guarantee of international acceptance (Weygandt, 1899; Kraepelin, 1904). Secondly, Kraepelin doubted that Kahlbaum's cyclothymia represented a separate illness but rather just a form of manic-depressive insanity in which there might be long lucid intervals between episodes. Today's *Diagnostic and Statistical Manual* (DSM) sees cyclothymic disorder as 'bipolar', yet as separate from the main bipolar disorders (I and II) because the mania and depression of cyclothymia both fall below the threshold of a full episode of mania or of major depression (American Psychiatric Association, 2000).

Kraepelin taught in Heidelberg and Munich. But the charge back towards bipolar disorder as a separate disease, *à la Française*, began in a different academic fortress entirely – Karl Kleist's university clinic in Frankfurt. Kleist owed nothing to Kraepelin and his circle but rather identified with the intensely biological approach to psychiatry of Carl Wernicke. It was actually Wernicke (1900) who adumbrated in Part 3 of his textbook, published in 1900, the first of these new bipolar entities: 'hyperkinetic and akinetic motility psychosis'.

For Wernicke, bipolarity was not a big deal. But for Kleist it was. Kleist's ambition was to continue the series of independent disease entities between manic-depressive illness and dementia praecox, which were the two great diseases that Kraepelin had established. Between these bookends, Kleist (1911) started to insert a number of diagnoses, some unipolar and some bipolar. It is thus Kleist who restored bipolar thinking to psychiatry in 1911, without challenging the existence of Kraepelin's manic-depressive illness (which was, of course, not a bipolar illness because Kraepelin did not conceptualise a separate unipolar depression).

In the following years, Kleist identified several other cyclical psychoses, including 'confusional psychoses' that alternate between 'agitated confusion' and 'stupor' (Kleist, 1926, 1928). The point was, for Kleist and other investigators in these years, to open up space in between Kraepelin's two great diseases, which were manic-depression and dementia praecox, and to find room in the middle for diagnoses with prognoses that were perhaps more benign than Kraepelin's terrible dementia praecox. Yet, against the great Kraepelinian 'two-disease' tide, Kleist's ideas made little headway at this point.

Kleist had two very productive students, Edda Neele and Karl Leonhard, who after the Second World War carried forward Kleist's teachings about bipolarity. In a 1949 study of all those with 'cyclical psychoses' admitted to the Frankfurt university clinic between 1938 and 1942, Neele (1949, p. 6) introduced the terms 'unipolar disorder' and 'bipolar disorder' (*einpolige und zweipolige Erkrankungen*). Kleist must have used these previously in a teaching setting but Neele's postdoctoral thesis (*Habilitation*) is their first major public airing.

Throughout the 1940s and 1950s, Leonhard burrowed away at the periodic and the cyclical psychoses – at Frankfurt until 1955, then at Erfurt and Berlin – trying to insert them in the larger scheme of psychiatric illness. In 1957, Leonhard's magisterial study – *The Classification of the Endogenous Psychoses* – appeared and definitively separated what we call bipolar affective disorder from 'pure depression'. This separation of depressive illness by polarity remains in force in most circles today. 'Undoubtedly there is a manic-depressive illness', wrote Leonhard (1957, pp. 4–5), 'having in its very nature the tendency to mania and melancholia alike. But next to this there are also periodically appearing euphoric and depressive states that show no disposition at all to change to the opposite form. Thus, there exists this basic and very important distinction between bipolar and monopolar psychoses.' This is the true birth, or rebirth if one will, of bipolar disorder in contemporary psychiatry. This is the part of Leonhard's work that went into the DSM of the American Psychiatric Association in 1980 (see below).

Yet for the most part, Leonhard did not use the terms unipolar or bipolar in describing manic-depressive illness or the 'pure' depressions and manias, even though they correspond nicely to our concepts of bipolar and unipolar today. Instead, in his detailed discussions he reserved bipolar and unipolar for the 'cyclic psychoses', such as 'anxiety-euphoria psychosis' and Wernicke's 'hyperkinetic-akinetic motility psychosis'. He stated that the 'cyclic psychoses are related to the phasic psychoses – indeed directly linked to them. [These are] the psychoses that Kleist brought together as cyclic. They are bipolar and multiform and never result in lasting disability' (Leonhard 1957, p. 120).

Leonhard's cyclic psychoses did not make it into the DSM system. He differentiated them from the 'periodic psychoses' (phasic psychoses) such as manic-depressive illness and pure depression and pure euphoria. Yet manic-depression is also cyclical, while pure depression and pure euphoria are not. These refinements would be almost too trivial to mention were it not for the fact that Leonhard's schema as a whole deserves a well-informed second look. The main point here is that Leonhard was the first author to separate depressions by polarity (though generally he reserved the polarity terms for other illnesses).

Leonhard's separation of manic-depressive illness from depression was taken up by a handful of scholars outside of Germany, and 1966 became 'a very good year' for the study of bipolar illness (for this phrase, see Winokur, 1991, p. 28). In that year, three studies appeared that distinguished among depressions by polarity, meaning the depression of bipolar disorder (manic-depressive illness) versus the unipolar depression termed 'melancholia' at that time. All three studies found greater family histories of mood disorder in bipolar patients than unipolar. However, as observed by Michael Alan Taylor: 'they and all others found that among the families of bipolar patients there was always more unipolar than bipolar illness' (Taylor, personal communication, 12 November, 2006).

In one of these studies, Jules Angst in Zurich compared patients with bipolar disorder to those with endogenous depression, involutional melancholia and mixed affective-schizophrenia. He ended up questioning 'the nosological unity of the (Kraepelinian) manic-depressive illness. The purely depressive monophasic and periodic psychoses are statistically differentiated from those that have a cyclic course' (Angst, 1966, p. 106).

Meanwhile, Carlo Perris in Sweden, adopting a specifically Leonhardian approach, compared bipolar and unipolar depressive patients at the Sidsjon Mental Hospital in Umea, arguing that 'they are two different nosographic entities' (Perris, 1966, p. 187). It is worth noting that some feel that Angst and Perris created a monster by permitting the use of terms such as bipolar depression and monopolar depression in suggesting the existence of fundamentally different entities, albeit of great commercial use in registering pharmaceutical agents for 'bipolar depression' and the like.

Finally, in 1966, Leonhard's distinction between monopolar and bipolar depression made its first American beachhead. In June 1966, at a meeting of the Society of Biological Psychiatry in Washington DC, George Winokur and Paula Clayton of Washington University in St. Louis, the then premier American institution for biological approaches to psychiatry, showed that 'the family background for manic-depressive patients differed from that of patients who showed only depression' (Winokur, 1991, p. 29; Winokur and Clayton, 1967). Interestingly, despite Winokur's presence on the team, manic-depressive illness did not make it into the so-called 'Feighner criteria', the attempt to recast psychiatric diagnosis launched at Washington University in the early 1970s, by Feighner *et al.* (1972).

In the 1970s, the evolution of bipolar disorder became a primarily American rather than a German story. In a reaction to the diagnostic indifference of psychoanalysis, these years saw a new fervour in nosological thinking in the USA. Led by Robert Spitzer, a group of researchers at the New York State Psychiatric Institute – that also included Eli Robins of Washington University – set about defining 'Research Diagnostic Criteria' (the RDC) as a way of recasting American psychiatric diagnoses. A preliminary paper produced by the group in the mid-70s (Spitzer *et al.*, 1975) included 'major depressive illness' (and 'minor depressive illness') but made no reference to bipolar disorder. Yet by the time a final version of the RDC was published in 1978, 'bipolar depression with mania (Bipolar I)' and 'bipolar depression with hypomania (Bipolar II)' had been added to the RDC, alongside 'major depressive disorder'. There were now two big depressions firmly fixed in American psychiatric nosology, one linked to mania as bipolar disorder and the other a unipolar depression called 'major depression', although the RDC system also included a host of other depressive subtypes and atypical forms of depression (Spitzer *et al.*, 1978).

The RDC became the template in 1978 for the dramatic reshaping of psychiatric diagnosis that took place 2 years later, also under the leadership of Robert Spitzer, in the American Psychiatric Association's DSM–III, the third edition of the APA's *Diagnostic and Statistical Manual* (American Psychiatric Association, 1980). DSM–III provided for a Leonhardian division between unipolar depression (called Major Depression), and bipolar manic-depression (called Bipolar Disorder). Although by this time everyone had forgotten who Leonhard was, DSM–III represented the international triumph of one of the core concepts of Leonhard's system. The distinction between major depression and bipolar disorder was preserved in subsequent editions of the DSM series. Both depressions were called 'major depression', but the latter was more severe in terms of chronicity and shorter length of time between episodes.

In the following years, a large body of clinical and pharmacological opinion upheld the distinction between bipolar and unipolar mood disorders, in other words, the distinction between two kinds of serious depression (Ban, 1990). Bernard Carroll called bipolar disorder 'the most extreme case of mood instability' and said that any theory of brain function would have to come to terms with, quoting Donald Klein, 'this striking phenomenon'. Carroll argued that there were fundamental biological differences between bipolar and unipolar disorders, in that although those with bipolar disorder had more lifetime episodes, the excess was 'entirely accounted for by the manias . . . in other words, manic depressive patients are not just more unstable than unipolar patients in mood regulation in both directions' (Carroll, 1994, p. 304). Yet there must be a pendular movement between the view that depression and mania are separate illnesses and the view that linked depression-mania constitutes an illness of its own. For, in the 1990s, the pendulum began to swing back from DSM–III and Leonhard to a more Kraepelinian view. This movement was initiated as early as 1980 by Michael Taylor and Richard Abrams, then at the Chicago Medical School, who wrote, after reviewing genetic and biological studies, 'These data suggest that the separation of affective disorders by polarity may have been premature' (Taylor and Abrams, 1980, p. 195). Unlike previous investigators, Taylor and Abrams based their work on well-defined rating scales and treatment response.

In 2006, Taylor, now at the University of Michigan, and Max Fink at SUNY's Stony Brook campus, in a major review of the diagnosis of melancholia, said of the bipolar versus unipolar dichotomy, 'The scientific evidence fails to distinguish unipolar and bipolar depressive disorders . . . bipolarity as a separate psychiatric disorder is not supported by psychopathology, family studies, laboratory tests, or treatment response' (Taylor and Fink, 2006, p. 24). What other people see as unipolar illness, Taylor and Fink consider to be non-melancholic depression and what is bipolar depression they consider melancholia.

As a historian, it is not my place to comment on the scientific merits of the polarity debate. Subsequent research may well establish that bipolar disorder is an illness in its own right, requiring a distinctive therapeutic approach involving mood stabilisation. Or bipolar disorder may join history's dust heap along with such discarded diagnoses as hysteria and madness. In the meantime, however, the frequency of bipolar disorders seems to be growing by leaps and bounds (Healy, 2006). It would be wise for patients and doctors to take with a grain of salt pharmaceutical claims of products having differential efficacy.

Acknowledgements

For comments on an earlier draft I should like to thank Thomas Ban, Tom Bolwig, Bernard Carroll, Max Fink and Michael Alan Taylor.

REFERENCES

American Psychiatric Association (1980). *Diagnostic and Statistical Manual of Mental Disorders*, 3rd edn. Washington, DC: APA.

American Psychiatric Association (2000). *Diagnostic and Statistical Manual of Mental Disorders*, 4th edn: Text Revision, DSM–IV–TR. Washington, DC: APA.

Angst, J. (1966). *Zur Ätiologie und Nosologie endogener depressiver Psychosen: Eine genetische, soziologische und klinische Studie*. Berlin: Springer.

Baillarger, J. (1854a). De la folie à double forme. *Annales Médico-psychologiques*, **6**, 369–91.

Baillarger, J. (1854b). (Response in discussion – no title). *Bulletin de l'Académie de Médecine*, **19**, 401–15.

Ban, T. (1990). Clinical pharmacology and Leonhard's classification of endogenous psychoses. *Psychopathology*, **23**, 331–8.

Carroll, B. (1994). Brain mechanisms in manic depression. *Clinical Chemistry*, **40**, 303–8.

Chiarugi, V. (1794). *Della Pazzia in Genere e in Specie. Trattato Medico-analitico*, Vol. 3. Florence: Carlieri.

Falret, J. P. (1854). Mémoire sur la folie circulaire. *Bulletin de l'Académie de Médecine*, **19**, 382–400.

Feighner, J., Robins, E., Guze, S., Woodruff, R., Winokur, G. and Munoz, R. (1972). Diagnostic criteria for use in psychiatric research. *Archive of General Psychiatry*, **26**, 57–63.

Flemming, C. (1844). Über Classification der Seelenstörungen. *Allgemeine Zeitschrift für Psychiatrie*, **1**, 97–130.

Healy, D. (2006). The latest mania: Selling bipolar disorder. *PLOS Medicine*, www.plosmedicine. org, **3**(4), e185.

Irschitzky (1838). Über psychische Krankheiten im Districts-Physikate Voitsberg. *Medicinische Jahrbücher des k. k. Österreichischen Staates*, **17**, 233–47.

Jackson, S. (1986). *Melancholia and Depression From Hippocratic Times to Modern Times*. New Haven, NJ: Yale.

Kahlbaum, K. (1882). Über cyklisches Irresein. *Der Irrenfreund*, **24**, 145–57.

Kirchhoff, T. (1924). *Deutsche Irrenärzte*, Vol. 2. Berlin: Springer.

Kirn, L. (1878). *Die Periodischen Psychosen*. Stuttgart: Enke.

Kleist, K. (1911). Die klinische Stellung der Motilitätspsychosen. *Zeitschrift für die gesamte Neurologie und Psychiatrie*, **3**, 914–17.

Kleist, K. (1926). Über zykloide Degenerationspsychosen, besonders Verwirrtheits- und Motilitätspsychosen. *Archiv für Psychiatrie und Nervenkrankheiten*, **78**, 416–21.

Kleist, K. (1928). Über zykloide, paranoide und epileptoide Psychosen und über die Frage der Degenerationspsychosen. *Schweizer Archiv für Neurologie und Psychiatrie*, **23**, 3–37.

Kraepelin, E. (1899). *Psychiatrie: ein Lehrbuch*, 6th edn, Vol. 2. Leipzig: Barth.

Kraepelin, E. (1904). *Psychiatrie: ein Lehrbuch*, 7th edn, Vol. 2. Leipzig: Barth.

Leonhard, K. (1957). *Aufteilung der Endogenen Psychosen*. Berlin: Akademie-Verlag.

Mendel, E. (1881). *Die Manie*. Vienna: Urban.

Neele, E. (1949). *Die phasischen Psychosen nach ihrem Erscheinungs- und Erbbild*. Leipzig: Barth.

Penrose, T. (1775). *Flights of Fancy*. London: Walter.

Perris, C. (1966). A study of bipolar (manic-depressive) and unipolar recurrent depressive psychoses. *Acta Psychiatrica Scandinavica*, **42** (Suppl. 194), S1–S189.

Shorter, E. (2005). *Historical Dictionary of Psychiatry*. New York: Oxford University Press.

Spitzer, R., Endicott, J., Robins, E., Kuriansky, J. and Gurland, B. (1975). Preliminary report of the reliability of Research Diagnostic Criteria applied to psychiatric case records. In *Predictability in Psychopharmacology: Preclinical and Clinical Correlations*, ed. A. Sudilovsky, S. Gershon & B. Beer, pp. 1–47. New York: Raven.

Spitzer, R., Endicott, J. and Robins, E. (1978). Research Diagnostic Criteria. *Archives of General Psychiatry*, **35**, 773–82.

Taylor, M. and Abrams, R. (1980). Reassessing the bipolar-unipolar dichotomy. *Journal of Affective Disorders*, **2**, 195–217.

Taylor, M. and Fink, M. (2006). *Melancholia: The Diagnosis, Pathophysiology, and Treatment of Depressive Illness*. New York: Cambridge University Press.

Wernicke, C. (1900). *Grundriss der Psychiatrie*, part 3. Leipzig: Thieme.

Weygandt, W. (1899). *Über die Mischzustände des manisch-depressiven Irreseins*. Munich: Lehmann.

Winokur, G. (1991). *Mania and Depression: A Classification of Syndrome and Disease*. Baltimore, MD: Johns Hopkins University Press.

Winokur, G. and Clayton, P. (1967). Family history studies I. Two types of affective disorders separated according to genetic and clinical factors. In *Recent Advances in Biological Psychiatry*, ed. J. Wortis, pp. 25–30. New York: Plenum.

Katzow, J. J., Hsu, D. J. and Ghaemi, S. N. (2003). The bipolar spectrum: a clinical perspective. *Bipolar Disorders*, **5**, 436–42.

Klerman, G. L. (1981). The spectrum of mania. *Comprehensive Psychiatry*, **22**, 11–20.

Leverich, G. S., Altshuler, L. L., Frye, M. A. *et al.* (2006). Risk of switch in mood polarity to hypomania or mania in patients with bipolar depression during acute and continuation trials of venlafaxine, sertraline, and bupropion as adjuncts to mood stabilizers. *American Journal of Psychiatry*, **163**, 232–9.

Mackinnon, D. F. and Pies, R. (2006). Affective instability as rapid cycling: theoretical and clinical implications for borderline personality and bipolar spectrum disorders. *Bipolar Disorders*, **8**, 1–14.

Mitchell, P., Goodwin, G., Johnson, G. and Hirschfeld, R. (2006). Diagnostic guidelines for Bipolar I depression: A probabilistic approach. *Bipolar Disorders*, in review.

Mondimore, F. M. (2005). Unipolar depression/bipolar depression: connections and controversies. *International Review of Psychiatry*, **17**, 39–47.

Moller, H. J. and Curtis, V. A. (2004). The bipolar spectrum: Diagnostic and pharmacologic considerations. *Expert Review of Neurotherapeutics*, **4** (Suppl. 2), S3–8.

Parker, G., Tully, L., Olley, A. and Hadzi-Pavlovic, D. (2006). SSRIs as mood stabilizers for Bipolar II Disorder? A proof of concept study. *Journal of Affective Disorders*, **92**, 205–14.

Phelps, J. (2005a). Using the MDQ in Primary Care: Predictive value of the test results. http://www.psycheducation.org/PCP/mdqSensSpec.htm, accessed 12/7/2006.

Phelps, J. R. (2005b). Agitated dysphoria after late-onset loss of response to antidepressants: a case report. *Journal of Affective Disorders*, **86**, 277–80.

Phelps, J. (2006). Depression is not a moral weakness. http://www.psycheducation.org/mechanism/MechanismIntro.htm, accessed 12/7/06.

Phelps, J. R., Angst, J., Katzow, J. and Sadler, J. (2006). Validity and utility of the Bipolar Spectrum. *Bipolar Disorders*, in review.

Phelps, J. R. and Ghaemi, S. N. (2006). Improving the diagnosis of bipolar disorder: predictive value of screening tests. *Journal of Affective Disorders*, **92**, 141–8.

Quitkin, F. M., Kane, J., Rifkin, A., Ramos-Lorenzi, J. R. and Nayak, D. V. (1981). Prophylactic lithium carbonate with and without imipramine for Bipolar I patients. A double-blind study. *Archives of General Psychiatry*, **38**, 902–7.

Skeppar, P. and Adolfsson, R. (2006). Bipolar II and the bipolar spectrum. *Nordic Journal of Psychiatry*, **60**, 7–26.

Wehr, T. and Goodwin, F. K. (1979). Tricyclics modulate frequency of mood cycles. *Chronobiologia*, **6**, 377–85.

3

Defining and measuring Bipolar II Disorder

Gordon Parker

Introduction

In the last decade many commentators have stated that Bipolar II Disorder (BP II) is under-diagnosed. Over the same period, many others have stated that it is over-diagnosed. Such contradictory views hint at problems with definition and diagnosis – and reflect the controversy as to whether it is a true condition or more a personality style. As it is also commonly viewed as lying along a spectrum of mood disorders bounded by Bipolar I Disorder (BP I) and unipolar depressive conditions (see Chapter 2), we can assume that 'boundary' problems (in differentiating one condition clearly from the other) also contribute to difficulties in diagnostic delineation.

In Chapter 2, Phelps well argued the salience of a 'spectrum' model. In this chapter, an opposing categorical model is offered for consideration. This does reflect a personal view that bipolar disorder is a categorical condition or an 'entity', and further, that if distinctive sub-set diagnoses (of BP I and BP II) exist, distinction between them must be meaningful (in inferring differing clinical pictures and causes, and/or salient differential treatments). Medicine advanced by distinguishing differing clinicopathological expressions of the 'pox' (i.e. small-pox and chickenpox), differing causes of 'dropsy' (e.g. renal and cardiac) and in distinguishing Type I and Type II diabetes. All three examples (i.e. the 'pox', 'dropsy' and diabetes) could have been dimensionally modelled, but explanatory power would have been less, while aetiological and treatment implications would have been obscured.

The bipolar disorders are either dimensional or categorical disorders. This chapter is underpinned by the working bias that they are categorically distinct from unipolar depressive disorders and that BP I and BP II are categorically

Note: This chapter extracts – with permission of the *Journal of Affective Disorders* – sections of a paper published by Parker, H., Hadzi-Pavlovic, D. and Tully, L. (2006). Distinguishing bipolar and unipolar disorders: An isomer model. *Journal of Affective Disorders*, **96**, 67–73.

distinct from each other. The task then is to consider how they can best be defined, circumscribed and distinguished. In essence, what are their characteristic or prototypic features and what 'model' best captures their entity status?

Currently, they are formally classified, and it is therefore important to overview the influential DSM and ICD diagnostic systems and identify intrinsic limitations before describing a model suggested by research at the Black Dog Institute.

The DSM system

DSM-IV informs us that Bipolar I Disorder (BP I) is characterised by either manic episodes or mixed episodes – with or without episodes of major depression. (A 'mixed episode' is defined by symptoms of both a manic episode and a major depressive episode 'nearly every day' for at least one week.) In contrast to BP I, Bipolar II Disorder (BP II) is characterised by one or more episodes of major depression, and at least one hypomanic episode. This would suggest that differentiation of bipolar from unipolar disorder requires, in effect, valid identification of a hypomanic or manic episode, and that BP I and BP II are distinguished from each other by the respective presence of manic and hypomanic episodes – and thus argues the need to distinguish mania from hypomania.

However, DSM–IV criterion features and cut-off criterion numbers are essentially the same for both mania and hypomania. Basically, Criterion A (for both mania and hypomania) is for a 'distinct period of abnormally and persistently elevated, expansive, or irritable mood'. Criterion B requires three or more (or four or more if the 'mood is only irritable') of the following summarised features: (i) inflated self-esteem or grandiosity; (ii) decreased need for sleep; (iii) being more talkative than usual; (iv) flight of ideas; (v) distractibility; (vi) increased goal-directed activity; and (vii) excessive involvement in pleasurable activities. While the DSM system imposes minimal durations of 7 days for mania and 4 days for hypomania, neither defined criterion period has been established empirically. Subsequently, Angst *et al.* (2003) established that (sub-threshold) brief hypomanic episodes (i.e. 1–3 days) were clinically comparable to (above threshold) hypomanic episodes with a minimum length of 4 days, while we have similarly identified (Tully and Parker, 2007) similar patterns of hypomanic symptoms in those with highs lasting minutes or hours as against 3–7 days. Returning to the DSM rules, if during such a mood state the individual requires hospitalisation, or if the individual experiences psychotic features, then irrespective of its duration, criteria for a manic episode are met. Thus, while psychotic features and need for hospitalisation are sufficient for defining BP I – they are not 'necessary'. In their absence, the only criterion difference to distinguish BP II is episode duration, a distinction that has not been empirically established.

It is important to note that DSM–IV criteria require 'impairment' for mania and an 'unequivocal change in functioning that is uncharacteristic of the person when not symptomatic' for hypomania, injunctions that assist delineation from non-clinical states. And further, that any such episodes are not 'caused by somatic antidepressant treatment' (e.g. drugs, ECT), and where any induced mood elevation (often termed 'Bipolar III') is not clearly part of an integral bipolar disorder. Thus, while DSM-IV criteria seek to differentiate mania and hypomania from normal mood states, and to differentiate one from the other, some of the decision rules lack precision while others (judgements of impairment and whether mood elevation is secondary to physical treatments) rely to a degree on subjective judgement.

While multiple examples could be provided of predictable boundary problems, distinguishing between mild 'true highs' and normal hedonistic states is possibly the most relevant issue. Imagine an individual who has just played in a winning football team, or an entrepreneur who has just cut a great deal, or a writer who has taken the embryo of an idea for *The Great Novel* forward and has the creative juices in full flow by the end of the first chapter. In such instances, we could envisage some inflation of self-esteem, a decreased need for sleep, being more talkative, flight of ideas, and possibly (at least for the winning footballer) involvement in at-risk hedonistic activities. My point: it is not always easy to determine if a 'high' is pathological (i.e. bipolar disorder) or not. Therefore, DSM-IV decision rules weighting impairment (or uncharacteristic functioning) and duration (4–7 days) have some practical utility, but in addition to requiring sophisticated clinical judgement, at times risk excluding those with 'true' bipolar disorder. This will also be considered more closely in relation to duration.

The ICD-10 system

ICD–10 has only one bipolar category ('bipolar affective disorder'), with a weighting to description rather than to a criteria-based diagnosis. It allows that, in the elevated mood phase, mania or hypomania may exist, while depression is also experienced. Hypomania should last 'at least several days', with the attendant mood and behavioural changes being 'too persistent and marked' to be included under cyclothymia, but not accompanied by psychotic features. Manic episodes are described as lasting from 2 weeks to several months, may or may not include psychotic features and, for any such psychotic features, these may or may not be specified as mood congruent or mood incongruent. Cyclothymia is defined as 'persistent instability of mood, involving numerous periods of mild depression and mild elation'. Cyclothymia is differentiated from bipolar affective disorder on the suggested basis of duration and severity – but without any duration or severity criteria being defined.

So the issue faced in this chapter is how can we distinguish true BP II from normal mood states, from 'cyclothymia' (whatever that state is) and from BP I. This issue has been a focus of our research in recent years, with some summary data now overviewed.

Questionnaire development

We sought to define and refine the quintessential or integral constructs under-pinning a hypomanic or manic mood state, and then focus on differentiating BP II 'highs' from both normal mood elevation and from BP I 'highs'. We developed a 46-item self-report measure – the Mood Swings Questionnaire – with items generated from a literature review and from clinical experience. Scoring options – in relation to provisional items – were: 'much more than usual' (scored 2); 'somewhat more than usual' (scored 1); and, 'no more than usual' (scored 0).

Subjects in the development studies were asked two probe screening questions:

'Do you ever have mood swings and, as part of such swings, have times when:
  (i) your mood is higher than your usual sense of happiness, and
 (ii) you feel quite 'wired', 'energised', 'elevated', 'expansive' and possibly 'irritable'?'

Study One

We posted the Mood Swings Questionnaire on our Black Dog Institute website, with relevant volunteers aged 18 years or older asked to complete the survey anonymously. Screening questions sought to limit respondents to those with a strong probability of their having had bipolar disorder. Subsidiary questions sought information on age, duration of initial highs, whether the individual had been hospitalised or received antipsychotic medication for a 'high', and sought information on their depression history and any family history.

Of the 460 eligible respondents, 299 (65%) had – when high – experienced psychotic features (i.e. delusions and/or hallucinations), and/or had been hospi-talised. These were regarded as provisionally having BP I (in meeting relevant DSM-IV psychotic feature and hospitalisation criteria for that condition). The residual subjects were putatively classified as having BP II, with 52 (11%) having had their longest high last 5 days or more, 61 (13%) having their highs last only 1–4 days, and 48 (10%) never having had a high last more than hours.

Forty of the 46 items returned differential scores across the four groups, warranting further analyses. Of these 40 items, 36 showed a linear trend (whereby scores decreased across the four respective groups). Not one item showed evidence of a 'trend break' (i.e. where scores increase non-linearly across the groups), though one would have anticipated such a break if there *was* a categorical distinction between groups (particularly, between the BP I and BP II groups).

As we did not formally establish the lifetime diagnosis of volunteer subjects, and were unable to clinically distinguish between those with BP I and BP II disorders, no firm conclusions can be drawn from these study results. If we assume for the moment, however, that all respondents had bipolar disorder and that the presence of psychotic features or requiring hospitalisation during a high efficiently differentiated BP I and BP II subjects, then two suggestions emerge. Firstly, that highs can be briefer than the four-day minimum imposed by DSM-IV – as has been argued previously (e.g. Angst *et al.*, 2003). Secondly, the linear trend in scores across the four groups for virtually all items suggests that the core mood/energy construct experienced during a high is likely to differ dimensionally (rather than categorically) across BP I and BP II disorders. Such findings encouraged a more detailed and extended study, elsewhere reported (Parker *et al.*, 2006), and now overviewed.

Study Two

The same Mood Swings Questionnaire was given to a sample of 157 of the author's unipolar and bipolar outpatients who had been referred for assessment and management of an episode of major depression. Logistical difficulties occasionally prevented consecutive recruitment, as individuals who were extremely distressed or who had severe psychomotor disturbance at initial assessment were not recruited at that time – to respect their clinical priority and to ensure that valid responses were not compromised.

Each had a detailed lifetime history review of their mood disorder to establish the probability of either a bipolar or unipolar course. Clinical screening questions for bipolar disorder included all seven DSM-IV criteria for manic and hypomanic episodes. Subsidiary questions clarified whether such mood states were observable, age of onset of both the highs and the depressive episodes, and whether there was a family history of depression or bipolar disorder. Referral information, treatment details from relevant therapists and hospital admissions, and corroborative histories from family members were available for many patients, and sought if there was any diagnostic difficulty.

Assignment of patients to the bipolar category required:
  (i) discrete periods of mood elevation (and distinctly different to normal mood swings – as judged by the clinician),
 (ii) meeting DSM-IV symptom criteria for manic or hypomanic episodes (but not, of necessity, duration criteria), and
(iii) a relatively clear lifetime onset of elevated mood states (to partially address risk of incorrect diagnosis).

Lifetime experience of any psychotic features during mood states was assessed. Patients hospitalised during an elevated mood state had their hospital files reviewed, establishing clear psychotic features in several who had not remembered or reported psychotic features at interview.

Those clinically diagnosed as having a bipolar disorder were divided into putative BP I and BP II sub-groups, with such decisions made prior to subjects completing the self-report questionnaire. Assignment to the BP I group largely respected DSM-IV decision rules, and occurred if the patient had ever (i) had psychotic features (delusions and/or hallucinations) during a high, (ii) been hospitalised for a manic episode, or (iii) been judged clinically as having severe highs that were also associated with distinct impairment (akin to the DSM-IV Criterion D impairment description). Length of highs (both 'on average' and 'for the longest episode') did not, however, influence assignment to BP I or BP II sub-groups.

Subjects first completed a questionnaire assessing socio-demographic variables, family history details and clinical information (e.g. episode duration and hospitalisation data) about mood states. They then completed the 46-item Mood Swings Questionnaire. Those diagnosed clinically with a bipolar disorder scored items in relation to manic or hypomanic episodes. As true unipolar subjects would be expected to score the two probe questions negatively, subjects with unipolar depression were given what was labelled a 'Happiness' questionnaire, and invited to think of 'times when you are really happy (e.g. your favourite sporting team has won, you are spending a weekend with long-lost friends)'. The same 46 items were presented identically across the two questionnaires.

Key study objectives were to (i) determine if the self-report questionnaire would differentiate BP I and BP II subjects from each other, and Bipolar and Unipolar subjects from each other, and (ii) determine if the DSM-IV-imposed criteria for duration of hypomania and mania could be supported empirically.

Of the 157 subjects assessed, 49 were assigned as BP I, 52 as BP II, and the residual 56 as having a unipolar (UP) depressive disorder. Respective mean ages (40.9, 37.5 and 43.0 years) and female representation rates (43%, 46% and 48%) were comparable. The BP I and BP II subjects were specifically compared on a number of variables in addition to age and gender. They did not differ on a six-point social class measure (4.4 vs 3.9), rates of a bipolar disorder family history (40.9% vs 38.1%), age of onset at initial high (24.4 vs 21.9 years) or age of onset of initial depressive episode (22.1 vs 19.7 years).

The next set of findings are worthy of emphasis. By our assignment rules, none of the BP II subjects, when high, had experienced psychotic features or had been hospitalised, whereas almost two-thirds of the BP I subjects (61.2%) had had psychotic features at such times, and one-third (36.7%) of our BP I subjects had required hospitalisation. While sub-group assignment was not dictated by the

Table 3.1. Comparison of subjects assigned as having Bipolar I and Bipolar II Disorders.

Duration data	BP I ($n = 49$)	BP II ($n = 52$)
Longest episode of a high		
Less than 1 day	2.1%	20.8%
1–2 days	16.7%	22.9%
2–4 days	8.3%	18.8%
5–7 days	18.8%	10.4%
More than 1 week	54.2%	27.1%
Average duration of highs		
Minutes	0.0%	2.1%
Hours	14.6%	27.7%
1–2 days	22.9%	27.7%
2–4 days	10.4%	19.1%
5–7 days	8.3%	2.1%
Weeks	25.0%	12.8%
Months	18.8%	6.4%
Years	0.0%	2.1%

presence of psychotic features during depressive episodes, 41% of the BP I subjects had experienced psychotic features when depressed as against none of the BP II subjects. More specifically, 78% of our BP I subjects had experienced psychotic features when either high or depressed. The specificity of psychotic features to BP I (whether high or depressed) is therefore noteworthy.

Duration data for highs are recorded in Table 3.1. The BP I subjects reported longer highs than those with BP II, both in relation to their longest episode ($\chi^2 = 15.2$, P < 0.01) and similarly trending ($\chi^2 = 11.9$, ns) for their average length high. While DSM-IV imposes a duration of one week for a manic episode and four days for a hypomanic episode, 46% of our BP I subjects had never had an episode last longer than one week, while 43% of our BP II subjects had never had an episode last longer than two days. Imposition of formalised DSM-IV duration criteria therefore risks not diagnosing those with bipolar disorder.

We compared scores on each of the Mood Swings Questionnaire items for those assigned to the bipolar and unipolar groups. While there was a general trend for BP I subjects to score higher than BP II subjects, mean scores did not differ significantly for any item. By contrast, the BP II group scored higher than the unipolar group on all items. Summing scores on all 46 items produced the following results:

- The composite bipolar group (i.e. BP I + BP II) scored distinctly higher than the unipolar group (means = 54.3 and 19.9 respectively, t = 12.0, P < 0.001).

Table 3.2. Mean group scores and contrast analyses.

Scale	BP I n = 49 Mean (SD)	BP II n = 52 Mean (SD)	UP n = 56 Mean (SD)	Contrast t values BP I + BP II vs UP	BP I vs BP II	BP II vs UP
Creativity	15.6 (5.0)	14.3 (5.1)	6.4 (4.1)	10.49*	1.30	8.33*
Disinhibition	6.8 (3.4)	6.5 (3.0)	2.4 (2.2)	8.62*	0.40	7.20*
Mysticism	4.6 (3.2)	3.8 (2.8)	1.4 (1.5)	6.50*	1.44	4.83*
Irritation	5.8 (2.5)	5.1 (2.9)	1.1 (1.3)	10.85*	1.35	8.61*
Total	32.7 (11.1)	29.7 (10.9)	11.2 (6.6)	12.07*	1.46	9.59*

BP I, Bipolar I; BP II, Bipolar II; UP, Unipolar;   *P < 0.001.

(Analysis of individual item differences established that the two groups differed most distinctly on high energy items.)

- The BP II group scored distinctly higher than the unipolar group (means = 52.0 vs 19.9, t = 10.2, P < 0.001).
- The BP I and BP II groups (means = 56.7 and 52.0, t = 1.1) did not differ.

The next task was to reduce the item set to a refined set of items that preserved discrimination. As some items overlapped conceptually (e.g. 'Sleep less and not feel tired' and 'Need less sleep'), we deleted 10 overlapping items and then undertook a factor analysis of the remaining 36 items. A four-factor solution appeared to have the greatest coherence, and derived factors were labelled 'Creativity', 'Disinhibition', 'Mysticism' and 'Irritation' respectively. We selected the highest-loading items from each factor until judging that the constituent constructs were appropriately represented, and this generated four scales – with 11, 6, 5 and 5 items respectively. Table 3.2 records mean scale scores across the three groups for the refined 27 items. Analyses indicated, firstly, that both the composite bipolar group and the BP II group returned higher scores on all scales (and a higher total score) than the UP group. Secondly, the BP I and BP II group did not differ on any of the four scale scores, nor on the total 27-item score. Importantly, within the BP I sample, total scores did not differ for those who reported psychotic features when high compared with those not so reporting (33.2 vs 32.9, t = 0.08).

We next sought to derive a cut-off score on the 27-item scale that would best differentiate BP and UP group members. For composite BP vs UP subjects, the area under the curve or AUC (95% CI) was 0.93 (0.89–0.97), the sensitivity (i.e. true positives) and specificity (i.e. true negatives) at the identified optimal cut-off score of ≥ 22 was 80.9% and 98.2% respectively, and the positive predictive value was high at 0.95. For distinguishing BP I vs BP II subjects from each other, the AUC was 0.59 (0.47–0.70), while the sensitivity was 53.5% and specificity 63.0% at the optimal cut-off of ≥ 34, and the positive predictive value modest at 0.57. For BP II vs UP subjects, the AUC was 0.92 (0.87–0.97), sensitivity 73.9% and specificity 98.1% at the cut-off of ≥ 22, and the positive predictive value high at 0.91.

Discussion

Study Two sought to develop and refine a self-report measure that would assist in clarifying the clinical boundary between mood elevation states, and so assist differentiation of those experiencing BP I from BP II disorders, as well as differentiate the elevated mood state experienced by those with BP II from 'normal' mood elevation or 'happiness' as experienced by those with unipolar disorders.

Our unrefined self-report measure comprised items capturing integral symptoms and behaviours associated with manic and hypomanic states – excluding psychotic features. Examined at the individual item level, those with bipolar disorder were most clearly distinguished from those with unipolar depression by high energy items. We had earlier suggested (Parker, 2000) that melancholic depression is as much a movement disorder as a mood disorder, with the former manifested by observable signs of psychomotor disturbance (PMD) and experienced symptomatically as a profound lack of energy. Thus, a central construct to bipolar states (high energy) appears the obverse of the anergia experienced in melancholia. It is intriguing then to contemplate whether the highs experienced in hypomanic and manic episodes reflect as much high energy states as elevated mood states.

Factor analysis identified four constructs subsumed by the total item set. Against expectation and the argument put in the previous paragraph, a distinct 'high energy' factor was not delineated as a pure factor. We interpret this finding – in conjunction with the dominance of high energy item discrimination in the univariate analyses – as suggesting that 'high energy' underpinned at least three of the four factors – especially 'mood elevation' and 'disinhibition', but even the 'irritability' construct.

Several sets of analyses – examining individual items, derived scales and the total measure – failed to establish any significant differences in scores returned by those with BP I and BP II disorders. While it had been anticipated that some items (e.g. 'Believe that you possess a 'special meaning''; 'Read special significance into things'; 'Notice lots of coincidences occurring') and scales (e.g. Mysticism) might more detect and assess over-valued ideas and even psychotic features than the underlying core state, and thus result in distinct differences between BP I and BP II subjects, such differences were not evident.

Thus, and in line with provisional Study 1 findings, results suggest that the severity of non-psychotic features may differ little between BP I and BP II states. Such an interpretation is at variance with clinical experience, where manifestations of BP I manic episodes (at least in hospitalised patients) are often extreme. Several possible explanations can be offered. Sampling an out-patient sample may have weighted inclusion to milder lifetime BP I conditions. However, more than a third of the subjects had been hospitalised when manic and nearly 60% when depressed, suggesting conditions of some gravity. Possibly, patients with BP I may only 'remember' their highs up to a certain level of severity, so that their ratings on any self-report measure may capture symptoms less severe than when they require hospitalisation. Finally, retrospective assessment of highs may be flawed for a range of additional reasons.

Nevertheless, the similar scores returned by the BP I and BP II subjects allow the possibility that the nature and severity of the core 'mood/energy' state differs only marginally. Thus, BP I and BP II disorders are unlikely to be successfully modelled or measured by any strategy that merely assesses the core construct – which would appear to differ only dimensionally and marginally.

How then might BP I and BP II states best be modelled and differentiated? We have previously proposed (Parker, 2000) a hierarchical model for conceptualising the depressive (i.e. psychotic, melancholic and non-melancholic) disorders, with psychotic depression and melancholic depression having class-specific features (i.e. psychotic symptoms and observable psychomotor disturbance respectively). We therefore suggest an 'isomer' model for BP I and BP II disorders that links with that structural model for melancholic and psychotic depression, with the isomer concept capturing polarised mood/energy states that are mirror images of each other.

The model – as illustrated in Figure 3.1 – assumes that the core construct to bipolar disorder is an elevated mood/energy state – being shared across both BP I and BP II states, but being somewhat more severe in BP I. Its converse expression (i.e. a depressed mood/anergic state) is again the core component for psychotic depression and melancholic depression, albeit somewhat more severe in psychotic depression. Thus, the model assumes that it is the presence of psychotic features (a psychotic 'mantle') that distinguishes BP I from BP II – in essence, a categorical and specific feature.

There are several advantages to the proposed model. Firstly, as a 'mirror imaging' isomer model it argues for polar expressions of both 'mood' (depression vs mood elevation) and 'energy' (anergia vs energised) as defining the core component of bipolar disorder – be it BP I or BP II. Secondly, it positions 'psychotic features' as having hierarchical and independent status at each pole

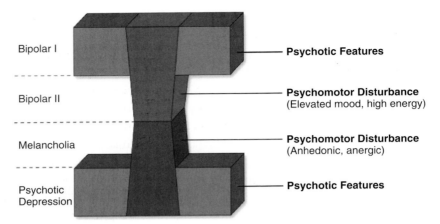

Figure 3.1.   An isomer model capturing psychotic and melancholic depression as mirror images of Bipolar I and Bipolar II Disorders respectively.

(i.e. alone defining psychotic depression and BP I status), and with psychotic features being experienced at one pole being associated with a distinctly greater chance of experiencing psychotic features at the other pole. Specifically, our data showed that psychotic features were experienced by only BP I subjects (in 61.2% when high and 40.8% when depressed) but not by any BP II subject when high (by definition) or (and here, more importantly) when depressed. This again fits to an isomer model, with mood/energy and psychotic components essentially being expressed as (non-psychotic and psychotic) mirror images. As our data were based on lifetime episodes, the model would be optimised by referencing lifetime clinical features. Thus, we would expect that individuals with BP I and who had experienced both psychotic manic and depressive episodes might still experience episodes of (say) non-psychotic depression at various times – whether attenuated by medication or other factors. Thus, decisions about bipolar status would require assessment of the individual's most severe episodes and, more importantly, inquiring whether they had ever had psychotic features while depressed or high.

This suggested specificity model for BP I delineation is at some variance with DSM-IV decision rules. Thus, psychotic features are not mandatory to the DSM definition of mania or Bipolar I Disorder. Next, hospitalisation – which can be subject to a range of secondary variables (such as access factors) – is sufficient to assign an individual to BP I status by DSM criteria. And also, DSM-IV manic episode criteria specify a minimum period of one week, whereas our diagnosed BP I subjects frequently reported episodes lasting less than a week (56% in relation to 'average duration' and 46% for their 'longest episode'). Similarly, the DSM-IV duration criterion of four days or more for a hypomanic episode would have excluded the majority of our BP II subjects. If disorders can be defined phenomenologically by their clinical features, this offers advantages over decision rules that are more facultative rather than obligatory (e.g. imposed duration criteria) or which can be more consequences (e.g. hospitalisation) of – rather than definitional components of – the disorder.

Clearly, the diagnosis of BP II is often intrinsically difficult. Our analyses failed to identify any significant differences in the core mood elevation/high energy state (as measured by scale and total measure scores) between BP I and BP II subjects. As noted, this argues for the need for a class-specific feature for BP I status (i.e. psychotic features). Thus, BP II status is defined by the absence of psychotic features in those who experience 'abnormally elevated mood states'. There is room for error in judging when such mood states are sufficiently abnormal – a task even more muddied when many individuals with BP II enjoy their highs. Thus, distinguishing the 'highs' experienced by those with diagnosed Bipolar II from states of normal 'happiness' (and so distinguishing BP II status from unipolar depressive disorders) was another key study objective, with the overall sensitivity and specificity – and positive predictive value – of our measure being impressive. Such results invite reference to comparison measures.

The Mood Disorder Questionnaire (MDQ) was developed by Hirschfeld *et al.* (2000). They had 198 patients attending five outpatient clinics for primary mood disorders complete the MDQ, which assesses 13 mood state items derived 'from DSM-IV criteria and clinical experience' (yes/no format), and 'functional impairment' (assessed on a 4-point scale). The reference diagnosis was made by telephone interview using the SCID (with 70 diagnosed as having BP I, 26 BP II and 13 BP 'not otherwise specified', and the remainder with unipolar disorder). An MDQ cut-off score of 7 or more was quantified as having a sensitivity of 73% and specificity of 90% in distinguishing bipolar and unipolar subjects, indicating that the MDQ had the capacity to correctly detect 7 out of 10 individuals with bipolar disorder. More recently, Angst *et al.* (2005) developed the Hypomanic Checklist, HCL-32, a self-report measure with similar objectives to the MDQ. In their study, scores were compared between 266 bipolar patients and 160 with major depression, with the HCL-32 showing sensitivity of 80% and specificity of 51%.

Our refined 27-item measure had – when our composite BP and UP groups were compared (akin to the MDQ development studies) – a sensitivity of 81% and specificity of 98%. This is an impressive performance by our Mood Swings Questionnaire, with the caveat being that we did not invoke strict DSM-IV criteria (both in terms of clinical symptoms and duration), and as sample nuances and stem questions could have contributed to study results. Thus, replication studies of inpatient and outpatient bipolar subjects, as well as general community studies, are required to test the model further. If the isomer model – with oscillating but independent mood/energy and psychotic feature components – is validated, application studies seeking to determine what factors might contribute to such oscillations would clearly be advanced – as would research into distinctions between BP I and BP II disorders.

Clinical definition of the bipolar disorders

Our clinical experience suggests some strategies for determining bipolar status. To begin with, we propose that all depressed patients should be screened for bipolar disorder, even if they offer no symptoms spontaneously. Patients rarely present complaining of manic or hypomanic symptoms – for such features are generally enjoyed – and are therefore of little relevance to the consultation. Bipolar disorder is more likely in those who report episodes of melancholic or psychotic depression when depressed, and particularly those who report their depression commencing before the age of 40.

Clinical screening might proceed as follows. First, rather than ask whether the individual has ever experienced 'highs' (as some people who do not wish to be diagnosed as having bipolar disorder will deny such a screening question), we prefer the following probe question: 'Apart from times when you are depressed, or when your mood is normal, do you have times when you feel more 'energised' and 'wired'?' If admitted to, representative screening questions pursue whether, at such times, the individual:

- talks more and/or over people
- is more loud
- is more creative
- needs less sleep and is not tired
- spends more money
- is verbally or socially indiscrete
- notices increased libido
- dresses more colourfully, and
- finds 'nature' (e.g. a beach, a park) more beautiful than usual.

One would expect at least 50% of such screening questions to be affirmed if the individual is likely to have bipolar disorder.

If positive on such screening questions, age of onset should be sought. Most people with true bipolar disorder will describe their highs coming on shortly before or after their first significant depression. While some individuals will describe highs from childhood, the likelihood of the diagnosis is advanced if a clear 'trend break' (i.e. onset of new mood states at a defined period) can be established – this distinguishing true highs from personality style or from ongoing conditions such as Attention Deficit Hyperactivity Disorder. Most with bipolar disorder will admit to a distinct change (and most commonly in adolescence).

Most patients with bipolar disorder – as do most individuals – have some level of anxiety. During a true high, anxiety tends to disappear ('like snow on a summer's day') or – for those with comorbid Obsessive Compulsive Disorder – be distinctly attenuated. This is often a key feature for diagnostic clarification.

Corroborative witness data from a parent or partner can assist – but not all hypomanic states are distinctly observable. A family history of bipolar disorder is generally obtained in only a minority – and a family history of depression in about a half – of true bipolar subjects, so that such data offer only slight value in making the diagnosis. At best, they support the possibility.

As noted earlier, most patients with bipolar disorder experience psychotic or melancholic depression when in a depressed phase, so that such features in a young person (i.e. adolescent or young adult) should be expected. Young bipolar individuals (i.e. under the age of 40) do not always show the characteristic features of melancholia (e.g. early morning wakening, appetite and weight loss, profound psychomotor disturbance). Many will report hypersomnia and hyperphagia (i.e. 'atypical' symptoms) instead. However, they generally do report significant cognitive impairment, difficulty in getting out of bed in the morning and anergia (reflecting some psychomotor disturbance). Such 'melancholic' features in a young person should encourage close questioning about the possibility of bipolar disorder.

We see many individuals (both with BP I and BP II) who report manic or hypomanic episodes lasting only hours. Thus we do not recommend a minimum duration to make such a diagnosis. The presence or absence of psychotic features during lifetime highs is used to determine BP I or BP II diagnoses respectively.

In distinguishing bipolar disorder from non-bipolar conditions, we find that those who have historically received a false positive diagnosis of bipolar disorder are most likely to have Attention Deficit Hyperactivity Disorder, a Borderline, or Explosive Personality style, or to be extremely creative individuals who hear the 'muse' more at times of creative endeavour. Creative individuals and hyperthymic entrepreneurs (who have sometimes been misdiagnosed as having bipolar disorder) rarely describe distinct periods of melancholic depression or even periods of substantive depression.

Self-testing for Bipolar Disorder

Our Institute's website (blackdoginstitute.org.au) allows direct, confidential and anonymous self-screening for bipolar disorder by use of the 27-item Mood Swings Questionnaire. To minimise the risk of a 'false positive' diagnosis of possible bipolar disorder, the first few questions seek to exclude those who are unlikely to have experienced clinical depression. At completion, the individual receives a score and a statement about the possibility of bipolar disorder. Our 27-item measure (and scoring instructions) is appended in this book (Appendix 1).

Conclusions

As noted at the beginning of this chapter, the DSM–IV and ICD–10 systems lack a clear model for distinguishing BP I and BP II disorders, while their actual decision rules lack sufficient or clear separation between those two conditions. Our data suggest that attempts to differentiate BP I and BP II disorders by severity (which underpins the so-called 'spectrum' model) will always risk misdiagnosis as the core energy/mood state is not distinctly different in severity, while both evidence a considerable and overlapping range in duration. By invoking a categorical model (involving the presence or absence of psychotic features over the lifetime course), then differentiation may be advanced. We suggest that a diagnosis of BP II Disorder – the focus of this chapter – is made first by judging whether bipolar disorder is categorically present and, if so, preserving this diagnosis for those who have not experienced psychotic features during such a mood swing.

REFERENCES

Angst, J., Adolfsson, R., Benazzi, F. *et al.* (2005). The HCL-32: Towards a self-assessment tool for hypomanic symptoms in patients. *Journal of Affective Disorders*, **88**, 217–33.

Angst, J., Gamma, A., Benazzi, F. *et al.* (2003). Toward a re-definition of sub-threshold bipolarity: Epidemiology and proposed criteria for Bipolar-II, minor bipolar disorders and hypomania. *Journal of Affective Disorders*, **73**, 133–46.

Hirschfeld, R. M. A., Williams, J. B. W., Spitzer, R. L. *et al.* (2000). Development and validation of a screening instrument for bipolar spectrum disorder: The Mood Disorder Questionnaire. *American Journal of Psychiatry*, **157**, 1873–5.

Parker, G. (2000). Classifying depression: should paradigms lost be regained? *American Journal of Psychiatry*, **157**, 1195–203.

Parker, G., Hadzi-Pavlovic, D. and Tully, L. (2006). Distinguishing bipolar and unipolar disorders: an isomer model. *Journal of Affective Disorders*, **96**, 67–73.

Tully, L. and Parker, G. (2007). How low do we go? Is duration of a 'high' integral to the definition of bipolar disorder? *Acta Neuropsychiatrica*, **19**, 38–44.

4

Bipolar II Disorder in context: epidemiology, disability and economic burden

George Hadjipavlou and Lakshmi N. Yatham

The beginning of wisdom is calling things by their right names. Confucius

Introduction

Writing in the late nineteenth century, the Prussian psychiatrist Ewald Hecker provided a clinical picture of a form of 'cyclothymic' illness manifesting in periods of depression and hypomania that bears a striking resemblance to the contemporary diagnostic category of Bipolar II Disorder (BP II) (Koukopoulos, 2003). Hecker and his senior colleague, Ludwig Kaulbaum, likely influenced Emile Kraepelin's seminal work on 'manic-depressive insanity' (Baethge et al., 2003). Kraepelin used the term 'hypomania' to refer to non-psychotic, milder forms of mania, which were expressed along a single continuum ranging from purely manic to recurring depressive states (Akiskal and Pinto, 1999; Koukopoulos, 2003). It is not difficult to imagine how a disorder similar to BP II would have fitted within this scheme (Akiskal and Pinto, 1999). Preceding such views by almost 2000 years, Aretaeus of Cappadocia is also known to have described a spectrum of bipolar illness with varying intensities of mania and depression in the first century AD (Goodwin and Jamison, 1990).

Despite these early, and perhaps even seemingly prescient advances, the modern concept of BP II was only first defined in the 1970s by Dunner and colleagues (Dunner et al., 1976). But it was not until the fourth edition of the *Diagnostic and Statistical Manual for Mental Disorders* (DSM–IV) in 1994 that BP II became officially recognised as a discrete, diagnostic entity (American Psychiatric Association, 1994). The current diagnosis of BP II is based on the presence or history of hypomania – a distinct period of persistently elevated, expansive or irritable mood lasting a minimum of 4 days – in conjunction with at least one major depressive episode. Interestingly, Dunner and colleagues' criteria for hypomania in the diagnosis of BP II required an elevated mood of greater than 2 days

Bipolar II Disorder. Modelling, Measuring and Managing, ed. Gordon Parker. Published by Cambridge University Press. © Cambridge University Press 2008.

(rather than 4) with at least 2 additional symptoms (rather than 3 or 4), making their original definition more aligned with recent proposals to revise the concept of hypomania (Benazzi, 2001b; Angst *et al.*, 2003a; Judd and Akiskal, 2003).

Given that the minimum symptom duration of 4 days stipulated by the DSM–IV is not based on data, it is not surprising that research efforts exploring its validity have argued for reducing this requirement, demonstrating that patients with shorter hypomanic episodes do not differ from those with longer episodes in other clinically meaningful ways (Akiskal *et al.*, 2000; Benazzi, 2001b; Angst *et al.*, 2003a; Judd and Akiskal, 2003). Some experts have also argued for a shift away from an emphasis on mood, suggesting that overactivity should be included as part of the stem criteria as it better reflects hypomanic presentations with their strongly associated elevated psychomotor drive (Angst *et al.*, 2003a, 2003b).

Such proposed modifications to the definition of hypomania and BP II are part of a broader movement to expand the classification of bipolar disorders to include more subtle expressions of hypomanic and depressive illness within the bipolar spectrum (see Chapters 2 and 3). Although studies addressing the epidemiology and natural history of bipolar disorders have been instructive in refining understandings of BP II, disagreement and changes to the definition of hypomania and BP II complicate efforts to fully understand the true scope of the illness, including its course, associated co-morbid conditions, epidemiology, and cost to society. This chapter reviews these issues.

Epidemiology

Despite ongoing disagreement, converging evidence from several community and clinical studies is resulting in an upward revision of the prevalence of bipolar spectrum disorders in general and BP II in particular (Angst, 1998; Akiskal *et al.*, 2000; Angst *et al.*, 2003a, 2003b; Judd and Akiskal, 2003). Clinical studies have suggested that approximately half (30–60%) of BP II patients are initially – and incorrectly – diagnosed with major depressive disorder (MDD) (Ghaemi *et al.*, 2002; Angst, 2006). In fact, even after the onset of their first hypomanic episodes, Ghaemi *et al.* (2002) report that it may still take more than a decade before patients are accurately diagnosed.

Why are episodes of hypomania so notoriously difficult to identify? Why does making a timely and accurate diagnosis of BP II seem so challenging? Several factors are implicated (Hadjipavlou and Yatham, 2004; Yatham, 2004; Ghaemi *et al.*, 2002; Angst, 2006). First, BP II tends to manifest initially and predominantly with depression. Second, patients usually have little insight into their hypomanic episodes and do not report them spontaneously when they seek treatment primarily for depression instead. Third, clinicians often fail to carefully screen depressed patients for symptoms of hypomania. Fourth, co-occurring disorders, such as substance abuse, as well as depressive mixed states, also frequently obscure diagnosis and complicate the illness course. In addition, current DSM criteria for hypomania require that symptoms are 'not severe enough to cause marked impairment in social or occupational functioning', which somewhat blurs the boundaries between illness and normality, making hypomania harder for some clinicians to identify with confidence (Ghaemi *et al.*, 2002; Goodwin, 2002).

However, there is evidence that experienced psychiatrists using semi-structured interviews can reliably diagnose BP II (Simpson *et al.*, 2002). Further, the diagnosis of BP II has been shown to remain stable over time, with only a small proportion (between 5% and 7.5%) of patients going on to experience a manic episode and convert to Bipolar I Disorder (BP I) (Coryell *et al.*, 1995; Joyce *et al.*, 2004). When clinicians systematically probe depressed patients for hypomania they are almost twice as likely to correctly identify BP II (Hantouche *et al.*, 1998). Screening instruments such as the Mood Disorders Questionnaire (MDQ) are useful tools for detecting disorders along the bipolar spectrum (Hirschfeld *et al.*, 2000; Isometsa *et al.*, 2003). Involving families in the diagnostic process further enhances recognition of hypomanic episodes (Katzow *et al.*, 2003). It is also important to probe for a family history of mood disorders as BP II patients are more likely to have BP II relatives compared with BP I or unipolar patients (Coryell *et al.*, 1984; Benazzi, 2004). BP II may also be the most common phenotype in families with bipolar disorder (Simpson *et al.*, 1993). Additional features shown to increase the likelihood that depressed patients are, in fact, suffering from a bipolar illness include 'atypical symptoms' of depression such as hypersomnia or hyperphagia, a positive family history of bipolar disorder, medication-induced hypomania, recurrent or psychotic depression, antidepressant refractory depression, and early or postpartum onset (Ghaemi *et al.*, 2002; Yatham, 2004).

Given the growing appreciation of the difficulties in timely and effective diagnosis, coupled with disagreement over what counts as a true hypomanic episode, it is not surprising that the epidemiology of BP II is complex and contested (Judd and Akiskal, 2003; Akiskal *et al.*, 2000; Angst *et al.*, 2003b; Angst, 1998; Ghaemi *et al.*, 2002; Angst, 2006; Yatham, 2004; Hadjipavlou and Yatham, 2004; Goodwin, 2002; Baldessarini, 2000). There is, however, increasing acceptance that the prevalence of bipolar disorders, including BP II, is higher than previously believed. The traditional epidemiology of bipolar disorders suggested that – compared with depressive or anxiety disorders – bipolar disorders were far less common.

As also considered in Chapter 5, the often cited and influential US National Epidemiological Catchment Area (ECA) Study, which surveyed over 18 000 participants, and the National Comorbidity Survey (NCS) yielded lifetime prevalence rates for all bipolar disorders (I and II) of 1.2% and 1.6%, respectively

(Ghaemi *et al.*, 2002; Bauer and Pfenning, 2005). A 2003 re-analysis of the ECA data which included patients within the bipolar spectrum and whose illness caused significant impairment but fell below the threshold for diagnosis based on DSM–IV criteria raised the prevalence of bipolar disorders to 6.4% (Judd and Akiskal, 2003). Similarly, a replication of the NCS study, though strictly implementing DSM–IV criteria for BP I and BP II, found a combined lifetime prevalence of 3.9% – more than double its previous report over a decade ago. Further, because of methodological issues, the authors believe their estimates are likely to have been conservative (Kessler *et al.*, 2005).

Lifetime prevalence rates reported specifically for BP II have ranged from 0.1% to 3.0%, with most studies hovering below the 1% mark (Bauer and Pfenning, 2005; Pini *et al.*, 2005). Some of the variance in these results is related to differences in study design and assessment strategies. These low estimates, all of which precede DSM–IV criteria, have been challenged both by the clinical studies of depressed patients found to be bipolar when carefully screened or followed longitudinally, and from epidemiological investigations intended to clarify the diagnostic classification of bipolar disorders (Angst, 1998; Akiskal *et al.*, 2000; Ghaemi *et al.*, 2002; Angst *et al.*, 2003b; Judd and Akiskal, 2003; Bauer and Pfenning, 2005; Angst, 2006).

Perhaps the most significant of these is a series of studies from Zurich, which followed almost 600 patients over 20 years and reported rates of 5.5% for hypomania or mania based on DSM–IV criteria, with an additional 2.8% of patients experiencing brief (1 to 3 days), recurrent episodes of hypomania (Angst, 1998). Similarly, a Hungarian study of patients from general medical clinics found that 5.1% of patients suffered from bipolar disorder (Szádóczky *et al.*, 1998). In another investigation exploring the validity of DSM–IV criteria for hypomania, the Zurich group modified the diagnostic criteria for hypomania and divided it into two subgroups, which were labelled as 'hard' or 'soft' (Angst *et al.*, 2003a, 2003b). Briefly, to diagnose 'hard' BP II, at least 3 of 7 DSM–IV symptoms were required (though overactive behaviour was added as a possible stem criterion), the episode must have resulted in observable consequences, and there was no minimum duration for hypomania. 'Soft' criteria simply allowed for any hypomanic symptoms. The authors reported prevalence rates of 5.3% and 5.7% for 'hard' and 'soft' BP II, respectively. They also showed that the two bipolar sub-groups differed significantly from MDD – but not from each other – on a number of clinical validators, thus supporting a broader definition of Bipolar II Disorder that could include both categories.

Another way to think about recent epidemiological data is in terms of the ratio of depressive to bipolar disorders. Upward revisions of the prevalence of bipolar spectrum disorders occur at the expense of unipolar depression. Although conventional wisdom suggests a 4:1 unipolar to bipolar ratio – some experts have indicated that, based on much broader definitions of bipolarity, there may be as many cases of bipolar spectrum disorders as there are of unipolar depression. On the current balance of evidence, taking into account issues of under-diagnosis, misdiagnosis and the arbitrary four-day cut-off for hypomania, a 2:1 unipolar to bipolar spectrum ratio may be more realistic, albeit not widely accepted (Ghaemi *et al.*, 2002). Accordingly, a reasonable overall figure for the prevalence of bipolar disorders is likely to be in the vicinity of 5%. (See Chapter 5 for a discussion regarding artefactual and real factors that might contribute to an increased prevalence of BP II in particular.)

Disability

The notion that BP II is simply a milder form of BP I is misleading. Although hypomania is, by definition, less severe and less impairing than mania, it is the overall chronic and highly comorbid course of BP II, dominated by recurrent symptoms of depression, that causes profound personal suffering and disability, arguably comparable (overall) to BP I (Benazzi, 2001a; Judd *et al.*, 2003, 2005; Joffe *et al.*, 2004). This is especially true when we consider the problem of suicide that haunts the course of bipolar illness.

There is some evidence that the suicide risk may be greater in BP II than in BP I or MDD. A review of suicidal behaviour across bipolar disorders found that patients with BP II attempted suicide more frequently than patients with BP I or MDD (24%, 17% and 12%, respectively) (Rihmer and Pestality, 1999). They were also more likely to employ more lethal means and have completed suicides (Rihmer and Pestality, 1999). Other studies have reported similar rates of suicidal behaviour. A recent study comparing suicidal ideation and attempts between BP I and BP II individuals found similar, albeit elevated rates, with 51% of patients attempting suicide at some point over their lifetime (Valtonen *et al.*, 2005). In addition to previous attempts, comorbidity, hopelessness and depression were identified as key indicators of risk (Valtonen *et al.*, 2005).

Findings from studies investigating the natural history of BP II indicate that patients spend a considerable proportion of their lives unwell, predominantly suffering from symptoms of depression (Benazzi, 2001a; Judd *et al.*, 2003, 2005). For instance, a prospective study following patients for an average of over 13 years found that they experienced syndromal or sub-syndromal symptoms – that is, were unwell – for over half (54%) of all follow-up weeks. Patients experienced depressive symptoms 39 times more often than hypomanic symptoms. The length of hypomanic episodes seems to have little bearing on the overall course of the illness, as patients with hypomania lasting 2–6 days were not measurably different from those with longer episodes.

Sub-syndromal symptoms are far more common than full major depressive episodes and are prominently implicated in the overall burden of psychosocial disability. Impairment in functioning has been shown to correspond directly to increasing increments of depressive symptoms, while conversely, purely sub-syndromal hypomanic symptoms may not be significantly disabling. That is, unlike for those experiencing true hypomania, the presence of only a few hypomanic symptoms was associated with mildly improved functioning (Judd *et al.*, 2005). These findings have important clinical implications: symptoms of depression that do not meet criteria for a DSM diagnosis still need to be urgently identified and treated until patients are euthymic. Although patients with BP II report good psychosocial functioning once they are in remission, they still do less well than healthy controls (Judd *et al.*, 2005). Indeed, there is evidence of some persistent, mild cognitive deficits in BP II patients even when euthymic (Torrent *et al.*, 2006).

Mixed symptoms and rapid cycling present additional common sources of disability. When not appropriately identified, patients with mixed symptoms are frequently treated as if they have unipolar depression – that is, they are prescribed antidepressants instead of mood stabilisers – potentially iatrogenically worsening the course of their illness. Both mixed states and rapid cycling have been linked to antidepressant use (Ghaemi *et al.*, 2002, 2003). Unfortunately, mixed symptoms and rapid cycling occur regularly in BP II. Full-blown rapid cycling may occur in 30% of patients, and mixed symptoms are even more common (Baldessarini *et al.*, 1998). A recent prospective study of 908 BP I and BP II patients found that 76% of BP II patients had experienced mixed symptoms on at least one follow-up visit. Although patients with BP I experienced hypomania more frequently than those with BP II, they were equally as likely to experience mixed depressive symptoms, which occurred on 57% of all hypomanic visits (Suppes *et al.*, 2005). Women with bipolar disorders are far more likely than men to experience mixed symptoms (70% vs 40%, respectively). It is worth noting that mixed symptoms and rapid cycling are both associated with increased suicide risk (Coryell *et al.*, 2003; Suppes *et al.*, 2005).

Comorbidity

Data from both epidemiological and clinical samples indicate that comorbidity is very common in the bipolar disorders (McElroy *et al.*, 2001; Simon *et al.*, 2004; Hirschfeld and Vornik, 2005; Krishnan, 2005). If not appropriately attended to, the presence of comorbid disorders may contribute to misdiagnosis and inappropriate treatment selection, potentially hampering treatment response. Further, co-occurring disorders have been associated with an earlier age of onset, worsening course of illness with rapid cycling, poorer functioning and increased risk of suicide (McElroy et al., 2001; Simon et al., 2004; Hirschfeld and Vornik, 2005; Krishnan, 2005).

A Stanley Foundation study that systematically evaluated 288 outpatients with BP I and BP II found that 57% of BP II patients had a lifetime co-occurrence of another DSM–IV Axis I disorder, while 24% met criteria for a current comorbid condition (McElroy et al., 2001). Overall rates of comorbid disorders did not differ significantly between BP I and BP II disorders (McElroy et al., 2001), while particularly common comorbid Axis I disorders in BP II included anxiety disorders (46%), substance and alcohol use disorders (31%) and eating disorders (12%). Epidemiological studies have also found high rates of anxiety and substance use disorders. For instance, the ECA survey reported that 56.1% of pooled BP I and BP II patients had alcohol or substance use disorders, while the lifetime rates for panic disorder and Obsessive Compulsive Disorder or OCD were 20.8% and 21.0%, respectively (compared with 0.8% and 2.6% in the general population, respectively) (Hirschfeld and Vornik, 2005). A second Stanley Foundation study exploring anxiety comorbidity in 500 BP I and BP II patients found similarly elevated lifetime rates of anxiety in both bipolar subtypes (Simon et al., 2004). When compared with the general population the prevalence of panic disorder (13.9%), OCD (7.0%) and generalised anxiety disorder or GAD (16.5%) were particularly pronounced (Simon et al., 2004). Similarly, BP II patients in the Zurich cohort were found to have a 10-fold increased risk of panic disorder (Pini et al., 2005). A considerable overlap between comorbid substance abuse and anxiety disorders in BP II has been observed (Simon et al., 2004; Krishnan, 2005). It has also been suggested that BP II may be the common link between social phobia and alcohol abuse (Krishnan, 2005). Although rapid cycling, mixed states and comorbidity (particularly anxiety and substance use disorders), are associated with a poorer prognosis, they can, on the other hand, also be considered as modifiable risk factors that – when properly addressed – may potentially improve outcomes. For instance, identifying and treating anxiety disorders concurrently may reduce suicide risk (Simon et al., 2004).

In addition to substance abuse and anxiety disorders, high rates of co-occurrence have also been reported for other psychiatric disorders, including impulse control disorders and Attention Deficit Hyperactivity Disorder (ADHD), binge-eating disorders and several personality disorders (Hirschfeld and Vornik, 2005; Krishnan, 2005). Some authors have argued that increased rates of comorbidity may be partially related to overlapping symptoms across disorders (Krishnan, 2005). For instance, distractibility and hyperactivity are core symptoms in both ADHD and BP II; the criteria for GAD overlap with symptoms of depression; and affective dysregulation and impulsivity are core components of

Borderline Personality Disorder (BPD). Data from genetics, neurobiology, neuro-imaging and long-term natural history studies will help clarify the extent of potentially shared underlying aetiological factors.

The relationship of BPD to BP II is a complex and controversial issue (Magill, 2004; Stone, 2006; Gunderson *et al.*, 2005; Yatham *et al.*, 2005; Benazzi, 2000). Although extreme and opposing positions – crudely oversimplified to polarising arguments that BPD is actually BP II dressed-up differently, or that borderline patients are regularly misdiagnosed with BP II – have been repeatedly voiced, there is sufficient evidence to suggest a more balanced view (Magill, 2004; Stone, 2006). Available data indicate that both disorders can occur in a sub-set of patients, with estimates ranging from 12–33% (MacQueen & Young, 2001; Joyce *et al.*, 2004). Findings from a recent, prospective four-year study evaluating the comorbidity of bipolar disorders in 629 patients with personality disorders (196 borderline patients) cast some light on this issue (Gunderson *et al.*, 2005). Interestingly, BP I co-occurred more frequently than BP II in those with a borderline personality disorder than BP II (11.7% vs 7.7%), and both were more common than other personality disorders. Over the 4 years of follow-up, 3.8% of borderline patients were diagnosed with a new onset of BP II (compared with 4.5% with BP I), compared with a 1.8% rate for other personality disorders. It is important to note that the authors required one week or more of hypomania for a diagnosis of BP II – a stringent requirement which may have improved specificity, making BP II easier to distinguish from BPD, at the cost of potentially underestimating the frequency of new occurrences. When looked at from the other direction, personality disordered patients with bipolar disorders were more likely to be newly diagnosed with BPD (25%) than those without bipolar disorder (10%).

Failing to identify BPD in BP II patients runs the risk of relying on medications and overlooking the potential benefits of targeted psychosocial interventions that may improve outcomes. Obtaining past history data from patients in a structured manner, with a careful assessment of phenomenology, development, longitudinal social history and familial psychiatric illnesses may help to differentiate between BPD and bipolar disorders (MacQueen & Young, 2001; Yatham *et al.*, 2005).

A wide range of medical problems have also been associated with bipolar disorders (Krishnan, 2005; Kupfer, 2005). Symptoms, both of the illness itself, and the medications that form the basis of psychiatric treatment (e.g. mood stabilisers and atypical antipsychotics), as well as associated comorbid conditions (e.g. substance abuse disorders) can all impact negatively on patients' physical health. This is especially true for cardiovascular disease, diabetes mellitus, obesity and thyroid disease – four of the most common medical illnesses in bipolar disorders that occur at significantly higher rates than in the general population

(Krishnan, 2005; Kupfer, 2005). Although data on medical comorbidities specifically for BP II are largely lacking, strikingly high rates (65–77%) of migraine headaches have been reported; BP II patients may be five times more likely to experience migraine (Krishnan, 2005).

Economic impact

Given its chronic course, increased rates of suicide and considerable physical and psychiatric comorbidities, it is not surprising that bipolar disorder is listed as one of the top 10 causes of disability worldwide (Kleinman *et al.*, 2003; Krishnan, 2005). Its overall economic burden includes both direct (e.g. hospitalisation, medications, psychiatric services, etc.) and indirect (e.g. loss of productivity or employment, caregiver burden, involvement with social welfare and criminal justice systems, etc.) costs. The most comprehensive study on this issue found that the total cost for bipolar disorder in the USA was $45 billion in 1991 (Kleinman *et al.*, 2003; Krishnan, 2005). By far the greatest proportion of this sum was attributed to indirect costs (83%), which amounted to $38 billion, with $8 billion accounting for the lost productivity of patients who committed suicide (Krishnan, 2005). Similarly, a UK study estimated that the annual cost in 1998 attributed to bipolar disorder was £2 billion, with 86% of that cost related to indirect costs (Das Gupta and Guest, 2002). Almost half (46%) of bipolar patients in the UK are unemployed, compared with 3% of the general population (Das Gupta and Guest, 2002). Unfortunately, these costs are likely underestimates, largely only reflecting the economic burden of BP I; there are no cost-of-illness studies that have focused specifically on BP II or the bipolar spectrum.

A 2006 analysis of a nationally representative sample of US workers who responded to the National Comorbidity Survey Replication found that bipolar disorder (I and II combined) resulted in 65.5 lost workdays per worker per year (compared with 27.2 for major depression) which, when projected to the total US workforce, accounted for 96.2 million lost workdays and $14.1 billion of lost productivity (Kessler *et al.*, 2006). One wonders how the projected costs might swell if both more impaired bipolar patients who are permanently unemployed and bipolar spectrum patients whose illness, though impairing, does not meet current DSM–IV criteria, were also included. It is also worth noting that the 12-month prevalence of bipolar disorder in this employed sample was 1.1%, a figure that is well below the more recent, revised lifetime rates, thus likely further underestimating the overall costs of BP II and bipolar spectrum disorders. This is supported by the re-analysis of the ECA data, which found significant degrees of impairment and associated costs in the sub-threshold bipolar patients (who comprised the majority of the 6.4% prevalence of bipolar spectrum disorders) compared with the general population (Judd and Akiskal, 2003). Further, comparable rates of total health service utilisation and public assistance (welfare and disability benefits) were reported across BP I and BP II conditions (Judd and Akiskal, 2003).

Another issue that contributes to the costs of BP II is misdiagnosis. Not only are patients with BP II who are misdiagnosed as having unipolar depression not counted in estimates of economic impact, the process of misdiagnosis itself results in additional costs as patients are likely to be treated sub-optimally (Hirschfeld and Vornik, 2005). For instance, a study analysing data from paid Medicaid claimants in California found that patients with unrecognised bipolar disorders (primarily BP I) incurred greater health care costs and were at higher risks for suicide attempts and hospitalisation than patients with recognised disorders (Li *et al.*, 2002; Shi *et al.*, 2004; Hirschfeld and Vornik, 2005). Health care costs were also significantly higher for patients who delayed or did not use mood stabilisers because they were not recognised as having bipolar disorder (Hirschfeld and Vornik, 2005; Li *et al.*, 2002).

Clearly, to accurately calculate the costs of bipolar disorders one must also have accurate figures regarding prevalence. Given that the prevalence of bipolar disorders, particularly BP II, is being upwardly revised, coupled with growing appreciation of the significant degree of disability among patients with non-manic bipolar illness, it is likely that the already daunting costs of bipolar disorder have been considerably underestimated.

Conclusions

The concept of BP II continues to be refined in light of recent clinical and epidemiological studies, which also indicate that its prevalence is likely to be higher than previously believed. Bipolar II Disorder tends to manifest with a chronic course dominated by symptoms of depression, causing considerable disability and frequently associated with other comorbid psychiatric and medical disorders. Rapid cycling is not uncommon, mixed symptoms occur regularly and the risk of suicide is significantly elevated. All of these factors contribute to its enormous costs to society.

REFERENCES

Akiskal, H. S. and Pinto, O. (1999). The evolving bipolar spectrum. Prototypes I, II, III, and IV. *Psychiatric Clinics of North America*, **22**, 517–34.

Akiskal, H. S., Bourgeois, M. L., Angst, J. *et al.* (2000). Re-evaluating the prevalence of and diagnostic composition within the broad clinical spectrum of bipolar disorders. *Journal of Affective Disorders*, **59** (Suppl. 1), S5–30.

American Psychiatric Association (1994). *Diagnostic and Statistical Manual of Mental Disorders*, 4th edn. Washington, DC: American Psychiatric Association.

Angst, J. (1998). The emerging epidemiology of hypomania and Bipolar II Disorder. *Journal of Affective Disorders*, **50**, 143–51.

Angst, J. (2006). Do many patients with depression suffer from bipolar disorder? *Canadian Journal of Psychiatry*, **51**, 3–5.

Angst, J., Gamma, A., Benazzi, F. *et al.* (2003a). Toward a re-definition of sub-threshold bipolarity: Epidemiology and proposed criteria for Bipolar II, minor bipolar disorders and hypomania. *Journal of Affective Disorders*, **73**, 133–46.

Angst, J., Gamma, A., Benazzi, F. *et al.* (2003b). Diagnostic issues in bipolar disorder. *European Neuropsychopharmacology*, **13** (Suppl. 2), S43–50.

Baethge, C., Salvatore, P. and Baldessarini, R. J. (2003). Introduction to Cyclothymia, a circular mood disorder, by Ewald Hecker. *History of Psychiatry*, **14**, 377–99.

Baldessarini, R. J. (2000). A plea for integrity of the bipolar disorder concept. *Bipolar Disorders*, **2**, 3–7.

Baldessarini, R. J., Tondo, L., Floris, G. and Hennen, J. (1998). Effects of rapid cycling on response to lithium maintenance treatment in 360 Bipolar I and II Disorder patients. *Journal of Affective Disorders*, **155**, 1434–6.

Bauer, M. and Pfenning, A. (2005). Epidemiology of bipolar disorders. *Epilepsia*, **46** (Suppl. 4), S8–13.

Benazzi, F. (2000). Borderline Personality Disorder and Bipolar II Disorder in private practice depressed outpatients. *Comprehensive Psychiatry*, **41**, 106–10.

Benazzi, F. (2001a). Course and outcome of Bipolar II Disorder: A retrospective study. *Psychiatry and Clinical Neurosciences*, **55**, 67–70.

Benazzi, F. (2001b). Is four days the minimum duration of hypomania in Bipolar II Disorder? *European Archives of Psychiatry and Clinical Neuroscience*, **251**, 32–4.

Benazzi, F. (2004). Bipolar II Disorder family history using the family history screen: findings and clinical implications. *Comprehensive Psychiatry*, **45**, 77–82.

Coryell, W., Endicott, J., Maser, J. D. *et al.* (1995). Long-term stability of polarity distinctions in the affective disorders. *American Journal of Psychiatry*, **152**, 385–90.

Coryell, W., Endicott, J., Reich, T., Andreasen, N. and Keller, M. A. (1984). A family study of Bipolar II Disorder. *British Journal of Psychiatry*, **145**, 49–54.

Coryell, W., Solomon, D., Turvey, C. *et al.* (2003). The long-term course of rapid-cycling bipolar disorder. *Archives of General Psychiatry*, **60**, 914–20.

Das Gupta, R. and Guest, J. F. (2002). Annual cost of bipolar disorder to UK society. *British Journal of Psychiatry*, **180**, 227–33.

Dunner, D. L., Gershon, E. S. and Goodwin, F. K. (1976). Heritable factors in the severity of affective illness. *Biological Psychiatry*, **11**, 31–42.

Ghaemi, S. N., Hsu, D. J., Soldani, F. and Goodwin, F. K. (2003). Antidepressants in bipolar disorder: the case for caution. *Bipolar Disorders*, **5**, 421–33.

Ghaemi, S. N., Ko, J. Y. and Goodwin, F. K. (2002). 'Cade's disease' and beyond: misdiagnosis, antidepressant use, and a proposed definition for bipolar spectrum disorder. *Canadian Journal of Psychiatry*, **47**, 125–34.

Goodwin, G. (2002). Hypomania: what's in a name? *British Journal of Psychiatry*, **181**, 94–5.

Goodwin, F. K. and Jamison, K. R. (1990). *Manic Depressive Illness*. New York: Oxford University Press.

Gunderson, J. G., Weinberg, I., Daversa, M. T. *et al.* (2005). Descriptive and longitudinal observations on the relationship of Borderline Personality Disorder and bipolar disorder. *American Journal of Psychiatry*, **163**, 1173–8.

Hadjipavlou, G. H. and Yatham, L. (2004). Bipolar II Disorder: an overview of recent developments. *Canadian Journal of Psychiatry*, **49**, 802–12.

Hantouche, E. G., Akiskal, H. S., Lancrenon, S. *et al.* (1998). Systematic clinical methodology for validating Bipolar II Disorder: Data in mid-stream from a French national multi-site study (EPIDEP). *Journal of Affective Disorders*, **50**, 163–73.

Hirschfeld, R. M. A. and Vornik, A. L. (2005). Bipolar disorder – costs and comorbidity. *American Journal of Managed Care*, **11** (Suppl. 3), S85–90.

Hirschfeld, R. M., Williams, J. B., Spitzer, R. L. *et al.* (2000). Development and validation of a screening instrument for bipolar spectrum disorder: the Mood Disorder Questionnaire. *American Journal of Psychiatry*, **157**, 1873–5.

Isometsa, E., Suominen, K., Mantere, O. *et al.* (2003). The Mood Disorder Questionnaire improves recognition of bipolar disorder in psychiatric care. *BMC Psychiatry*, **3** (1), 8.

Joffe, R. T., MacQueen, G. M., Marriott, M. and Young, L. T. (2004). A prospective, longitudinal study of percentage of time spent ill in patients with Bipolar I or Bipolar II disorders. *Bipolar Disorders*, **6**, 62–6.

Joyce, P. R., Luty, S. E., McKenzie, J. M. *et al.* (2004). Bipolar II Disorder: personality and outcome in two clinical samples. *Australian and New Zealand Journal of Psychiatry*, **38**, 433–8.

Judd, L. L. and Akiskal, H. S. (2003). The prevalence and disability of bipolar spectrum disorders in the US population: re-analysis of the ECA database taking into account sub-threshold cases. *Journal of Affective Disorders*, **73**, 123–31.

Judd, L. L., Akiskal, H. S., Schettler, P. J. *et al.* (2003). A prospective investigation of the natural history of the long-term weekly symptomatic status of Bipolar II Disorder. *Archives of General Psychiatry*, **60**, 261–9.

Judd, L. L., Akiskal, H. S., Schettler, P. J. *et al.* (2005). Psychosocial disability in the course of Bipolar I and II Disorders. A prospective, comparative, longitudinal study. *Archives of General Psychiatry*, **62**, 1322–30.

Katzow, J. J., Hsu, D. J. and Nassir, G. S. (2003). The bipolar spectrum: a clinical perspective. *Bipolar Disorders*, **5**, 436–42.

Kessler, R. C., Akiskal, H. S., Ames, M. *et al.* (2006). Prevalence and effect of mood disorders on work performance in a nationally representative sample of U.S. workers. *American Journal of Psychiatry*, **163**, 1561–8.

Kessler, R. C., Berglund, P., Demler, O. *et al.* (2005). Lifetime prevalence and age-of-onset distributions of DSM-IV disorders in the national comorbidity survey replication. *Archives of General Psychiatry*, **62**, 593–602.

Kleinman, L. S., Lowin, A., Flood, E. *et al.* (2003). Costs of bipolar disorder. *Pharmacoeconomics*, **21**, 601–22.

Koukopoulos, A. (2003). Ewald Hecker's description of cyclothymic mood disorder: its relevance to the modern concept of Bipolar II. *Journal of Affective Disorders*, **73**, 199–205.

Krishnan, K. R. R. (2005). Psychiatric and medical comorbidities of bipolar disorder. *Psychosomatic Medicine*, **67**, 1–8.

Kupfer, D. J. (2005). The increasing medical burden of bipolar disorder. *Journal of the American Medical Association*, **293**, 528–30.

Li, J., McCombs, J. S. and Stimmel, G. L. (2002). Cost of treating bipolar disorder in the California Medicaid (Medi-Cal) program. *Journal of Affective Disorders*, **71**, 131–9.

McElroy, S. L., Altshuler, L. L., Suppes, T. *et al.* (2001). Axis I psychiatric comorbidity and its relationship to historical illness variables in 288 patients with bipolar disorder. *American Journal of Psychiatry*, **158**, 420–6.

MacQueen, G. M. and Young, L. T. (2001). Bipolar II Disorder: symptoms, course, and response to treatment. *Psychiatric Services*, **52**, 358–61.

Magill, C. A. (2004). The boundary between Borderline Personality Disorder and bipolar disorder: Current concepts and challenges. *Canadian Journal of Psychiatry*, **49**, 551–6.

Pini, S., de Queiroz, V., Pagnin, D. *et al.* (2005). Prevalence and burden of bipolar disorders in European countries. *European Psychopharmacology*, **15**, 425–34.

Rihmer, Z. and Pestality, P. (1999). Bipolar II Disorder and suicidal behavior. *Psychiatric Clinics of North America*, **22**, 667–73.

Shi, L., Thiebaud, P. and McCombs, J. S. (2004). The impact of unrecognized bipolar disorders for patients treated for depression with antidepressants in the fee-for-services California Medicaid (Medi-Cal) program. *Journal of Affective Disorders*, **82**, 373–83.

Simon, N. M., Otto, M. W., Wisniewski, S. R. *et al.* for the STEP-BD Investigators (2004). Anxiety disorder comorbidity in bipolar disorder patients: data from the first 500 participants in the systematic treatment enhancement program for bipolar disorder (STEP-BD). *American Journal of Psychiatry*, **161**, 2222–9.

Simpson, S. G., Folstein, S. E., Meyers, D. A. *et al.* (1993). Bipolar II: the most common bipolar phenotype? *American Journal of Psychiatry*, **150**, 901–3.

Simpson, S. G., McMahon, F. J., McInnis, M. G. *et al.* (2002). Diagnostic reliability of Bipolar II Disorder. *Archives of General Psychiatry*, **59**, 736–40.

Stone, M. H. (2006). The relationship of Borderline Personality Disorder and bipolar disorder. *American Journal of Psychiatry*, **163**, 1126–8.

Suppes, T., Mintz, J., McElroy, S. L. *et al.* (2005). Mixed hypomania in 908 patients with bipolar disorder evaluated prospectively in the Stanley Foundation Bipolar Treatment Network. *Archives of General Psychiatry*, **62**, 1089–96.

Szádóczky, E., Papp, Z., Vitrai, J., Rihmer, Z. and Füredi, J. (1998). The prevalence of major depressive and bipolar disorder in Hungary. Results from a national epidemiologic survey. *Journal of Affective Disorders*, **50**, 153–62.

Torrent, C., Martinez-Aran, A., Daban, C. *et al.* (2006). Cognitive impairment in Bipolar II Disorder. *British Journal of Psychiatry*, **189**, 254–9.

Valtonen, H., Suominen, K., Mantere, O. *et al.* (2005). Suicidal ideation and attempts in Bipolar I and II disorders. *Journal of Clinical Psychiatry*, **66**, 1456–62.

Yatham, L. (2004). Diagnosis and management of patients with Bipolar II Disorder. *Journal of Clinical Psychiatry*, **66** (Suppl. 1), S13–17.

Yatham, L. N., Kennedy, S. H., O'Donovan, C. *et al.* (2005). Canadian Network for Mood and Anxiety Treatments (CANMAT) guidelines for the management of patients with bipolar disorder: Consensus and controversies. *Bipolar Disorders*, **7** (Suppl. 3), S5–69.

5

Is Bipolar II Disorder increasing in prevalence?

Gordon Parker and Kathryn Fletcher

Introduction

Until the last decade, epidemiological studies have suggested a relatively consistent and low lifetime risk of bipolar disorder in the order of 0.2–0.8% (for manic illness) and some 1% for bipolar spectrum disorders (Goodwin and Jamison, 1990). In the last decade, distinctly higher lifetime community prevalence rates have been reported, as shortly detailed. Any increase is likely to reflect a number of factors, including broadening of disorder boundaries imposed by the 'bipolar spectrum' concept, shortening of duration criteria for 'highs', as well as greater community and clinician awareness and improved detection of the bipolar disorders.

Many clinicians suggest that, in addition to such factors, there appears to have been an increase in patients presenting with bipolar disorders – and Bipolar II (BP II) in particular. If not an artefact of improved awareness and modified detection and diagnostic processes, any true increase should be identifiable in community studies undertaken over time. The limitation to this argument is that, while there have been a number of relevant community studies over the last quarter-century, few have captured BP II, while the case-finding diagnostic tools have also varied considerably.

Epidemiological studies

Several US community studies illustrate a focus on Bipolar I Disorder (BP I). In the Epidemiologic Catchment Area (ECA) study (Robins *et al.*, 1984), where DSM–III diagnoses were generated by the Diagnostic Interview Schedule (DIS),

Note: This chapter extracts – with permission of the *Journal of Affective Disorders* – modified sections of a paper published by Parker, G., Brotchie, H. and Fletcher, K. (2006). An increased proportional representation of bipolar disorder in younger depressed patients: Analysis of two clinical databases. *Journal of Affective Disorders*, **95**, 141–4.

the lifetime rate of a 'manic episode' was 0.92%, and represented 11.8% of the overall affective disorders group (i.e. manic episode, major depressive episode, dysthymia). In the NCS (National Comorbidity Study) – where the study report was published a decade later by Kessler *et al.* (1994) – DSM–III–R diagnoses were generated by the Composite International Diagnostic Interview (CIDI). Here the lifetime prevalence of 'manic episodes' was quantified at 1.6%, and represented 8.3% of the 'any affective disorders' group (constituted similarly to the ECA overall group). Thus, while the lifetime rate of a manic episode had nearly doubled (from 0.9% to 1.6%), other depressive conditions were also more likely to be rated as distinctly increased (e.g. major depression increasing from 5.2% to 17.1%), arguing against any increase being unique to bipolar disorder.

In the US National Comorbidity Survey Replication (NCS-R), involving more than 9000 individuals, DSM–IV diagnoses were generated by the World Health Organization Composite International Diagnostic Interview (WMH-CIDI) system. As documented by Kessler *et al.* (2005), the rate of lifetime BP I and BP II disorders was 3.9% – representing 18.7% of the 'any mood disorder' category (comprising bipolar, major depression and dysthymia). In an even larger US community study (the National Epidemiologic Survey on Alcohol and Related Conditions or NESARC) comprising more than 40 000 individuals, a purpose-designed structured diagnostic measure generated DSM–IV diagnoses, and with a lifetime prevalence of 3.3% being quantified for BP I Disorder (Grant *et al.*, 2005) – a considerable increase on the BP I rates quantified in the earlier ECA and NCS studies (0.9% and 1.6% respectively for BP I). In a recent New Zealand study (Oakley-Browne *et al.*, 2006), as in the NCS-R survey, the WMH-CIDI strategy was used to generate DSM–IV diagnoses and with a lifetime rate of 3.8% being derived for bipolar disorder – quite comparable to the NCS-R estimate of 3.9%.

Thus, the only large community study including BP II was the NCS-R survey but, in reporting a consolidated 'Bipolar I–II Disorder' category, it gave no information on the prevalence or relative proportion of BP II subjects.

Nevertheless, there are smaller community studies suggesting a high prevalence of BP II. Much-quoted is the Zurich Cohort Study (Angst, 1998) of a community sample of more than 4000 subjects. Lifetime prevalence rates using DSM–IV criteria were 0.55% for BP I, 1.65% for BP II and 20.7% for unipolar depression, so that the bipolar disorders constituted 9.6% of that total affective disorder group. Quantification of hypomania (for BP II estimation) respected DSM–IV criteria of a minimum duration of 4 days and at least 4 of the 7 criterion features. When, however, duration criteria were reduced to episodes lasting 1–3 days, Angst estimated that an additional 1.5% had 'recurrent brief hypomania', 1.3% had 'sporadic brief hypomania' and 11.3% had 'subdiagnostic hypomanic' symptoms. Angst reported data indicating that all three hypomanic sub-groups (i.e. DSM-defined, recurrent and sporadic brief) had similar symptom profiles and 'comparable validity in terms of positive family history of depression, treatment for depression and lifetime history of suicide attempts' (p. 149). Thus, he argued for the 'existence of a broad spectrum of hypomanic symptoms' and that the 'Zurich study demonstrates the high prevalence' (p. 149) of such states.

While earlier studies suggested that bipolar disorder represented some 10% of the consolidated mood disorder category, most recent studies report a distinctly higher representation. For example, Angst *et al.* (2003) reported a cumulative prevalence rate in the community study of 24.2% for bipolar spectrum disorders and 24.6% for depressive spectrum disorders. In their review, Akiskal *et al.* (2000) stated that 'the bipolar spectrum in studies conducted during the last decade accounts for 30–55% of all major depressions'.

The data reviewed so far allow several conclusions. Firstly, that the bipolar disorders and the softer bipolar spectrum disorders, in particular, have a higher prevalence than previously judged. Secondly, and as a corollary, that if the definitional criteria are loosened (i.e. by reducing the duration of 'highs' and the number of necessary criterion symptoms), lifetime prevalence rates and the proportion of bipolar disorder within any overall mood disorder group increases. However, while demonstrating a clear impact of definition on prevalence estimates, the key community surveys do not allow us to conclude whether the lifetime true prevalence of bipolar disorder (BP I or BP II) is increasing or not.

The community studies do, however, allow another analytic approach to the question – in that we can examine for any evidence of a 'cohort effect'. If bipolar disorder has a stable incidence, its lifetime prevalence should increase with age unless confounded by methodological nuances (e.g. subjects 'forgetting' episodes with time) or if there is differential mortality affecting older subjects. Ignoring such methodological limitations for the moment, if a condition's lifetime rate actually decreases with age, we should suspect an increasing incidence in younger subjects who have been exposed to the onset age of risk – in essence, a 'cohort effect'.

In the ECA, NCS, NCS-R and New Zealand studies, distinct cohort effects are suggested for bipolar disorder but, as they are also suggested (albeit less distinctly) for many other diagnostic conditions, a general methodological artefact is likely to have contributed – perhaps individuals forgetting episodes with age. As the NCS-R survey was the only US community study overviewed earlier to include BP II Disorder, we shall focus on age effects quantified there. In effect, data analyses demonstrate a general curvilinear phenomenon for conditions other than for the 'Bipolar I–II Disorder' category, with prevalence rates increasing and then decreasing across the four age bands (18–29 years, 30–44 years, 45–59 years, and 60 years and over). However, the data indicate a different pattern for the Bipolar I–II

Disorder category, with lifetime prevalence decreasing linearly across those four age bands (i.e. 5.9%, 4.5%, 3.5% and 1.0% respectively). Further, if one calculates the proportion of those with Bipolar I–II Disorder – as against major depression alone – there is a similar decrease with age in the proportion of those with bipolar disorder (i.e. 27.7%, 18.5%, 15.7% and 8.4% respectively) across the four age bands. Thus, an increase in bipolar disorder in younger subjects is unlikely to be determined merely by a general increase in those with those principal mood disorders. The standardised methodology across the sample (and the differing age bands) again supports a true increase in bipolar disorder in younger individuals.

Black Dog Institute studies

Clarification of any true increase is limited when comparative studies use differing case finding techniques over time, when the diagnostic category is redefined and broadened, and when diagnostic awareness is increased. There is an advantage then to examining databases where standardisation of diagnostic assessment and definition of bipolar disorder occurs. We therefore undertook analyses of two appropriate clinical datasets, and overview those previously reported studies (Parker *et al.*, 2006), while also reporting some new analyses.

Sample 1 comprised 157 consecutively referred patients to our tertiary referral Depression Clinic at the Black Dog Institute in 2005, and with 64 (41%) receiving a diagnosis of Bipolar II Disorder. Standardised screening for bipolar disorder included all DSM–IV diagnostic criteria (apart from duration), additional probe questions and (where possible) corroborative witness interviews. Lifetime polarity judgement was undertaken by two assessing psychiatrists for each patient.

Sample 2 comprised a near-consecutive sample of 492 outpatients referred to the author over a 4-year period ('Personal Clinic') and with a primary depressive disorder. Assessment was standardised in terms of the clinician's probe and criterion questions for assessing lifetime bipolar disorder, again including all DSM–IV criteria and additional probe questions. Those who had 'highs' only on commencement or cessation of antidepressant drugs were not included in the final sample. Reflecting current difficulties in differentiating BP I and BP II, we aggregate both conditions within a 'bipolar' category for comparison against a residual category of primary unipolar depressive disorders.

Across the two samples, the proportion of those with bipolar disorder was quantified as 48% for Depression Clinic and 51% for Personal Clinic subjects. We then sub-divided patient groups using the same age bands employed in the NCS-R study. The age-band percentage representation of bipolar disorder for the Depression Clinic and Personal Clinic respectively were 58% and 63% (aged 29 years and under), 51% and 57% (30–44 years), 44% and 41% (45–59 years) and

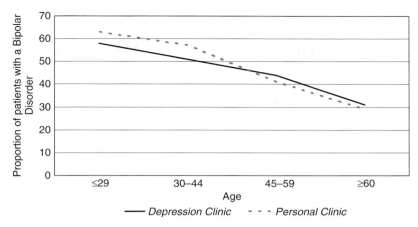

Figure 5.1.   Proportion of bipolar disorder in two clinical samples of unipolar and bipolar depressed patients, across four age bands.
Republished with permission from the *Journal of Affective Disorders* (Parker *et al.*, 2006).

31% and 29% (60 years and over). Thus, as age increased, the bipolar representation decreased from some 60% to some 30% and with the pattern (see Figure 5.1) showing distinct consistency across the two samples.

In our report (Parker *et al.*, 2006), we suggested that it is difficult to envisage any referral bias that might have shaped a differential proportion of bipolar patients across the age bands. Study strengths included two independent samples and standardised assessment procedures being used over time for each sample. The similar (proportional bipolar:unipolar) pattern across two distinct samples and the linear trajectory are all consistent with the hypothesis of a 'cohort effect'. Regrettably these studies aggregated those with BP I and BP II.

In preparing this chapter, we elected to analyse data from a third sample of unipolar and bipolar individuals recruited from the Depression Clinic in 2005 and 2006. The sample comprised 30 BP I subjects, with a mean age of 39.2 (SD 13.7) years, and 125 BP II subjects who had a mean age of 39.6 (SD 15.0) years, while the 212 unipolar depressed subjects had a mean age of 43.6 (SD 13.2) years.

Examining BP I data first, Figure 5.2 suggests a slightly higher proportion of BP I to unipolar patients in the youngest age band (i.e. 29 years or less) but then a relatively consistent proportion over the next three age bands, with the overall chi-square linear test for trend being non-significant (χ^2 for trend $= 1.4$, df $= 1$, $P = 0.23$). Turning to BP II subjects, Figure 5.2 data indicate a linear decrease with age for three of the four time points and then a stabilising proportion in the oldest age band for the BP II subjects. A chi-square linear test for trend revealed a statistically significant decrease in the proportion of BP II Disorder representation with age (χ^2 for trend $= 7.6$, df $= 1$, $P = 0.006$).

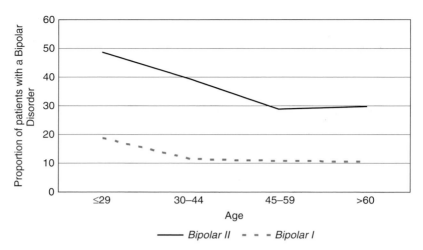

Figure 5.2.   Proportion of 2005–2006 Depression Clinic sample depressed patients with BP I and BP II Disorders across four age bands.

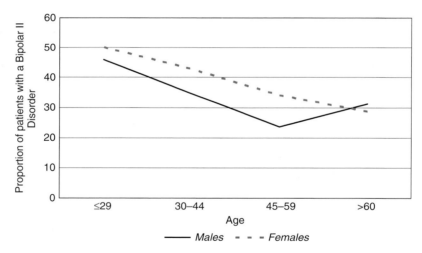

Figure 5.3.   Proportion of BP II Disorder subjects in the sample, by age and sex.

We next examined (see Figure 5.3) for any influence of gender in the BP II subjects (the sample numbers for BP I being too low for analysis). While a chi-square test examining for proportional differences in BP II by gender across the four age bands was not significant ($\chi^2 = 1.2$, df $= 3$, P $= 0.76$), there is the sugges-tion of a differential pattern in the oldest age band. Thus, while the proportional rate decreases linearly across all four age bands for females, the flattened proport-ion graphed in the overall sample in those aged over 60 appears to reflect a curvilinear pattern in males, where the linear decrease over three age bands is reversed in those over the age of 60 years. As sample numbers were few in the last age band (i.e. five males and six females), the curvilinear trajectory may purely reflect chance.

Conclusions

As there have been no large community studies measuring the lifetime prevalence of BP II consistently – both over reasonable time periods and with identical or similar diagnostic measures – it is impossible to determine if the condition is increasing as observed by many clinicians. Even if the proportion of depressed patients meeting criteria for Bipolar II Disorder has increased in overall samples of depressed subjects (as quantified earlier), such a change could reflect referral, definitional, awareness and detection influences, as well as other artefactual determinants noted earlier.

While not conclusive, demonstration of a cohort effect offers an indirect argument. While a paradoxical decrease in lifetime risk is theoretically counter-intuitive for any mood disorder, it is partly explainable by confounding factors (e.g. elderly people forgetting earlier episodes) and real factors (e.g. differential mortality). However, its magnitude for bipolar disorder in large scale US studies in comparison to other conditions does support a phenomenon whereby the condition may be increasing in younger people and so shaping such a profile. The 2005–06 data from our Depression Clinic is the first examination of a cohort effect in a restricted sample of BP II subjects, and should encourage other studies. While formal analyses suggested a significant change in the proportion of BP II patients with age – and a non-significant trend for those with BP I – numbers of the latter group were small. It would therefore be unwise to conclude that the BP I and BP II sub-sets showed distinctly differing patterns. Nevertheless, the data set for those with diagnosed BP II did show evidence of a cohort effect.

There is a need then for a range of epidemiological strategies to pursue the suggested possibility of an increased incidence of BP II Disorder in younger patients. If confirmed, pursuit of candidate determinants (e.g. greater use of illicit – or even antidepressant drugs; dietary changes) would be advanced.

REFERENCES

Akiskal, H. S., Bourgeois, M. L., Angst, J. *et al.* (2000). Re-evaluating the prevalence of and diagnostic composition within the broad clinical spectrum of bipolar disorders. *Journal of Affective Disorders*, **59**, S5–30.

Angst, J. (1998). The emerging epidemiology of hypomania and Bipolar II Disorder. *Journal of Affective Disorders*, **50**, 143–51.

Angst, J., Gamma, A., Benazzi, F. *et al.* (2003). Toward a re-definition of sub-threshold bipolarity: epidemiology and proposed criteria for Bipolar II, minor bipolar disorders and hypomania. *Journal of Affective Disorders*, **73**, 133–46.

Goodwin, F. K. and Jamison, K. R. (1990). *Manic-Depressive Illness*. New York: Oxford University Press.

Grant, B. F., Stinson, F. S., Hasin, D. S. *et al.* (2005). Prevalence, correlates, and comorbidity of Bipolar I Disorder and Axis I and II disorders: results from the National Epidemiologic Survey on Alcohol and Related Conditions. *Journal of Clinical Psychiatry*, **66**, 1205–15.

Kessler, R. C., Berglund, P., Demier, O. *et al.* (2005). Lifetime prevalence and age-of-onset distributions of DSM-IV disorders in the National Comorbidity Survey Replication. *Archives of General Psychiatry*, **62**, 593–602.

Kessler, R. C., McGonagle, K. A., Zhao, S. *et al.* (1994). Lifetime and 12-month prevalence of DSM-III-R psychiatric disorders in the United States. Results from the National Comorbidity Survey. *Archives of General Psychiatry*, **51**, 8–19.

Oakley-Browne, M. A., Wells, J. E., Scott, K. M. and McGee, M. A. (2006). Lifetime prevalence and projected lifetime risk of DSM-IV disorders in Te Rau Hinengaro: The New Zealand Mental Health Survey. *Australian and New Zealand Journal of Psychiatry*, **40**, 865–74.

Parker, G., Brotchie, H. and Fletcher, K. (2006). An increased proportional representation of bipolar disorder in younger depressed patients: analysis of two clinical databases. *Journal of Affective Disorders*, **95**, 141–4.

Robins, L. N., Helzer, J. E., Weissman, M. M. *et al.* (1984). Lifetime prevalence of specific psychiatric disorders in three sites. *Archives of General Psychiatry*, **41**, 949–58.

6

The neurobiology of Bipolar II Disorder

Gin S. Malhi

Introduction

As discussed elsewhere in this book, bipolar disorder is categorically distinguished from unipolar recurrent depression by the presence of mania or hypomania. Bipolar illness is further divided into Bipolar I Disorder (BP I) and Bipolar II Disorder (BP II) generally on a dimensional basis of severity and symptom duration. While clinically useful, such dimensional distinction has limited the capacity to identify differing neurobiological markers, thereby contributing to a common non-specific approach to conceptualising and managing the two bipolar disorders.

Of the growing number and variety of studies pursuing neurobiological markers, most have not considered BP I and BP II separately and, of those that have attempted this distinction, few have achieved satisfactory partitioning. Consequently, there is a paucity of relevant information especially in regards to the neurobiology of BP II. Hence, this chapter focuses on the few promising findings that may eventually provide insights into the neural underpinnings of bipolar disorder, and especially BP II.

The approaches that investigators have used can, broadly, be considered chronologically. Neurobiological approaches that have been employed most widely and thus far yielded interesting results in patients with bipolar disorder include the direct sampling of blood and brain chemistry, and the assessment of brain function using neurocognitive tests coupled with neuroimaging. Post-mortem studies have also been useful, as have studies exploring the complex genetics of bipolar disorder.

The chemistry of bipolar disorder

Metabolic differences across subtypes of bipolar disorder should be detectable (if the subtypes are categorically distinct) and have been sought amongst central and

Bipolar II Disorder. Modelling, Measuring and Managing, ed. Gordon Parker. Published by Cambridge University Press. © Cambridge University Press 2008.

peripheral neurotransmitters, second messenger systems and cellular components such as calcium.

3-Methoxy-4-hydroxyphenylglycol (MHPG)

A number of studies have attempted to measure 3-methoxy-4-hydroxyphenylglycol (MHPG) concentrations in the peripheral body fluids (plasma, CSF and urine) of healthy subjects and patients with bipolar disorder. It is the principal metabolite of noradrenaline in the brain and MHPG levels in peripheral body fluids are thought to correlate to cerebral levels (Redmond and Leonard, 1998), however the coupling of the two systems is not well characterised.

An early study reported that depressed bipolar patients secrete less urinary MHPG compared with bipolar patients when euthymic or manic (Deleon-Jones et al., 1973). This is more pronounced in depressed BP I patients compared with depressed BP II patients, and in both treated and untreated depressed bipolar patients when compared with patients with unipolar depression (Beckmann et al., 1975; Schildraut et al., 1978). Note, however, that some of the reported differences may be a consequence of differences in patient sampling and not of contrasts across subtypes. Interestingly, in one of the studies, depressed BP I and BP II lithium responders had higher urinary MHPG levels than did lithium non-responders (Beckmann et al., 1975). In another study comparing untreated BP I and BP II patients, both urinary and plasma MHPG concentrations did not differ significantly from healthy subjects (Grossman and Potter, 1999; Shiah et al., 1999). Similarly, studies comparing CSF MHPG levels across euthymic BP I and BP II patients and healthy subjects did not find any significant differences (Berrettini et al., 1985).

Taken altogether, the evidence in favour of MHPG concentration differences in bipolar disorder is unconvincing, especially if seeking differences between bipolar subtypes. The approach is nevertheless interesting, and perhaps can be refined in terms of sensitivity if coupled with modern-day techniques such as ligand binding neuroimaging (Yatham and Malhi, 2003).

Protein kinase C (PKC)

Protein kinase C (PKC) is an intracellular mediator of receptor signalling. Akin to the role of G-proteins and cyclic adenosine monophosphate (AMP), it is integral to the modulation of neurotransmission at the synaptic level. Postmortem studies of patients with bipolar disorder suggest that PKC function is altered to the degree that it may help differentiate bipolar disorder from other neuropsychiatric illnesses (Dean et al., 1997), however, the extent of these changes – and their causes – remain to be determined.

Postmortem studies of bipolar disorder brain tissue report increased levels of PKC activity (Wang and Friedman, 1996), whereas normal levels of PKC have been found in patients with major depression (Hrdina *et al.*, 1998). A significant confound amongst these studies is that of medication, necessitating studies of un-medicated bipolar subjects. Nevertheless, the role of PKC appears to be relevant and it is a worthy candidate of future research, especially as there is indirect corroborative evidence from platelet studies that also suggests it has a role in bipolar disorder. In a series of innovative studies examining the ratio of active PKC in platelets, there appeared to be differences between patients with bipolar disorder (Wang *et al.*, 1999) and major depression (Pandey *et al.*, 1998), but no study has explicitly examined bipolar subtypes, so that it is unclear whether these putative differences between the two major mood disorders further sub-divide bipolar disorder.

Calcium

Changes in the concentration of intracellular calcium can alter cellular processes such as neurotransmitter synthesis and release. Hence, it has been suggested that changes in intracellular calcium concentration regulation may contribute to certain psychiatric disorders such as bipolar disorder (Dubovsky and Franks, 1983). A number of studies that have measured blood cell calcium concentrations in bipolar disorder patients have found markedly elevated basal levels in both BP I and BP II subjects. Specifically, elevated levels of basal calcium have been identified in lymphoblasts and platelets in lithium-medicated euthymic bipolar disorder patients (Berk *et al.*, 1994), and in bipolar disorder patients when either manic or depressed (Emamghoreishi *et al.*, 1997). Furthermore, the levels of basal calcium in bipolar disorder patients are elevated when compared with patients with major depression (Dubovsky *et al.*, 1989). In both BP I and BP II patients, lithium normalises basal calcium levels (Wasserman *et al.*, 2004), however, some studies do not show any significant changes in basal calcium levels with changes in mood state or in response to medication (Berk *et al.*, 1994). Therefore, the implications as regards cellular calcium levels in bipolar disorder remain inconclusive and more specific comparisons between subtypes of bipolar disorder have yet to be conducted.

A more robust finding in bipolar disorder is that of a heightened calcium response to agonist stimulation. This is more pronounced during depressed and manic phases (as compared to when euthymic) and the response normalises in bipolar patients medicated with lithium (Berk *et al.*, 1995; Yamawaki *et al.*, 1998). Differences in the calcium response within phenotypic comparisons do not hold across subtypes of bipolar disorder, with consistency of findings in BP I and BP II patients, and similar responses when compared to patients with major depression.

In sum, there is evidence of an increased cell calcium response in patients with bipolar disorder that is discernibly greater than that in patients with major depression, however, it is unsuccessful in distinguishing BP I from BP II patients.

Neuroimaging research

Neuroimaging strategies have provided a novel means of examining the brain. Both structure and brain function can be tapped using techniques such as magnetic resonance imaging (MRI) and magnetic resonance spectroscopy (MRS). The latter samples the chemical composition of targeted brain regions, whereas MRI provides precise structural information. Additional technologies and modifications of MRI permit the in vivo assessment of brain function. Findings from studies that have used these technologies to examine bipolar disorder are briefly overviewed.

Structural neuroimaging studies

Those that have compared bipolar disorder patients with healthy subjects and patients with major depression have reported an array of findings involving a number of brain structures, in particular within prefrontal and temporal brain regions and the basal ganglia. In general, certain brain structures have been found to be diminished in size in both major depression and bipolar disorder as compared with healthy subjects, although some studies of bipolar patients have also noted increases in size in specific subcortical structures. Some of these changes – for instance, smaller amygdalae – may be specific to bipolar disorder, and provide clues about the development of the illness (Brambilla *et al.*, 2002; McDonald *et al.*, 2004). However, few studies have attempted to separate bipolar disorder into clinical subtypes, and those which have done so have failed to identify any significant differences (Sassi *et al.*, 2001; Brambilla *et al.*, 2004).

Functional neuroimaging studies

Such studies rely on proxy measures of brain activity such as total or regional cerebral blood flow (CBF) and glucose metabolism – measured by positron emission tomography (PET) and single photon emission computed tomography (SPECT). Functional MRI (fMRI) exploits the unique properties of haemoglobin (blood oxygen level-dependent (BOLD) effect) to identify changes that are thought to reflect neural responses. These technologies have provided a substantive advance in accessing the working brain, however, it is important to note that functional imaging studies remain constrained by methodological limitations, and many findings require replication.

SPECT and PET studies that have examined cerebral blood flow (CBF) in bipolar disorder suggest differences across contrasting mood states. Ambitious studies that have scanned bipolar patients during manic/hypomanic episodes report increased temporal and limbic brain region CBF with reductions in the frontal and prefrontal regions as compared with healthy subjects (Gyulai *et al.*,

1997; Rubinzstein *et al.*, 2001). Studies that have compared the pattern of CBF in depressed BP II patients with that of healthy subjects have found reductions involving, once again, fronto-temporal and limbic regions (Drevets *et al.*, 1997). As yet no studies have investigated for possible differences in CBF in BP I and BP II patients.

Studies mapping glucose metabolism in patients with BP I, BP II and major depression have generally found this to be reduced in comparison to healthy subjects. Interestingly, though, there are subtle differences between bipolar subtypes, with increased metabolism demonstrated in the prefrontal cortex of BP I patients with mania, and in the limbic system of BP II patients (Drevets *et al.*, 1997; Ketter *et al.*, 2001). Studies that have directly compared BP I and BP II patients reported that glucose metabolism in BP I patients is increased in the limbic region and prefrontal regions of the brain as compared to BP II patients (Baxter *et al.*, 1989; Ketter *et al.*, 2001) and that some of these differences are further enhanced by changes in mood. This suggests that functional differences as gauged by measuring glucose metabolism may have some salience to partitioning BP I and BP II disorders. However, these preliminary findings await further study and replication.

There is a growing fMRI literature specifically examining patients with bipolar disorder, though it is important to note that most fMRI studies have small sample size and thus findings are tentative at best. Few fMRI studies have attempted to compare BP I and BP II patients, with the majority of studies lumping the two subtypes together and some failing to note whether patients belong to a particular subtype.

Studies of depressed and euthymic BP I and BP II patients have shown increased frontal lobe and basal ganglia activation as compared with controls (Lawrence *et al.*, 2004; Malhi *et al.*, 2004a; Strakowski *et al.*, 2004; Blumberg *et al.*, 2003). Increased limbic and basal ganglia activation are also reported in bipolar patients with hypomania (Malhi *et al.*, 2004b). Frontal lobe changes appear to be less consistent, especially in patients with hypomania/mania (Caligiuri *et al.*, 2004) and, in many studies, are not that dissimilar to activation in healthy subjects (Malhi *et al.*, 2004c). Recent evidence suggests that these differences across mood states may reflect a bipolar trait (Blumberg *et al.*, 2003; Strakowski *et al.*, 2004; Malhi *et al.*, 2007a) both involving cortical brain regions (frontal and temporal) and subcortical limbic structures (Malhi *et al.*, 2007b). However, in the absence of any direct comparisons between BP I and BP II patients using fMRI, a functional distinction cannot be supported between these subtypes.

MR Spectroscopy

This strategy samples brain regions for specific metabolites that are detectable using MRI 'probes' (Malhi *et al.*, 2002). The metabolites that can be sampled using proton spectroscopy, for instance, include myo-inositol, N-acetylasparate (NAA), choline and glutamate. These are 'measured' in relation to other metabolites or water and the relative concentrations can then be quantified and compared. This technique has become increasingly popular and is now widely used; but few studies to date have specifically examined BP I and BP II subtypes.

The metabolite myo-inositol is integral to the phosphoinositol second messenger system – whose functioning has been shown to be altered by medications such as lithium. It is suggested that myo-inositol may have a specific role in bipolar disorder (Friedman *et al.*, 2004) though studies examining this further with respect to BP I and BP II have not been conducted (Yildiz-Tesiloglu and Ankerst, 2006).

The metabolite N-acetylaspartate (NAA), found predominantly intraneuronally, is used as an indicator of neuronal integrity (Malhi *et al.*, 2002), and decreases of brain NAA in psychiatric disorders are thought to reflect neuronal degeneration. Some studies examining NAA in BP I and BP II patients as compared with healthy subjects have found reduced prefrontal and frontal lobe concentrations, while other studies have failed to find significant differences (Bertolino *et al.*, 2003; Chang *et al.*, 2003), and definitive changes are yet to be determined. A study that directly compared basal ganglia NAA in BP I and BP II patients also failed to discriminate between the two subtypes suggesting that such NAA differences, if any, may not be sufficient to separate bipolar disorder subtypes, or that they are difficult to identify because of confounds such as medication (Hamakawa and Kato, 1998; Malhi *et al.*, 2007d).

In proton spectroscopy, choline is sometimes used as a comparison metabolite. It is a precursor of acetylcholine and is integral to cell membrane structure. It is thus thought to be important in the aetiology of mood disorders and has been examined in studies of bipolar disorder patients. However, the findings are inconclusive. Diminished frontal concentrations and increases in basal ganglia levels have been reported in both BP I and BP II patients, with some changes associated with mood symptoms (Kato *et al.*, 1996; Hamakawa and Kato, 1998; Moore *et al.*, 1999; Davanzo *et al.*, 2001). In general, nonetheless, the changes are inconsistent and non-specific, and cannot be relied on to define bipolar disorder subtypes.

Neurocognition

Neurocognitive deficits have long been identified in mood disorders, especially during periods of illness. In bipolar disorder, both depression and mania/hypomania have been shown to be associated with deficits of executive and mnemonic functioning (for review, see Olley *et al.*, 2005). Also, recent studies, in both cross-sectional and longitudinal comparisons, have identified euthymic bipolar patients as being cognitively compromised (Malhi *et al.*, 2007c). This is of particular interest, as it suggests a trait deficit that can perhaps be pursued as a marker of diagnosis or treatment responsiveness. A recent study (Summers *et al.*, 2006) has specifically examined BP I and BP II patients with respect to cognition. Surprisingly, this report found that BP II patients were more impaired than BP I patients on IQ, memory and executive measures. Further, another recent study suggests that cholinesterase inhibitors such as donepezil may have differential effects on improving cognition across BPI and BPII subtypes, favoring the latter (Kelly, 2007). This offers some promise in pursuing the neurobiology of bipolar subtypes, especially if these findings can be coupled with neuroimaging and genetic studies.

Genetics

The genetics of bipolar disorder has emerged as far more complex than initially anticipated (McGuffin *et al.*, 2003). It is clear that, clinically, bipolar disorder is the result of gene–environment interactions, and that genetic vulnerability is likely to be polygenic. Researchers, with some success, are conducting candidate gene association studies in an attempt to link bipolar disorder and its subtypes to gene loci (McQueen *et al.*, 2005); however, in general the results from genome-wide scans, although promising, are as yet inconclusive. Family studies comparing BP I and BP II probands suggest some degree of distinction, in that BP II disorder appears to breed true, with relatives of BP II patients more likely to suffer from the same bipolar subtype, or major depression, rather than developing BP I (Gershon *et al.*, 1982; Heun and Maier, 1993; Hasler *et al.*, 2006). This builds to the possibility of a BP II endophenotype that warrants further inquiry (Gottesman and Gould, 2003).

Discussion

Readers are well aware of the many studies that have been conducted in patients with depression, and that much is known about the neurobiology of depressive disorders. In comparison, bipolar disorder remains largely a mystery in terms of its neurobiological underpinnings and very little is known specifically with respect to BP II. It is clear from the bipolar studies reviewed in this chapter that few researchers have focused on Bipolar II Disorder or limited their studies to BP II subjects. The findings from the few robust studies that suggest some differences await replication. It is important, therefore, to question whether the separation of BP I and BP II disorders along symptomatological boundaries is neurobiologically meaningful and whether the differences observed clinically have a pathophysiological basis. It is possible – and quite likely – that the 'true' neurobiology of bipolar disorder does not reflect any currently employed diagnostic classification. Nevertheless, it is important to pursue the neural substrates of bipolarity to assist in redefining and thus better managing of the illness in all its clinical manifestations. However, an agreed nosology is essential, along with a more systematic and integrated approach.

REFERENCES

Baxter, L., Schwartz, J., Phelps, M. and Mazziotta, J. G. (1989). Reduction of prefrontal cortex glucose metabolism common to three types of depression. *Archives of General Psychiatry*, **46**, 243–50.

Beckmann, H., St Laurent, J. and Goodwin, F. (1975). The effect of lithium on urinary MHPG in unipolar and bipolar depressed patients. *Psychopharmacologia*, **42**, 277–82.

Berk, M., Bodemer, W., van Oudenhove, T. and Butkow, N. (1994). Dopamine increases platelet intracellular calcium in bipolar affective disorder and control subjects. *International Clinical Psychopharmacology*, **9**, 291–3.

Berk, M., Bodemer, W. and van Oudenhove, T. (1995). The platelet intracellular calcium response to serotonin is augmented in bipolar manic and depressed patients. *Human Psychopharmacology*, **10**, 189–93.

Berrettini, W., Nurnberger, J. R., Scheinin, M. *et al.* (1985). Cerebrospinal fluid and plasma monoamines and their metabolites in euthymic bipolar patients. *Biological Psychiatry*, **20**, 257–69.

Bertolino, A., Frye, M., Callicott, J. *et al.* (2003). Neuronal pathology in the hippocampal area of patients with bipolar disorder: A study with proton magnetic resonance spectroscopic imaging. *Biological Psychiatry*, **53**, 906–13.

Blumberg, H., Leung, H-C., Skudlarski, P. *et al.* (2003). A functional magnetic resonance imaging study of bipolar disorder. State- and trait-related dysfunction in ventral prefrontal cortices. *Archives of General Psychiatry*, **60**, 601–9.

Brambilla, P., Nicoletti, J., Harenski, K. *et al.* (2002). Anatomical MRI study of subgenual prefrontal cortex in bipolar and unipolar subjects. *Neuropsychopharmacology*, **27**, 792–9.

Brambilla, P., Nicoletti, M., Sassi, R. *et al.* (2004). Corpus callosum signal intensity in patients with bipolar and unipolar disorder. *Journal of Neurology, Neurosurgery and Psychiatry*, **75**, 221–5.

Caligiuri, M., Brown, G., Meloy, M. *et al.* (2004). A functional magnetic resonance imaging study of cortical asymmetry in bipolar disorder. *Bipolar Disorders*, **6**, 183–96.

Chang, K., Adelman, N., Dienes, K. *et al.* (2003). Decreased N-acetylaspartate in children and familial bipolar disorder. *Biological Psychiatry*, **53**, 1059–65.

Davanzo, P., Thomas, M., Yeu, K. *et al.* (2001). Decreased anterior cingulate myo-inositol/creatine spectroscopy resonance with lithium treatment in children with bipolar disorder. *Neuropsychopharmacology*, **24**, 359–69.

Dean, B., Opeskin, K., Pavey, G., Hill, C. and Keks, N. (1997). Changes in protein kinase C and adenylate cyclase in the temporal lobe from subjects with schizophrenia. *Journal of Neural Transmission*, **104**, 1371–81.

Deleon-Jones, F., Maas, J. and Dekermenjian, H. (1973). Urinary catecholamine metabolites during behavioral changes in patients with manic-depressive cycles. *Science*, **179**, 300–2.

Drevets, W., Price, J., Simpson, J. Jr. *et al.* (1997). Subgenual prefrontal cortex abnormalities in mood disorders. *Nature*, **386**, 824–7.

Dubovsky, S. and Franks, R. (1983). Intracellular calcium ions in affective disorders: A review and a hypothesis. *Biological Psychiatry*, **18**, 781–97.

Dubovsky, S., Christiano, J., Daniell, L. *et al.* (1989). Increased platelet intracellular calcium concentration in patients with bipolar affective disorder. *Archives of General Psychiatry*, **46**, 632–8.

Emamghoreishi, M., Schlichter, L., Li, P. P. *et al.* (1997). High intracellular calcium concentrations in transformed lymphoblasts from subjects with Bipolar I Disorder. *American Journal of Psychiatry*, **154**, 976–82.

Friedman, S. D., Dager, S. R., Parow, A. *et al.* (2004). Lithium and valproic acid treatment effects on brain chemistry in bipolar disorder. *Biological Psychiatry*, **56**, 340–8.

Gershon, E., Hamovit, J., Guroff, J. *et al.* (1982). A family study of schizoaffective, Bipolar I, Bipolar II, unipolar and normal control probands. *Archives of General Psychiatry*, **39**, 1157–67.

Gottesman, I. I. and Gould, T. D. (2003). The endophenotype concept in psychiatry: etymology and strategic intentions. *American Journal of Psychiatry*, **160**, 636–45.

Grossman, F. and Potter, W. (1999). Catecholamines in depression: a cumulative study of urinary norepinephrine and its major metabolites in unipolar and bipolar depressed patients versus healthy volunteers at the NIMH. *Psychiatry Research*, **87**, 21–7.

Gyulai, L., Alavi, A., Broich, K. *et al.* (1997). I-123 iofetamine single-photon computed emission tomography in rapid-cycling bipolar disorder: A clinical study. *Biological Psychiatry*, **41**, 152–61.

Hamakawa, H. and Kato, T. (1998). Quantitative proton magnetic resonance spectroscopy of the basal ganglia in patients with affective disorders. *European Archives of Psychiatry and Clinical Neuroscience*, **248**, 53–8.

Hasler, G., Drevets, W. C., Gould, T. D., Gottesman, I. I. and Manji, H. K. (2006). Toward constructing an endophenotype strategy for bipolar disorders. *Biological Psychiatry*, **60**, 93–105.

Heun, R. and Maier, W. (1993). The distinction of Bipolar II Disorder from Bipolar I and recurrent unipolar depression: results of a controlled family study. *Acta Psychiatrica Scandinavica*, **87**, 279–84.

Hrdina, P., Faludi, G. L., Li, Q. *et al.* (1998). Growth associated protein (GAP-43), its mRNS, and protein kinase C (PKC) isoenzymes in brain regions of depressed suicides. *Molecular Psychiatry*, **3**, 411–18.

Kato, T., Hamakawa, H., Shioiri, T. *et al.* (1996). Choline-containing compounds detected by proton magnetic resonance spectroscopy in the basal ganglia in bipolar disorder. *Journal of Psychiatry and Neuroscience*, **21**, 248–53.

Kelly, T. (2007). Is donezepil useful for improving cognitive dysfunction in bipolar disorder? *Journal of Affective Disorders*, in press. DOI: 10.106/j.jad.2007.07.027.

Ketter, T., Kimbrell, T., George, M. *et al.* (2001). Effects of mood and subtype on cerebral glucose metabolism in treatment-resistant bipolar disorder. *Biological Psychiatry*, **49**, 97–109.

Lawrence, N., Williams, A., Surguladze, S. *et al.* (2004). Subcortical and ventral prefrontal cortical neural responses to facial expressions distinguish patients with bipolar disorder and major depression. *Biological Psychiatry*, **55**, 578–87.

Malhi, G., Valenzuela, M., Wen, W. and Sachdev, P. (2002). Magnetic resonance spectroscopy and its application in psychiatry. *Australian and New Zealand Journal of Psychiatry*, **36**, 31–43.

Malhi, G., Lagopoulos, J., Ward, P. *et al.* (2004a). Cognitive generation of affect in bipolar depression: an FMRI study. *European Journal of Neuroscience*, **19**, 741–54.

Malhi, G., Lagopoulos, J., Sachdev, P. *et al.* (2004b). Cognitive generation of affect in hypomania: an fMRI study. *Bipolar Disorders*, **6**, 271–85.

Malhi, G. S., Lagopoulos, J., Owen, A. M. and Yatham, L. N. (2004c). Bipolaroids: functional imaging in bipolar disorder. *Acta Psychiatrica Scandinavica*, **422**, 46–54.

Malhi, G. S., Lagopoulos, J., Owen, A., Ivanovski, B. and Sachdev, P. (2007a). Reduced activation to implicit affect induction in euthymic bipolar patients: an fMRI study. *Journal of Affective Disorders*, **97**, 109–22.

Malhi, G. S., Lagopoulos, J., Sachdev, P. *et al.* (2007b). Is a lack of disgust something to fear? An fMRI facial emotion recognition study in euthymic bipolar disorder patients. *Bipolar Disorders*, **9**, 345–57.

Malhi, G. S., Ivanovski, B., Hadzi-Pavlovic, D. *et al.* (2007c). Neuropsychological deficits and functional impairment in bipolar depression, hypomania and euthymia. *Bipolar Disorders*, **9**, 114–25.

Malhi, G. S., Ivanovski, B., Wen, W. *et al.* (2007d). Measuring mania metabolites: a longitudinal protonspectroscopy study of hypomania. *Acta Psychiatrica Scandinavica*, **116**(Suppl.434), 57–66.

McDonald, C., Zanelli, J., Rabe-Hesketh, S. *et al.* (2004). Meta-analysis of magnetic resonance imaging brain morphometry studies in bipolar disorder. *Biological Psychiatry*, **56**, 411–17.

McGuffin, P., Rijsdijk, F., Andrew, M. *et al.* (2003). The heritability of bipolar affective disorder and the genetic relationship to unipolar depression. *Archives of General Psychiatry*, **60**, 497–502.

McQueen, M. B., Devlin, B., Faraone, S. V. *et al.* (2005). Combined analysis from 11 linkage studies of bipolar disorder provides strong evidence of susceptibility loci on chromosome q and 8q. *American Journal of Human Genetics*, **77**, 582–95.

Moore, G., Bebchuk, J., Parrish, J. *et al.* (1999). Temporal dissociation between lithium-induced changes in frontal lobe myo-inositol and clinical response in manic-depressive illness. *American Journal of Psychiatry*, **156**, 1902–8.

Olley, A., Malhi, G. S., Mitchell, P. *et al.* (2005). When euthymia is just not good enough: The neuropsychology of bipolar disorder. *Journal of Nervous and Mental Disease*, **193**, 323–30.

Pandey, G., Dwivedi, Y., Kumari, R. and Janicak, P. G. (1998). Protein kinase C in platelets of depressed patients. *Biological Psychiatry*, **44**, 909–11.

Redmond, A. and Leonard, B. (1998). An evaluation of the role of the noradrenergic system in the neurobiology of depression: a review. *Biological Psychiatry*, **46**, 247–55.

Rubinzstein, J., Fletcher, P., Rogers, R. *et al.* (2001). Decision-making in mania: A PET study. *Brain*, **124**, 2550–63.

Sassi, R., Nicoletti, J., Brambilla, P. *et al.* (2001). Decreased pituitary volume in patients with bipolar disorder. *Biological Psychiatry*, **50**, 271–80.

Schildraut, J., Orsulak, P., Schatzberg, A. *et al.* (1978). Toward a biochemical classification of depressive disorders. I. Differences in urinary excretion of MHPG and other catecholamine metabolites in clinically defined subtypes of depression. *Archives of General Psychiatry*, **35**, 1427–33.

Shiah, I-S., Ko, H-C., Lee, J-F. and Lu, R-B. (1999). Platelet 5-HT and plasma MHPG levels in patients with Bipolar I and Bipolar II depression and normal control subjects. *Journal of Affective Disorders*, **52**, 101–10.

Strakowski, S., Adler, C., Holland, S., Mills, N. and DeBello, M. (2004). A preliminary fMRI study of substained attention in euthymic, unmedicated bipolar disorder. *Neuropsychopharmacology*, **29**, 1734–40.

Summers, M., Papdopoulou, K., Bruno, S., Cipolotti, L. and Ron, M. A. (2006). Bipolar I and Bipolar II disorder: cognition and emotion processing. *Psychological Medicine*, **36**, 1799–809.

Wang, H-Y., and Friedman, E. (1996). Enhanced protein kinase C activity and translocation in bipolar affective disorder brains. *Biological Psychiatry*, **40**, 568–75.

Wang, H-Y., Markowitz, P., Levinson, D., Undie, A. and Friedman, E. (1999). Increased membrane-associated protein kinase C activity and translocation in blood platelets from bipolar affective disorder patients. *Journal of Psychiatric Research*, **33**, 171–9.

Wasserman, M., Corson, T., Sibony, D. *et al.* (2004). Chronic lithium treatment attenuates intracellular calcium mobilization. *Neuropsychopharmacology*, **29**, 759–69.

Yamawaki, S., Kagaya, A., Tawara, Y. and Inagaki, M. (1998). Extracellular calcium signaling systems in the pathophysiology of affective disorders. *Life Sciences*, **62**, 1665–70.

Yatham, L. N. and Malhi, G. S. (2003). Neurochemical brain imaging studies in bipolar disorder. *Acta Neuropsychiatry*, **15**, 381–7.

Yildiz-Yesiloglu, A. and Ankerst, D. P. (2006). Neurochemical alterations of the brain in bipolar disorder and their implications for pathophysiology: a systematic review of the in vivo proton magnetic resonance spectroscopy findings. *Progress in Neuropsychopharmacology and Biological Psychiatry*, **30**, 969–95.

7

The role of antidepressants in managing Bipolar II Disorder

Joseph F. Goldberg

Introduction

Depression is the most common mood state among individuals with Bipolar II (BP II) Disorder. Indeed, much of the historical under-recognition of bipolar illness, and its misdiagnosis as unipolar disorder, stems from the overwhelming predominance and severity of depressive rather than manic symptoms. As described in Chapter 4, depression, far more than hypomania, accounts for the excess morbidity, functional disability and mortality from suicide in BP II patients. Because hypomanic periods are by definition non-disabling, with symptoms often ego-syntonic to patients, clinicians and patients alike often fail to distinguish BP II depression from unipolar depression. Differences in medication response, course, prognosis and outcome of unipolar versus BP II depression make this nosologic distinction far from academic. Hence, the optimal strategy for BP II depression assumes particular importance.

Traditional antidepressants represent the most obvious and relevant pharmacotherapy strategy for BP II depression, although clinical practice relies heavily on assumptions and inferences from the treatment of unipolar depression, and even Bipolar I Disorder (BP I) depression – rightly or wrongly – to guide decision-making. Choosing to treat BP II depression with antidepressants hinges on the two most fundamental concerns of any medical intervention: is it safe? And, is it effective? Moreover, because alternative pharmacotherapy strategies exist to treat bipolar depression, as discussed in other chapters, it is worthwhile first to consider the existing evidence, gaps in evidence, and clinical judgements that can best inform decisions about when antidepressants should (and should not) be used.

Defining the pathology and delineating the clinical status

Before deciding to implement an antidepressant, or any other treatment, a necessary first step involves accurate recognition of the disease state, symptom profile,

Bipolar II Disorder. Modelling, Measuring and Managing, ed. Gordon Parker. Published by Cambridge University Press. © Cambridge University Press 2008.

and context of presentation. In many ways, BP II here poses an especially formidable challenge, since as an illness construct it is more heterogeneous and nascent than other established forms of affective disorder such as BP I, or unipolar depression. Elsewhere in medicine, clinicians rely on modifying characteristics of a disease entity to help guide treatment decisions, as occurs when oncologists choose from among antineoplastic chemotherapy options based on factors such as tumour grade and stage, presence of hormonal receptor subtypes, primary occurrence versus recurrence, and extent of local versus systemic involvement. Such corroborative markers for estimating response to psychotropic drugs are presently unavailable in the pharmacotherapy of mood disorders, although clinicians can nevertheless rely on clinical (rather than laboratory) features relevant to clinical outcome.

Differential diagnosis is perhaps the most essential component in the treatment of both BP II and BP I depression. Apart from the absence of psychosis – by definition, non-characteristic of BP II – depressive symptoms of BP I and BP II episodes per se may be qualitatively indistinguishable. Melancholic features, atypical (i.e. reversed neurovegetative) signs, and suicidality are as prevalent if not even more extensive in BP II than BP I depression (Rihmer and Pestality, 1999). Symptom targets for pharmacotherapy, in this respect, may be similar in both conditions. The chronicity of depression in BP II appears more distinctive than in BP I depression, and those with BP II Disorder spend a greater proportion of time with depressive symptoms than with euthymia (Judd *et al.*, 2003). Treatment of BP II depression, whether with antidepressants or alternative psychotropics, is typically the major focus of long-term disease management.

Apart from cataloguing DSM–IV symptoms of current depression and past hypomanic episodes, a number of additional relevant clinical factors warrant consideration when diagnosing BP II depression. First, given the high prevalence of comorbid psychopathology in both BP I and BP II – especially alcohol or drug abuse/dependence, and anxiety disorders – recognising the context in which affective symptoms arise can be essential. For example, in the case of drug or alcohol misuse, preliminary findings from the Affective Disorders Research Program at Silver Hill Hospital in New Canaan, CT, suggest that diagnoses of BP I or BP II cannot be validated in the context of active substance misuse – even with collateral historians – in up to three-quarters of individuals within the community suspected of having bipolar disorder. Importantly, despite the high prevalence of depressive features coexistent with alcohol or other substance misuse, antidepressant use has been associated with a substantially increased risk for induction of mania in patients with dual-diagnosis bipolar/substance use disorders (Goldberg and Whiteside, 2002; Manwani *et al.*, 2006).

Anxiety represents another, particularly under-studied comorbid diagnosis in bipolar disorder, and frequently poses further differential diagnostic challenges.

Lifetime prevalence rates of anxiety disorders in general, and social or simple phobias in particular, appear higher in BP II than BP I Disorder (Judd *et al.*, 2003). Anxiety features may colour the presentation of BP II depression – as when differentiating depression with hypomania from depression with anxiety – and can perhaps entirely obscure the ability to discriminate previous hypomanic episodes from anxiety states. In this respect, the autonomic hyperarousal, psychomotor agitation, or inner tension associated with panic attacks, social phobia or generalised anxiety disorder may at times resemble hypomania but lack the rate acceleration, sleep disturbances and goal-directedness of increased activity more specific to hypomania.

When depressive features accompany anxiety states such as these, the presence of signs related to psychomotor acceleration may be key determinants for choosing to intervene with an antidepressant versus other psychotropic drug classes. Past history, including prior medication outcomes (such as non-response to multiple antidepressant trials, or prior evidence of psychomotor activation with past anti-depressants) may be useful for guiding initial therapies.

Beyond establishing the presence of a lifetime hypomania by DSM–IV criteria, supportive signs of a diagnosis of bipolar illness described previously in the literature include prepubescent onset of depression, bipolar disorder in first-degree relatives, patterns of brief and recurrent depression, 'fade off' effects of antidepressants after an initial response (possibly suggestive of cyclicity), and atypical depressive features such as hypersomnia or hyperphagia (Goldberg and Truman, 2003).

Depression with anxiety in Bipolar II Disorder

In patients with identified BP II, little is known about whether or not traditional antidepressants exert anxiolytic effects that are comparable to those seen in uni-polar depression. Before choosing to implement an antidepressant for depression coexistent with presumed anxiety, clinical experience would suggest the value of first screening out the presence of signs related to psychomotor acceleration – such as a diminished need for sleep to feel rested, and increased productivity or goal-directed activity – to help discern anxious depression from depression with hypo-mania. Similarly, when questioned about hypomanic symptoms, patients may sometimes endorse terms such as 'racing thoughts' in an imprecise manner – they may more accurately be identifying anxious ruminations. Thus it is often useful for clinicians not to take patients' use of terminology for granted, and experienced practitioners expend greater effort to ensure that patients who use phrases such as 'racing thoughts' are indeed referring to an accelerated rate of thoughts and ideas speeding through their mind – as if watching multiple television channels simultaneously or in rapid succession, with inability to focus on any one.

Antidepressants likely offer less value in such instances than might traditional mood-stabilising agents.

In the absence of frank signs of hypomania during depression, there may indeed be value in using standard antidepressants for anxious depression, particularly selective serotonin reuptake inhibitors (SSRIs), with careful attention paid to ensure that suspected anxiety symptoms do not worsen and that probable hypomanic symptoms do not emerge. Clinical deterioration may then reflect either an adverse, iatrogenic reaction or else lack of antidepressant efficacy due to the natural course of illness. Antidepressant dosage reductions – or discontinuation altogether – typically helps to resolve such uncertainties.

For many reasons, close monitoring in the days and weeks following antidepressant initiation is perhaps one of the most fundamental yet easily overlooked elements of quality care. In particular, depressive symptoms may worsen either as a result of an intervention or from the natural course of illness. Suicide risk may change, particularly when there are concerns that adding an antidepressant could increase impulsivity or the emotional energy needed to act on existing suicidal thoughts. In patients who experience increased energy, motivation and spontaneity with antidepressants, careful evaluation is often needed to differentiate improvement and normalisation of mood from affective cycling.

Antidepressant safety

Perhaps the most common safety consideration regarding the use of antidepressants for bipolar depression in general involves concern about their potential risk for inducing mania or hypomania, and their potential to accelerate cycling frequency. Some clinicians believe that abnormal mood elevation induced by antidepressants more often entails hypomanic than manic features, although the empirical literature on this issue is sparse (Goldberg and Truman, 2003). Based largely on this controversial phenomenon, practice guidelines vary in their enthusiasm or caution for antidepressant use in general for bipolar disorder. The risk for antidepressant-induced mania or hypomania appears to be confined to a subgroup of probably about 15–30% of individuals with bipolar disorder (Goldberg and Truman, 2003). Recent observations from the Stanley Bipolar Network suggest that the time until switch to mania or hypomania is significantly slower in patients with BP II than BP I disorder (Altshuler *et al.*, 2006; Leverich *et al.*, 2006). These findings would suggest that, all else being equal, concerns about the potential for antidepressants to induce mania or hypomania for patients with BP II depression may be considerably smaller than the risk in BP I depression.

However, all else is seldom equal. In addition to clarifying a BP I versus BP II subtype, other *patient-specific factors* are likely to bear on the relative risk for antidepressants to induce mania or hypomania. As noted above, the presence of comorbid alcohol or substance misuse may elevate the risk for antidepressant-associated mania/hypomania, as does a history of prior antidepressant-induced hypomania (Goldberg and Truman, 2003). Antidepressants have never been shown to improve depression symptoms when they co-occur with hypomanic features. In frank mixed states (which, technically, apply solely to Bipolar I Disorder in DSM–IV, due to the absence of a DSM–IV nosologic category for 'mixed hypomania'), antidepressants are eschewed by some practice guidelines and indeed have no demonstrated prophylactic value (Prien et al., 1988). In bipolar rapid cycling, antidepressants have been suggested as increasing cycling frequency and rendering mood-stabilising agents less effective (Wehr et al., 1988). Recent mania or hypomania (i.e. during the two months preceding a current depressive episode) has also been associated with an elevated risk for affective polarity switch when antidepressants are added to mood stabilisers (MacQueen et al., 2002). In data from the Stanley Bipolar Network, risk for antidepressant-induced mania or hypomania also was higher in Bipolar (I, II or NOS) depressed patients without a family history of affective disorder (Leverich et al., 2006).

New findings from the National Institute of Mental Health Systematic Treatment Enhancement Program for Bipolar Disorder (NIMH STEP-BD) indicate that in Bipolar (I or II) patients with full depressive episodes plus any concurrent manic/hypomanic symptoms, the addition of antidepressants to mood-stabilising agents holds no value for hastening improvement, but does increase mania symptom severity. Hence, antidepressants likely would not be considered either safe or useful for depressive features present in conjunction with even sub-syndromal hypomania. The STEP-BD database also identifies a greater risk for antidepressant-induced mania in younger patients, regardless of age at illness onset, further pointing to the importance of close monitoring when giving antidepressants to children or adolescents.

With respect to antidepressant-specific factors related to treatment-emergent mania/hypomania, risk may be intrinsically greater with noradrenergic agents such as tricyclics as compared to SSRIs (Peet, 1994) or bupropion. Rates of switch from depression to mania or hypomania appear higher with the serotonergic/noradrenergic agent, venlafaxine, relative to SSRIs (Vieta et al., 2002; Leverich et al., 2006; Post et al., 2006) or bupropion (Leverich et al., 2006; Post et al., 2006). Notably, randomised data from the Stanley Bipolar Network found a 3.5-fold increased risk for switches to mania or hypomania evident during 10 weeks of acute treatment with venlafaxine as compared to sertraline or bupropion, particularly among subjects with a history of rapid cycling (Leverich et al., 2006; Post et al., 2006). Other serotonergic/noradrenergic mixed agonists, such as duloxetine or mirtazapine, have not been studied specifically in bipolar depression, although clinicians sometimes think of this drug class – especially the combination of venlafaxine and mirtazapine, given their complementary receptor profiles – for highly severe, melancholic or treatment-resistant depression in general. Such high-potency strategies, while conceptually appealing and often clinically tempting, should be undertaken with caution if used in severe forms of BP II depression, with recognition of a possibly increased risk for induction of hypomania or cycle acceleration.

In an early study, the monoamine oxidase inhibitor (MAOI) tranylcypromine was associated with a greater risk for antidepressant-induced mania or hypomania in BP II than BP I depression, despite comparable efficacy in both bipolar subtypes (Himmelhoch *et al.*, 1991). By contrast, in the NIMH STEP-BD programme, a somewhat *lower* rate of antidepressant-associated mania or hypomania was identified during treatment with MAOIs than with other antidepressants. Disparate findings across studies may owe in part to differences in the extent and dosing of concomitant mood stabilisers, as well as distribution and accounting of other aforementioned *patient-specific factors* related to antidepressant-induced mood switching, such as BP I versus BP II depression, or the presence of rapid cycling.

A further safety concern with antidepressants involves the controversial relationship between antidepressant use and the emergence or exacerbation of suicidal features, particularly in children and adolescents. Issues related to suicide prevention and management are of special importance in patients with BP II in light of reports of higher risk for suicidal behaviour than are seen in BP I or unipolar depression (Rihmer and Pestality, 1999). Some clinicians have raised concerns that the intensification of suicidal features during antidepressant treatment could bear on heightened activation and impulsivity in depressed patients with a bipolar diathesis, or depressed patients with sub-syndromal hypomanic features. However, in observational findings from the National Institute of Mental Health Systematic Treatment Enhancement Program for Bipolar Disorder (STEP-BD), Bauer and colleagues (2006) found no discernible increase in suicidal ideation or behaviour associated with antidepressant use – although the lack of statistical control for potential confounding factors makes the generalisability of findings from that study contingent on replication from randomised trials.

Are traditional antidepressants efficacious for Bipolar II depression?

Drug safety and efficacy together represent the cornerstones of any pharmacotherapy. While much attention has been paid in recent years to concerns about the safety of antidepressants in bipolar disorder (potential for induction of mania or precipitation of impulsive suicidal behaviours), clinicians and patients may often take as a given the efficacy of antidepressants for bipolar depression. Some

clinicians have raised concerns that antidepressants in general may be less efficacious for bipolar than unipolar depression, although such hypotheses have thus far
not been borne out by large-scale naturalistic studies in BP I depression (Moller
et al., 2001).

From the standpoint of evidence-based medicine, data from controlled trials
examining the utility of traditional antidepressants specifically for BP II depression
are exceedingly rare. Many practice guidelines acknowledge this shortcoming by
advising extrapolation from the literature regarding BP I depression. Perhaps the
largest randomised study specifically reporting on BP II depression is the sub-
group of BP II depressed patients within the Stanley Bipolar Network. This study
compared sertraline (n = 14), bupropion (n = 13), or venlafaxine (n = 15) added
to traditional mood stabilisers (Leverich et al., 2006), although acute and long-
term efficacy in that study was not reported separately for BP II and BP I subjects.
In the total sample of Bipolar I, II and NOS disorder subjects, all three pharma-
cotherapies showed similar rates of acute (10-week) response (49–53%) and
remission (34–41%). However, the absence of a placebo plus mood stabiliser
group in this study renders the findings somewhat provisional.

Himmelhoch and colleagues (1991) described a unique role for monoamine
oxidase inhibitors in anergic bipolar depression, regardless of diagnostic I or II
subtype. Overall, acute antidepressant response with tranylcypromine was superior to that seen with imipramine (81% versus 48%, respectively), although
separate response rates were not reported for BP II versus BP I patients. Little if
any information exists about other MAOIs, such as phenelzine, or the newly
available transdermal preparation of the irreversible MAOI-B inhibitor selegeline,
for bipolar depression.

While there currently are no large-scale randomised placebo-controlled trials of
antidepressants specifically for BP II depression, open data exist with the use of
venlafaxine and fluoxetine (Amsterdam and Brunswick, 2003). In one open trial
(Amsterdam et al., 2004) of fluoxetine monotherapy dosed at 20 mg/day, response
(defined as > 50% reduction in Hamilton Depression scale scores from baseline)
occurred in 11 of 37 subjects (intent-to-treat sample, 30%; 11/23 completers, or
48%). In addition, efficacy with escitalopram monotherapy has been suggested
from a proof of concept double-blind, randomised crossover study involving
10 BP II subjects, in which Parker and colleagues (2006) found significantly
fewer periods of either depression or mood elevation during 9 months of treatment with escitalopram than placebo.

To the extent one can extrapolate from findings of studies in BP I depression,
two randomised controlled trials challenge the presumed efficacy of traditional
antidepressants relative to mood stabilisers alone. In one 10-week study, Nemeroff
and colleagues (2001) found that the addition of either paroxetine or imipramine

to therapeutically dosed lithium offered no antidepressant advantage over thera-peutically dosed lithium plus placebo. Another study by Young and colleagues (2000) found similar acute antidepressant response rates with the combination of lithium and divalproex (n = 16), or paroxetine added to either lithium or dival-proex (n = 11).

Possible novel antidepressants

While it is beyond the scope of this chapter to discuss the variety of novel psychotropics with possible antidepressant efficacy in BP II depression, mention is warranted for two agents that have demonstrated at least preliminary evidence from placebo-controlled trials. First, the dopamine agonist pramipexole was described in a preliminary trial (n = 22) by our group as showing greater efficacy than placebo for treatment-resistant BP I or BP II depression (Goldberg et al., 2004), and in a separate study solely of BP II depression (n = 21) by Zarate and colleagues (2004). Both studies reported response rates of approximately 60% when added to standard mood stabilisers, significantly greater than placebo, at doses of approximately 1.7 mg/day. The rationale for dopamine agonism in bipolar depression bears on theories of putative hypodopaminergic tone in meso-cortical tracts, suggesting a perhaps unique benefit in anergic, psychomotor retarded presentations of depression, involving diminished attention, and an absence of agitated or psychotic features. Hypomania emerged in one of 10 subjects taking pramipexole in the BP II depression study by Zarate and colleagues, and in 1 of 12 in the study by Goldberg et al. (2004). Other common adverse effects included nausea, sedation and headache, though seldom did drug intolerance lead to premature discontinuation.

A second promising agent for bipolar depression is the novel psychostimulant modafinil. In a 6-week study, Frye and colleagues (2005) compared a standard mood stabiliser plus either modafinil (mean dose of 175 mg/day) or placebo in 90 BP I or BP II depressed-phase outpatients. Significantly greater reductions from baseline were observed, using the Inventory for Depressive Symptoms (IDS), with modafinil than with placebo.

Is co-administration with mood stabilisers necessary for Bipolar II depression?

Most contemporary practice guidelines advise against the use of antidepressant monotherapies for BP I, and suggest that mood stabilisers be used prior to antidepressants (both for their possible antidepressant efficacy as well as a pre-sumed protection against induction of mania should an antidepressant later become added). In BP I depression, traditional mood stabilisers (i.e. lithium, divalproex or carbamazepine) appear to reduce the risk for mania induced by tricyclic antidepressants, but such protection may be less robust against other antidepressant classes. In BP II depression, comparatively little empirical information exists about whether or not mood stabilisers are needed to protect against antidepressant-associated hypomania. Some authorities advise that antidepressant monotherapies may be reasonable first-line treatments for BP II depression, particularly in the absence of rapid cycling.

A small body of evidence supports this position, as summarised by Amsterdam and Brunswick (2003). For example, in a small (n = 23) open trial of fixed dose fluoxetine (20 mg/day) for major depression in BP II or Bipolar Disorder Not Otherwise Specified (NOS), at least a 50% improvement from baseline depression severity scores was seen in nearly half of subjects completing 8 weeks of treatment, with 7.3% showing signs of emerging hypomania. A subsequent placebo-controlled 6-month randomised substitution study found a statistically non-significant, but numerically greater, risk for subsequent depressive relapse with placebo than fluoxetine. This latter study also reported a statistically significant, though clinically modest, increase in mania symptom severity scores during 6 months of continuation treatment with fluoxetine than placebo. Fluoxetine monotherapy was further supported by findings from an 8-week study of fluoxetine or olanzapine monotherapy versus their combination in BP I (n = 34) or BP II (n = 2) depressed patients (Amsterdam and Shults, 2005a, 2005b). Significant reductions occurred for depression symptoms in all treatment groups, with no significant elevation of mania symptoms. Venlafaxine monotherapy (up to 225 mg/day) also has been studied by this same research team in 15 women with BP II depression for up to 6 weeks, with comparable efficacy to that seen in a comparison group of women with unipolar depression, and no switches to hypomania (Amsterdam and Brunswick, 2003). Finally, the aforementioned proof of concept study with escitalopram monotherapy (Parker *et al.*, 2006) provides additional preliminary evidence of the possible bimodal efficacy of SSRIs for acute as well as longer-term treatment of BP II depression.

From the standpoint of clinical management, mood stabilisers would seem to be appropriate components of a pharmacotherapy regimen for BP II when there is evidence of high cyclicity (i.e. frequent episodes, regardless of polarity), a proneness toward hypomania, hypomanic symptoms coexistent with current depression, and/or a poor or inadequate response to antidepressant monotherapies.

Loss of antidepressant efficacy

A number of authors have identified the 'fading off' of antidepressants after an initial response as potentially suggestive of cyclicity, and hence bipolarity. Such speculations derive partly from observations that tolerance to antidepressants may be more common among individuals with bipolar (58%) than unipolar (18%) depression (Ghaemi *et al.*, 2004). The so-called 'poop-out' phenomenon of some antidepressants has been described from one perspective as a strictly pharmaco-dynamic event that reflects tachyphylaxis, or physiological tolerance. Others have suggested that the early rapid response to an antidepressant may actually be a non-enduring placebo effect, and that 'poop out' after several weeks or months is merely the loss of initial placebo responsiveness. Taken in the context of other indicators of a diagnosis of bipolar disorder, the frequent loss of efficacy after an initial apparent response to antidepressants may usefully prompt clinicians to consider the possibility of a cyclical process for which ongoing antidepressants may be inadvisable.

Dosing

It is also unknown whether modal dosing of antidepressants tends to differ for patients with BP II than BP I depression, or for BP II than unipolar depression. In the randomised flexible-dose antidepressant trial by Altshuler and colleagues previously mentioned, modal dosing of bupropion was somewhat higher in sub-jects with BP II (400 mg/day) than BP I (300 mg/day) disorder, although sertraline doses tended to be lower in those with BP II (100 mg/day) than BP I (200 mg/day) subdiagnoses. Venlafaxine doses in this study were roughly comparable between BP II and BP I subjects (200 mg/day and 175 mg/day, respectively). In the ran-domised comparison of paroxetine and venlafaxine by Vieta and colleagues (2002), venlafaxine was administered at a mean dose of 179 mg/day, as compared to a mean paroxetine dose of 32 mg/day. Preclinical evidence suggests a predom-inantly SSRI effect with venlafaxine when dosed at less than 150 mg/day, with serotonergic-noradrenergic reuptake inhibition (SNRI) properties at higher doses. It is unknown whether or not risks for antidepressant-induced mania may be dose-dependent with venlafaxine, or other antidepressants.

Do antidepressants prevent recurrence in Bipolar II Disorder?

Long-term antidepressant continuation and maintenance therapy remains the subject of considerable debate, in part due to concerns about long-term cycle acceleration but also because there are no large-scale randomised placebo-controlled trials with any modern antidepressants to assess relapse prevention with, versus without antidepressants. Open trials have described – in those who have had an acute remission – an association between subsequent antidepressant cessation and high rates of depression relapse in BP I or BP II patients (Altshuler *et al.*, 2003), although the non-controlled, non-randomised nature of such studies precludes drawing causal inferences about the consequences of antidepressant continuation or cessation – that is, subjects may have stopped their antidepressants and therefore relapsed, or relapsed and therefore stopped their antidepressants; and those who remained on antidepressants may have done so because they were euthymic, rather than having stayed euthymic because they remained on antidepressants.

One-year data exist from the randomised comparison of bupropion, sertraline or venlafaxine added to a traditional mood stabiliser for patients with Bipolar Disorder Type I, II or NOS, as reported by Leverich and colleagues (2006), with relapse rates ranging from 29.0% to 37.5%. However, the absence of a placebo plus mood stabiliser comparison group makes it difficult to know the extent to which antidepressants added to mood stabilisers may have increased or decreased relapse rates.

Summary

In the absence of sufficiently large or numerous clinical trials of antidepressants for BP II depression, assumptions about their efficacy should be made with caution. It would seem prudent before initiating an antidepressant trial for BP II depression to assure the absence of current or recent concomitant hypomanic symptoms, evaluate historical response to past mood-stabilising agents as well as antidepressants, and affirm the absence of any previous switch to hypomania in the recent aftermath of antidepressant exposure. Particular caution should be exercised in giving antidepressants to BP II patients with rapid cycling. In general, one might favour antidepressants that have been studied in BP II depression (bupropion, sertraline, fluoxetine, escitalopram) and have relatively low reported switch rates, before choosing other antidepressants with no reported safety or efficacy data in BP I or BP II disorders.

Long-term antidepressant pharmacotherapy for bipolar disorder remains controversial, although there are provisional data to support the long-term utility of some antidepressants in patients with BP II. Finally, decisions about the role of an antidepressant must be made relative to the utility of alternative interventions, such as psychotherapy (see Chapter 12), mood-stabilising agents alone (see Chapter 9), atypical antipsychotics such as quetiapine (see Chapter 10), and novel agents that have been studied for BP II depression such as pramipexole or modafinil added to traditional mood stabilisers.

REFERENCES

Altshuler, L. L., Suppes, T., Black, D. *et al.* (2003). Impact of antidepressant discontinuation after acute bipolar depression remission on rates of depressive relapse at one-year follow-up. *American Journal of Psychiatry*, **160**, 1252–62.

Altshuler, L. L., Suppes, T., Black, D. O. *et al.* (2006). Lower switch rate in depressed patients with Bipolar II than Bipolar I Disorder treated adjunctively with second-generation anti-depressants. *American Journal of Psychiatry*, **163**, 313–15.

Amsterdam, J. D. and Brunswick, D. J. (2003). Antidepressant monotherapy for Bipolar Type II major depression. *Journal of Affective Disorders*, **5**, 388–95.

Amsterdam, J. D. and Shults, J. (2005a). Fluoxetine monotherapy of Bipolar II and Bipolar NOS major depression: a double-blind, placebo-substitution, continuation study. *International Clinical Psychopharmacology*, **20**, 257–64.

Amsterdam, J. D. and Shults, J. (2005b). Comparison of fluoxetine, olanzapine, and combined fluoxetine plus olanzapine initial therapy of Bipolar Type I and Type II major depression – lack of manic induction. *Journal of Affective Disorders*, **87**, 121–30.

Amsterdam, J. D., Shults, J., Brunswick, D. J. and Hundert, M. (2004). Short-term fluoxetine monotherapy for Bipolar Type II or Bipolar NOS major depression – low manic switch rate. *Bipolar Disorders*, **6**, 75–81.

Bauer, M. S., Wisniewski, S. R., Marangell, L. B. *et al.* for the STEP-BD Investigators (2006). Are antidepressants associated with new-onset suicidality in bipolar disorder? A prospective study of participants in the systematic treatment enhancement program for bipolar disorder (STEP-BD). *Journal of Clinical Psychiatry*, **67**, 48–55.

Frye, M. A., Grunze, H., Suppes, T. *et al.* (2005). Modafinil in the treatment of bipolar depression: a placebo-controlled trial. New research abstract presented at the ACNP Annual Meeting, 11–15 December, Hilton Waikoloa Village, Hawaii.

Ghaemi, S. N., Rosenquist, K. J., Ko, J. Y. *et al.* (2004). Antidepressant treatment in bipolar versus unipolar depression. *American Journal of Psychiatry*, **161**, 163–5.

Goldberg, J. F., Burdick, K. E. and Endick, C. J. (2004). Preliminary randomized, double-blind, placebo-controlled trial of pramipexole for treatment-resistant bipolar depression. *American Journal of Psychiatry*, **161**, 564–6.

Goldberg, J. F. and Truman, C. J. (2003). Antidepressant-induced mania: An overview of current controversies. *Bipolar Disorders*, **5**, 407–20.

Goldberg, J. F. and Whiteside, J. E. (2002). The association between substance abuse and antidepressant-induced mania in bipolar disorder: A preliminary study. *Journal of Clinical Psychiatry*, **63**, 791–5.

Himmelhoch, J. M., Thase, M. E., Mallinger, A. G. and Houck, P. (1991). Tranylcypromine versus imipramine in anergic bipolar depression. *American Journal of Psychiatry*, **148**, 910–16.

Judd, L. L., Akiskal, H. S., Schettler, P. J. *et al.* (2003). A prospective investigation of the natural history of the long-term weekly symptomatic status of Bipolar II Disorder. *Archives of General Psychiatry*, **60**, 261–9.

Leverich, G. S., Altshuler, L. L., Frye, M. A. *et al.* (2006). Risk of switch in mood polarity to hypomania or mania in patients with bipolar depression during acute and continuation trials of venlafaxine, sertraline, and bupropion as adjuncts to mood stabilizers. *American Journal of Psychiatry*, **163**, 232–9.

MacQueen, G. M., Young, L. T., Marriott, M. *et al.* (2002). Previous mood state predicts response and switch rates in patients with bipolar depression. *Acta Psychiatrica Scandinavica*, **105**, 414–18.

Manwani, S. G., Pardo, T. B., Albanese, M. J. *et al.* (2006). Substance use disorder and other predictors of antidepressant-induced mania: a retrospective chart review. *Journal of Clinical Psychiatry*, **67**, 1341–5.

Moller, H. J., Bottlender, R., Grunze, H., Strauss, A. and Wittmann, J. (2001). Are antidepressants less effective in the acute treatment of Bipolar I compared to unipolar depression. *Journal of Affective Disorders*, **67**, 141–6.

Nemeroff, C. B., Evans, D. L., Gyulai, L. *et al.* (2001). Double-blind, placebo-controlled comparison of imipramine and paroxetine in the treatment of bipolar depression. *American Journal of Psychiatry*, **158**, 906–12.

Parker, G., Tully, L., Olley, A. and Hadzi-Pavlovic, D. (2006). SSRIs as mood stabilizers for Bipolar II Disorder? A proof of concept study. *Journal of Affective Disorders*, **92**, 205–14.

Peet, M. (1994). Induction of mania with selective serotonin re-uptake inhibitors and tricyclic antidepressants. *British Journal of Psychiatry*, **164**, 549–50.

Post, R. M., Altshuler, L. L., Leverich, G. S. *et al.* (2006). Mood switch in bipolar depression: comparison of adjunctive venlafaxine, bupropion and sertraline. *British Journal of Psychiatry*, **189**, 124–31.

Prien, R. F., Himmelhoch, J. M. and Kupfer, D. J. (1988). Treatment of mixed mania. *Journal of Affective Disorders*, **15**, 9–15.

Rihmer, Z. and Pestality, P. (1999). Bipolar II disorder and suicidal behavior. *Psychiatry Clinics of North America*, **22**, 667–73.

Vieta, E., Martinez-Aran, A., Goikolea, J. M. *et al.* (2002). A randomized trial comparing paroxetine and venlafaxine in the treatment of bipolar depressed patients taking mood stabilizers. *Journal of Clinical Psychiatry*, **63**, 508–12.

Wehr, T. A., Sack, D. A., Rosenthal, N. E and Cowdry, R. W. (1988). Rapid-cycling affective disorder: contributing factors and treatment responses in 51 patients. *American Journal of Psychiatry*, **145**, 179–84.

Young, L. T., Joffe, R. T., Robb, J. C. *et al.* (2000). Double-blind comparison of addition of a second mood stabilizer versus an antidepressant to an initial mood stabilizer for treatment of patients with bipolar depression. *American Journal of Psychiatry*, **157**, 124–6.

Zarate, C. A. Jr., Payne, J. L., Singh, J. *et al.* (2004). Pramipexole for Bipolar II depression: A placebo-controlled proof of concept study. *Biological Psychiatry*, **56**, 54–60.

8

The use of SSRIs as mood stabilisers for Bipolar II Disorder

Gordon Parker

Introduction

The general role of antidepressants in managing depression in those with bipolar disorder ('bipolar depression') attracts views and management strategies that are poles apart, as detailed by Goldberg in Chapter 7 and debated closely in the commentaries published in this book. The 'bipolar' positioning of expert opinion on this topic can be briefly illustrated.

While the British Association of Psychopharmacology (Goodwin, 2003) guide-lines note that antidepressants 'are effective for treating depression in bipolar disorder' (p. 162), such guidelines – as for all others written for bipolar disorder – explicitly or implicitly refer to the management of Bipolar I Disorder (BP I). Nevertheless, there are substantive concerns about using antidepressants alone in managing episodes of bipolar depression. Essentially, most formal treatment guide-lines argue against using antidepressants as monotherapy in bipolar patients – due to concerns about antidepressant drugs inducing switching and rapid cycling. In Chapter 7, Goldberg also notes some data arguing against any effectiveness of antidepressants as combination therapies (with mood stabilisers). In terms of what might be considered as the current representative view, Gijsman *et al.* (2004) informed us that all major reviews and guidelines for managing bipolar depression over the past decade have instead recommended that a mood stabiliser should be prescribed alone or before prescribing (after a significant interval) any antidepres-sant drug, to prevent risks of switching and rapid cycling.

However, and as noted by Gijsman *et al.* (2004), antidepressants *are* commonly prescribed by clinicians for patients with bipolar depression without any mood stabiliser cover. In their review of 12 randomised controlled trials of the efficacy

Note: This chapter extracts – with permission of the *Journal of Affective Disorders* – sections of a paper published by Parker, G., Tully, L., Olley, A. and Hadzi-Pavlovic, D. (2006). SSRIs as mood stabilizers for Bipolar II Disorder? A proof of concept study. *Journal of Affective Disorders*, **91**, 149–59.

and safety of short-term antidepressant use in managing bipolar depression, they concluded that antidepressant drugs were effective, and that switching was not a common early treatment complication. In fact, the overall switch rate of those prescribed an antidepressant was 3.8%, and thus comparable to the 4.7% switch rate for those receiving a placebo. However, the rate of switching was higher in those receiving a tricyclic antidepressant than for all other antidepressants combined (i.e. 10.0% vs 3.2%). The authors pose a number of intriguing questions, including challenging (a) whether short-term antidepressant use actually does cause subsequent mood instability or cycling and (b) whether there is any disadvantage to the long-term use of non-tricyclic antidepressants for the prevention of depressive relapse. Their conclusions are compatible with two previous reviews of antidepressant-induced switching (Peet, 1994; Parker and Parker, 2003), in suggesting that the narrow-action antidepressant drugs (especially the SSRIs) may not be associated with any increased switch rate. However, all three studies examined data from randomised controlled studies almost invariably undertaken by pharmaceutical companies – and where switching was not necessarily formally examined across the trial and only when nominated or identified as an adverse event. Even given that limitation, a revisionist position is still suggested. In essence, while there is no effective antidepressant drug that has not been described in case reports as inducing manic switching (including SAMe, St John's wort and Omega-3 – as well as formalised antidepressants) in individual patients, group data argue against switching being necessarily increased. Recent reviews suggest, however, that antidepressant-induced switching is not as common as generally believed (particularly for the SSRIs) and that, when it does occur, it is more likely to reflect the 'natural' cyclicity of the bipolar disorder rather than be a side-effect of the antidepressant drug.

For nearly a decade, we have prescribed SSRIs and the dual action antidepressant venlafaxine as monotherapy in patients with Bipolar II Disorder (BP II) presenting with an episode of clinical depression. This initially reflected concerns about waiting for a mood stabiliser to achieve a therapeutic level in a patient with a severe depression before prescribing such antidepressants. However, when such bipolar patients were reviewed over subsequent months, very few reported or admitted to worsening of their highs – in fact, the opposite. Thus, when specifically asked, many patients stated that, in addition to experiencing an improvement in their depression, they had had fewer, less severe and less persistent hypomanic episodes. In reporting a case series of BP II patients who had benefited from an SSRI or venlafaxine (Parker, 2002), the suggestion was put that those medications might have mood-stabilising propensities, in that they appeared – in many BP II patients – to attenuate or curb mood swings.

Such a hypothesis prompted a formal proof of concept study of the SSRI antidepressants as mood stabilisers in those with BP II. In this chapter, study components that have been more extensively detailed elsewhere (Parker et al., 2006) are overviewed. The study was designed to assess whether a standard dose of an SSRI antidepressant was more effective than placebo in reducing the frequency, severity and duration of both depressive and hypomanic episodes in those with BP II.

Methods

Study subjects were recruited by media advertisements. Eligibility criteria comprised being aged 18–65 years; a minimum 2-year history of both depressive and hypomanic episodes; and hypomanic or depressive episodes occurring at least monthly. Subjects were required to meet DSM-IV criteria for Bipolar II Disorder (but not necessarily meet the minimum 4-day duration criterion for hypomanic episodes), and to have never previously received any antidepressant, mood-stabilising or neuroleptic medication, firstly as we wished to preempt a situation of subjects having to cease medication. Secondly, we wished to avoid any bias emerging from previous medication exposure – where subjects might have either previously benefited from or preferentially failed to respond to an SSRI.

Exclusion criteria included a history of psychotic symptoms; current suicidal behaviours or ideation; current substantive illicit drug use or alcohol consumption (>30 g/day); significant personality disorder (assessed clinically); women who were breastfeeding, pregnant or intending to become pregnant over the study period; and several medical conditions. The study was funded by an NHMRC Program Grant, designed independently of any pharmaceutical company input and the only assistance sought from the SSRI manufacturer was the provision of identical presentation capsules of escitalopram and placebo.

The study was a randomised, double-blind, placebo-controlled, 9-month cross-over trial of escitalopram (10 mg) versus placebo, commencing with a no-treatment baseline period of 3 months (Baseline Phase) to ensure that subjects met criteria for episode frequency. Subjects compliant with baseline phase requirements were then randomised to receive escitalopram or placebo for three months (Phase 2), and then crossed over to receive the alternative compound for the final three-month period (Phase 3). Prior to drug cross-over, there was a two-day taper period to avoid potential withdrawal effects, followed by a 7-day wash-out period to avoid carry-over effects from drug to placebo. Investigators were blind to drug assignment, with randomisation and drug dispensing managed by the hospital pharmacy.

Subjects rated their mood states using a daily rating schedule (Patient Mood Chart or PMC) developed at our Institute, marking the PMC at the end of each day, with recordings representing their mood over the day, and with three categories: 'OK' (denoting euthymia), 'low' (depression) and 'high' (hypomania). If they felt 'low' or 'high', they charted whether their mood was mild (rated 1), moderate (rated 2) or severe (rated 3, where 'severe' was defined as 'the worst you have ever been for any episode'). If experiencing a high and a low in one day, they rated the severity of both mood states. Subjects also rated functional impairment daily, quantifying any impact of their mood on their ability to work, and to interact with colleagues, family and friends (0 for no functional impairment, 1 for slight impairment, 2 for moderate impairment, and 3 for severe impairment). We established (Parker *et al.*, 2007) the validity of the PMC measure by correlating generated scores with clinician-rated measure scores.

For each of the three study phases, the PMC allowed us to quantify:

 (i) average severity of highs, lows and impairment
 (ii) percentage of days rated high, low and impaired
(iii) percentage of days rated ill (high or low)
(iv) average severity of days rated ill
 (v) number of episodes of highs, lows and impairment
(vi) number of episodes rated as ill (high or low), and
(vii) longest episode of highs, lows and impairment.

Subjects also completed the Beck Depression Inventory or BDI (Beck *et al.*, 1961) assessing depression severity over the previous week, and on a monthly basis, and a 21-item checklist assessing the presence and severity ('mild', 'moderate' or 'severe') of drug or placebo side-effects over the previous month. At monthly intervals, a research psychologist or psychiatrist completed the Hamilton Depression Rating or HAMD (Hamilton, 1960), Young Mania Rating Scale or YMRS (Young *et al.*, 1978) and the DSM–IV Social and Occupational Functioning Assessment Scale (SOFAS) based on functioning over the previous week. Scores on the HAMD, YMRS, SOFAS and PMC measures were averaged across the three time points for each phase of the study (i.e. Baseline, Phase 2 and Phase 3).

We screened 320 volunteers by telephone, with the majority excluded on the basis of previously receiving psychotropic medication or not being in the Sydney area and therefore not readily able to attend for review over the 9 months. Forty-one subjects met eligibility criteria. After initial interview by a research psychologist, a psychiatrist undertook a comprehensive clinical assessment to confirm BP II Disorder – with four individuals excluded by failing to meet diagnostic criteria. Seventeen eligible participants did not attend the initial appointment. Of the remaining 20 subjects, 10 withdrew during the baseline three months of mood charting, leaving 10 subjects to be randomised to active drug or placebo. Subjects were reviewed by a psychiatrist prior to randomisation, and at months 4, 6, 7 and 9 to check on progress and to discuss SSRI side-effects and withdrawal symptoms. At each monthly assessment, compliance was determined by counting returned tablets. All 10 patients completed each of the nine monthly assessments.

The principal analyses involved repeated measures Analysis of Covariance (ANCOVA) with group (SSRI first vs placebo first) and phase (means of phase 2 and phase 3) as the predictor independent factors, mean baseline scores on each measure as the covariate, and with patient- and clinician-rated measures of mood and impairment as the outcome dependent variables.

Results

The ten subjects (five female) had a mean age of 29 years and an average of 14 years of education. At study entry, six subjects were depressed and four were euthymic. Subjects reported having experienced depressive episodes over a mean interval of 12.9 years and hypomanic episodes for a mean interval of 12.2 years. A family history of depression was acknowledged by three, of bipolar disorder by two and a family history of both bipolar disorder and depression by one.

While remaining blind to drug order, nine of the ten subjects reported at the end of the study that their overall mood was best when on the active drug, while one reported their mood as best on placebo. Two of the ten subjects breached the study protocol (one by taking high levels of alcohol and marijuana, while the second consulted a psychiatrist and was commenced on sodium valproate late in the study). While neither showed any evidence of improvement across the study, their data were included in all analyses, reflecting the 'intention to treat' study design. Rates of compliance were estimated by counting returned tablets. In Phase 2 of the study there was a mean medication compliance rate of 93.5%, and in Phase 3, a mean of 83.8%.

Figure 8.1 plots PMC severity ratings for highs and lows over the 9 months of the study for each of the 10 subjects, presented according to the suggested impact of the active drug. Scores above the midpoint represent highs (mild, moderate and severe), while those below the midpoint capture depression severity. Four patterns of response are suggested: distinctly superior response to the SSRI than to the placebo (subjects 1, 2, 4 and 7), a moderately superior SSRI response (subject 5), a marginally superior SSRI response (subject 9), and no differentiation (protocol violators 3 and 6, and subjects 8 and 10) on the SSRI.

Our journal account of this study (Parker *et al.*, 2006) reports means, standard deviations, treatment effects and effect sizes for each of the variables at each phase of the study for the SSRI first and placebo first groups. In this report, we summarise these findings.

In terms of impact on depression:

- A significant 'group by phase' interaction and a large effect size was found for the HAMD measure, with mean depression severity scores significantly lower when subjects received SSRI than placebo for both groups.
- The interaction for the PMC-rated percentage of days depressed approached significance in favour of receiving the SSRI, and with a medium effect size quantified.

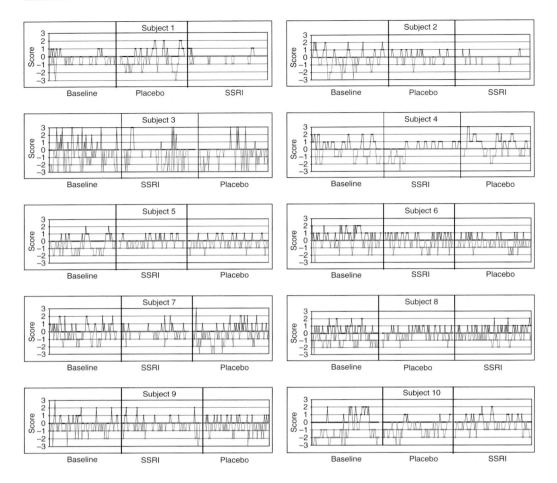

Figure 8.1.   Graphs of severity of depressive and hypomanic episodes over the three phases of the study for each of the ten subjects. Dashed lines = lows, full lines = highs.
(Reprinted from Parker *et al.* (2006) with permission from the *Journal of Affective Disorders*.)

- For the BDI, the interaction was not significant and a small effect size was found, while for the remaining three PMC depression variables the interactions were not significant.
  In terms of hypomania:
- There was no significant group by phase interaction or main effects for the YMRS or for any of the PMC variables.
- Only one small effect size was observed – for mean longest episode of impairment.

In terms of days ill (whether hypomanic or depressed) as rated on the PMC:

- The percentage of days ill showed a significant group by phase interaction, and moderate effect size, with subjects reporting fewer days ill when receiving the SSRI.
- The interactions for mean severity of illness and number of episodes ill did not reach significance, but moderate effect sizes were found. Again, no group or phase effects emerged.

In terms of functional impairment:

- As measured by the SOFAS, significantly higher functioning was reported when subjects were receiving the SSRI, and with a medium effect size quantified.
- For the PMC variables, a significant interaction and large effect size emerged for the percentage of days impaired, while the interaction approached significance for fewer episodes being reported when receiving the SSRI.

In Figures 8.2–8.5, data are plotted on principal variables for subjects during the baseline 3-month phase, and irrespective of whether they received SSRI or placebo first for the two 3-month periods on SSRI and placebo. Figure 8.2 reports data for key depression variables, demonstrating the greater improvement on Hamilton depression (HAMD) and PMC-defined 'percentage of days low' variables when in receipt of the SSRI (Figure 8.3). Figure 8.4 plots data for 'highs' as quantified by the Young Mania Rating Scale (YMRS) and Figure 8.5 PMC-defined 'percentage of days high' variables. Figure 8.6 plots data for PMC-defined 'percentage of days ill' and Figure 8.7 plots functional impairment data, as measured by the SOFAS and PMC measures (Figure 8.8). There is a consistent trend for less severe mood perturbation and for less impairment while in receipt of the SSRI although, as quantified above, not all trends were significant.

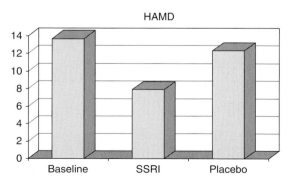

Figure 8.2.   Hamilton depression score means for Baseline, SSRI and Placebo phases.

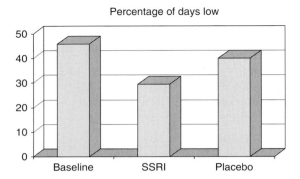

Figure 8.3.   Percentages of days depressed across Baseline, SSRI and Placebo phases.

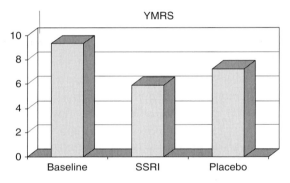

Figure 8.4.   YMRS means for Baseline, SSRI and Placebo phases.

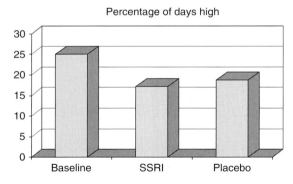

Figure 8.5.   Percentage of days high for Baseline, SSRI and Placebo phases.

Side-effects were quantified during the study. Six symptoms (loss of appetite, somnolence, nausea, sexual dysfunction, decreased libido and headaches) tended to be reported more commonly by subjects when on SSRI medication than on placebo (and when compared with baseline), although none were significantly

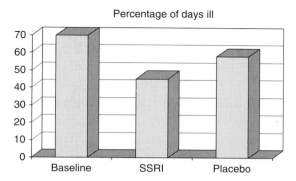

Figure 8.6.   Percentage of days ill (depressed or high) across Baseline, SSRI and Placebo phases.

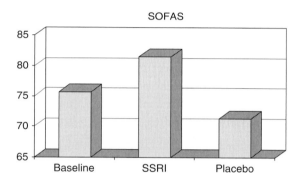

Figure 8.7.   SOFAS scores for functioning across Baseline, SSRI and Placebo phases.

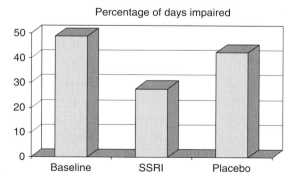

Figure 8.8.   Percentage of days impaired across Baseline, SSRI and Placebo phases.

increased in the SSRI phase. No patient required a dose reduction of drug nor required discontinuation from the study because of side-effects or adverse events.

Discussion

A number of studies have examined the efficacy of antidepressant monotherapy (including SSRI medication) for those with BP II depression, as detailed in Chapter 7 of this book. Several (e.g. Amsterdam and Brunswick, 2003) have reported data supporting the efficacy of antidepressants for the depressed phase of bipolar disorder – and examined whether there is any increased rate in switching. However, no previous study has examined whether the SSRI antidepressants might have benefits for both the highs and the lows of bipolar disorder and thus have mood stabiliser propensities.

A number of study limitations require noting. Firstly, the study was under-powered – although not by design. Onerous study requirements – particularly in recruiting those who had never received any psychotropic drug (i.e. antidepressant, antipsychotic or mood-stabilising medication) previously, as well as the projected 9-month period, made recruitment difficult. Nevertheless, there were a number of study strengths, allowing several preliminary conclusions. The daily self-report measure provided more detailed information than that generated by interval cross-sectional measures of a cycling disorder, where chance may well dictate whether (at any one review) the individual is high, low or euthymic. We suggest that the plot for individual subjects (Figure 8.1) allows fine-focused pattern analyses (of frequency, duration, severity and cyclicity of symptoms) to be undertaken that enhance the formal quantitative analyses. The inclusion of a baseline monitoring period identified all subjects as experiencing mood swings on a relatively frequent basis, and well above the study pre-entry criterion rate of one mood swing episode per month. DSM–IV defines 'rapid cycling' as four or more mood episodes in the preceding 12 months, with the implicit suggestion that this is not the common pattern. Our subjects' plots identified ultra-rapid cycling for all, which we suggest is not unusual for those with BP II and may represent the commonest pattern – but which is only evident on mood charting as patients tend to focus only on the more substantive episodes when reporting to their physician. Thus, such data again emphasise the importance of obtaining data on a regular – if not constant – basis rather than relying on weekly or monthly measurement.

Our data suggest that receipt of SSRI medication was associated with (i) an improvement in depression (reduced severity and percentage of days depressed), (ii) improved functioning (severity, number and percentage of days impaired), (iii) a weak overall trend (but distinct for four of the ten patients) for reduction in hypomania and (iv) a significant reduction in the percentage of days ill (whether high or low). In addition to those quantitative analyses, the Figure 8.1 graphs suggest some degree of benefit from the SSRI in seven of the ten subjects for depression, while four of the ten showed some attenuation of their highs while on the SSRI. Further, after completion of the 9-month study and, while remaining blind to drug order, nine of the ten subjects judged that their mood was better on the SSRI than the placebo. Finally, apart from the two protocol violators who were referred back to a treating clinician, following unblinding, six of the eight other subjects stated that they would wish to have their condition continue to be treated with an SSRI.

Concerns that prescription of antidepressants to those with bipolar disorder may cause switching or rapid cycling were not supported by formal analyses nor is there any such suggestion when Figure 8.1 plots are inspected.

Results from this proof of concept study were consistent with our earlier clinical judgement that the SSRIs, and possibly venlafaxine, have mood-stabilising properties. We suggest that our formal study analyses offer indicative support for the potential utility of SSRI medication in those with BP II, and provide no evidence that such drugs worsen the course of the illness. Clearly, adequately powered replication studies are required to clarify whether the SSRIs can be regarded as formal mood stabilisers (in impacting on highs as well as on lows) or merely have antidepressant properties in those with BP II and then attenuate any rebound highs. Further, as the individual SSRIs differ quite considerably, there is a need to determine whether any mood-stabilising potential is an SSRI class effect specific to those SSRIs that are highly serotonergic.

Clinical conclusions

As noted frequently in this book, there are no formal guidelines for managing BP II and most clinicians assume that management strategies can be extrapolated from BP I management guidelines. For the latter condition, most guidelines recommend commencing with a mood stabiliser. However, most current mood stabilisers have a number of side-effects that can be quite troubling and concerning to patients over time (e.g. weight gain, tremor). While recognising that SSRI drugs can also have significant side-effects, we would suggest that, *overall*, the side-effect profile of SSRI medication is less troubling to patients than that of the formal mood stabilisers.

Thus, as noted in the Commentary section, my clinical custom is to commence management of those with BP II with an SSRI and recommend that the patient plot progress with a daily mood chart. In line with results from this study, some 40–50% of patients report an improvement in their mood swings – and again, most distinctly for their depression. However, of such 'improvers', about one-half report a progressive 'poop out' effect in a period of several months to several years. To maintain benefit, I increase the SSRI dose progressively, generally observing temporary improvement (for weeks or months) but progressive continuation of the 'poop out' phenomenon. Once the maximum dose has been achieved and benefit not sustained, I then initiate and trial a formal mood stabiliser. A percentage will report more rapid cycling and mixed states (particularly at higher doses of the SSRI or of venlafaxine, while the latter drug does appear to have a higher intrinsic rate of rapid cycling and mixed states developing over time). If such is reported – or observed – the dose of the antidepressant drug is lowered or the drug ceased, and generally a mood stabiliser introduced at that time. Nevertheless, some 20% of those with BP II can be maintained for long periods and with benefit on an SSRI alone.

There is another possible comparative advantage to use of SSRIs (in addition to the better side-effect profile) as against use of a formal mood stabiliser. Many patients with a bipolar disorder are concerned about treatment removing their enjoyable highs. My clinical observation is consistent with findings from this study in suggesting that, when effective, the SSRIs tend to have distinctly greater benefit for the depressed features and tend only to attenuate the highs rather than eliminate them. The ideal mood stabiliser for many individuals with Bipolar II Disorder would be one that prevented depressive episodes and rather 'tweaked' the highs to remove their more severe components. For a percentage of those with BP II, the SSRIs appear to achieve such a profile.

Acknowledgements

As noted, this chapter overviews a study reported recently (Parker *et al.*, 2006). Co-authors Lucy Tully, Amanda Olley and Dusan Hadzi-Pavlovic are thanked for their contribution to the study, as is Caryl Barnes for rating assistance, and the subjects who participated in this study.

REFERENCES

Amsterdam, J. D. and Brunswick, D. J. (2003). Antidepressant monotherapy for Bipolar Type II major depression. *Bipolar Disorders*, **5**, 388–95.

Beck, A. T., Ward, C. H., Mendelson, M., Mock, J. and Erbaugh, J. (1961). An inventory for measuring depression. *Archives of General Psychiatry*, **4**, 561–71.

Gijsman, H. J., Geddes, J. R., Rendell, J. M., Nolen, W. A. and Goodwin, G. M. (2004). Antidepressants for bipolar depression: a systematic review of randomized, controlled trials. *American Journal of Psychiatry*, **61**, 1537–47.

Goodwin, G. M. (2003). Evidence-based guidelines for treating bipolar disorder: recommendations from the British Association for Psychopharmacology. *Journal of Psychopharmacology*, **17**, 149–73.

Hamilton, M. (1960). A rating scale for depression. *Journal of Neurology, Neurosurgery and Psychiatry*, **23**, 56–62.

Parker, G. (2002). Do the newer antidepressants have mood stabilizing properties? (letter). *Australian and New Zealand Journal of Psychiatry*, **36**, 427–8.

Parker, G. and Parker, K. (2003). Which antidepressants flick the switch? *Australian and New Zealand Journal of Psychiatry*, **37**, 464–8.

Parker, G., Tully, L., Olley, A. and Hadzi-Pavlovic, D. (2006). SSRIs as mood stabilizers for Bipolar II Disorder? A proof of concept study. *Journal of Affective Disorders*, **92**, 205–14.

Parker, G., Tully, A., Olley, A. and Barnes, C. (2007). The validity and utility of patient's daily ratings of mood and impairment in clinical trials of bipolar disorder. *Acta Psychiatrica Scandinavica* (in press).

Peet, M. (1994). Induction of mania with selective serotonin reuptake inhibitors and tricyclic antidepressants. *British Journal of Psychiatry*, **164**, 549–50.

Young, R. C., Biggs, J. T., Ziegler, V. E. and Meyer, D. A. (1978). A rating scale for mania: reliability, validity and sensitivity. *British Journal of Psychiatry*, **133**, 429–35.

9

Mood stabilisers in the treatment of Bipolar II Disorder

George Hadjipavlou and Lakshmi N. Yatham

Introduction

We first raise two questions. Are mood stabilisers underused in the treatment of patients with Bipolar II Disorder (BP II)? Secondly, and perhaps more centrally, do all BP II patients need to be treated with mood stabilisers?

While mood stabilisers are integral to the evidence-based management of Bipolar I Disorder (BP I), there are no large, well-designed, controlled trials specifically tailored to help guide treatment decisions about mood stabilisers for BP II patients – and so there are no definitive answers to these questions. Despite this dearth of data to guide therapy, clinicians often rely on mood stabilisers when treating patients with BP II. For instance, a study describing prescription patterns for 500 bipolar patients in a US psychiatric academic setting showed that lithium and anticonvulsants play a prominent role in the treatment of BP II patients referred from the community (Ghaemi *et al.*, 2006a). Lithium was prescribed in 36% of that sample, while 30% had been treated with valproate or carbamazepine, and 34% had received second-generation anticonvulsants such as lamotrigine, topiramate or gabapentin (Bauer and Mitchner, 2004; Ghaemi *et al.*, 2006a).

In this chapter we review the evidence for lithium and anticonvulsants specifically for the treatment of BP II Disorder. Though we consider studies that included both BP I and BP II conditions, those studies reporting separate results for BP II are highlighted. We make it a rule *not* to generalise from studies with only BP I patients as such generalisations may prove hasty and inappropriate; for instance, some studies that have conducted subgroup analyses of BP I and BP II subjects have shown meaningful differences in treatment response (Hadjipavlou and Yatham, 2004; Yatham, 2004). Bipolar II patients are likely a heterogeneous group; some members are more likely to resemble BP I patients in their response to treatment while others might be more similar to patients with unipolar depression (Yatham, 2004; Yatham *et al.*, 2005). Increasing awareness that patients with BP II may require treatment approaches distinct from those with BP I has led to the

Bipolar II Disorder. Modelling, Measuring and Managing, ed. Gordon Parker. Published by Cambridge University Press. © Cambridge University Press 2008.

inclusion of separate, albeit inevitably limited, recommendations for managing BP II in the most recent available guidelines (Yatham *et al.*, 2005; NICE, 2006). This chapter takes such guidelines into consideration.

From the outset, we want to be clear that if our goal is to identify data that can be confidently applied to the management of BP II, then all of the studies mentioned in this chapter have methodological shortcomings. Most offer only preliminary findings, are derived from small samples, and lack blinded randomisation and placebo controls, while those that are randomised controlled trials (RCTs) either lump BP II together with BP I patients or analyse them separately, when their sample sizes are sufficient, after the fact. Although not the sort of studies that inspire much confidence, they do provide an encouraging starting base. We should all be aware of the knowledge base our treatment decisions draw on, however shaky.

There is no consensus definition of the term, 'mood stabiliser'. Nor is there universal agreement about what agents count as mood stabilisers (Bauer and Mitchner, 2004; Malhi *et al.*, 2005). A stringent proposal would be to include only medications that stabilise mood both from 'above' (during mania or hypomania) and from 'below' (during depression), while also preventing relapses of both mania and depression without destabilising the course of the disorder. Alternatively, any medication that prevents the likelihood of a mood episode, either depression or mania, but not both, or any medication that treats mania or depression without destabilising the course of the disorder, could count as a 'mood stabiliser'. In this chapter we use the term loosely and inclusively to refer to lithium and anticonvulsant medications used in the treatment of bipolar disorder. Anticonvulsants that have some data supporting their therapeutic role in BP II include valproate (for simplicity, we use valproate to refer to any of its preparations – valproic acid, divalproex sodium, etc.), lamotrigine, carbamazepine, and less so, topiramate and gabapentin.

Mood stabilisers in the management of hypomania

Hypomania poses both a diagnostic and therapeutic challenge (Judd *et al.*, 2005). Pure hypomania in BP II is relatively infrequent compared to depression; patients experience depressive symptoms 39 times more often than hypomanic symptoms (Judd *et al.*, 2003). Hypomanic episodes may also be quite brief, lasting much less than the DSM-defined 4-day criterion. The hypomania in BP II may require a different management approach than in BP I, in which 'highs' are more impairing and may develop into full-blown mania (Judd *et al.*, 2005). Although untreated hypomania may be associated with marital, financial, legal, occupational and other psychosocial problems (Yatham *et al.*, 2005), there is also evidence to suggest that functioning may be neither impaired nor cause significant distress. Indeed, sub-syndromal symptoms of hypomania have actually been shown to slightly improve functioning in some patients (Judd *et al.*, 2005).

This clearly begs the question: Should hypomania always be treated in BP II? There is no universal answer to this question. We would recommend carefully considering hypomania in the context of each patient's life and pattern of illness as the necessary first step. Paying particular attention to collateral data from family and friends about its observable impact or associated consequences is often instructive, as patients tend to lack insight into such matters (Yatham *et al.*, 2005). If there is no evidence of disruption or distress, if symptoms are very mild or if patients are unwilling to have their hypomanic symptoms treated, ongoing assessment with close follow-up may be adequate short-term management. It is also necessary to evaluate hypomanic patients for the presence of mixed symptoms or a pattern of rapid cycling. If either of these is present, initiating treatment with a mood stabiliser earlier may be more appropriate.

Lithium and valproate are firmly established first-line options in the treatment of acute mania, with proven efficacy in double-blind, placebo-controlled trials, and without a propensity to switch patients into depression (Bauer and Mitchner, 2004; Yatham, 2004; Yatham *et al.*, 2005). However, the specific treatment of hypomania in BP II has largely escaped attention in the clinical trials literature. As detailed in Chapter 10, with the exception of an open-label trial of risperidone, there have been no other studies specifically focusing on the management of hypomania (Hadjipavlou and Yatham, 2004; Yatham, 2004; Yatham *et al.*, 2005).

Since hypomanic episodes for many patients with BP II are occasional elevations in a landscape of depression, choosing a medication to treat hypomania is also potentially about choosing an effective treatment for maintenance that protects against depression, as patients are likely to continue with the treatment that worked in the acute phase (Yatham, 2004; Ghaemi *et al.*, 2006a). Although valproate and lithium are both effective anti-manic agents, given that lithium has somewhat stronger evidence in the maintenance treatment of BP II (see below), it is arguably a better choice in patients presenting with hypomania who are not on any medications. Patients already on lithium or another anti-manic agent should have that medication optimised before changing the course of treatment. If monotherapy with an appropriately dosed mood stabiliser is insufficient, the next step – for which there is no evidence-based guidance – might include switching to another anti-manic agent such as valproate or combining the mood stabiliser with an atypical antipsychotic (see Chapter 10). A small open-label study that included 15 hypomanic BP II patients also found benefit in topiramate as adjunctive therapy (Vieta *et al.*, 2003).

Management of acute depression

The management of mania has drawn far more attention in therapeutic trials than bipolar depression. Bipolar depression, from BP I across the bipolar spectrum, has arguably been relatively understudied (Bauer and Mitchner, 2004; Thase, 2005). And so, though discouraging, it is not surprising that there is inadequate evidence to convincingly establish any medication as first-line therapy in acute BP II depression (Yatham *et al.*, 2005). Whether treatment should be initiated with mood stabilisers as monotherapy, in conjunction with antidepressants, or if antidepressants can be used effectively and safely on their own, has yet to be determined by compelling data. Hence there is no universally agreed-upon strategy. Because of high rates of mixed symptoms and concerns about rapid cycling – both of which may go unrecognised – as well as frequent comorbidities such as substance abuse, we would recommend a cautious approach which favours initiating therapy with mood stabilisers rather than antidepressants (see Chapters 7 and 8 for discussion of antidepressants in BP II). Again, paying attention to the mood episode in the context of the overall illness course is very helpful. If hypomanic episodes are mild and infrequent, if depression is not accompanied by mixed symptoms, and if there is no history of rapid cycling, judicious use of antidepressants instead of mood stabilisers may be appropriate (Yatham, 2004; Thase, 2005). Conversely, antidepressants are best avoided in patients whose depressive episodes are marked by mixed hypomanic symptoms.

If an initial mood stabiliser trial is insufficient, combining mood stabilisers (e.g. valproate plus lithium), may be an appropriate next step in depressed BP II patients with significant, mixed hypomanic symptoms. Adding an atypical antipsychotic may also be an option in such patients, though neither of these strategies has been properly studied. In a recent review of bipolar depression, Thase argues that there is a 3-fold rationale underlying the near-universal endorsement of mood stabilisers as first-line management of BP I patients with milder untreated episodes of depression (Thase, 2005). Mood stabilisers have modest antidepressant effects, they are not typically associated with cycle acceleration or switching, and – even if they do not work as monotherapy acutely – they may still have a subsequent, prophylactic role (Thase, 2005). In the faint light of available data, this rationale can be tentatively applied to the management of BP II. There is also the added benefit that, if antidepressants are to be used, having mood stabilisers on board may potentially confer some protection against the induction of rapid cycling or switching into hypomania.

An extensive review of controlled trials of medications used to treat any phase of bipolar disorder concluded that only lithium had sufficient data supporting its role as a mood stabiliser that is also effective in the treatment of acute depression

(Bauer and Mitchner, 2004). Support for lithium in acute bipolar depression is largely derived from several small trials conducted in the 1970s, three of which were placebo-controlled, double-blind studies that included both BP I and BP II patients (Bauer and Mitchner, 2004). Its role in depression is further supported by long-term maintenance studies and data on suicide prevention, discussed below. Given the paucity of data in acute BP II depression, initiating treatment with lithium may be a reasonable choice. It is worth optimising lithium therapy prior to augmenting with an antidepressant, another mood stabiliser, or abandoning lithium for another agent. The value of ensuring adequate doses of lithium is well illustrated by an RCT in which 117 patients with BP I, stratified according to whether they had high (above 0.8 meq/L) or low (below or equal to 0.8 meq/L) serum lithium levels, were randomised to receive either additional paroxetine, imipramine or placebo (Nemeroff *et al.*, 2001). While patients with low serum lithium levels improved when augmented with paroxetine or imipramine compared with placebo, there was no additional benefit from antidepressants in patients tolerating high serum lithium levels – which is consistent with previous findings of lithium's antidepressant effect and highlights the need for adequate dosing. Further, there are data to support the combination of lithium with valproate in the treatment of acute depression. A small double-blind RCT of 27 patients with BP I or BP II (n = 16) who experienced an acute depressive relapse while on maintenance therapy with lithium or valproate found that adding a second mood stabiliser – specifically valproate or lithium – was similarly efficacious to adding paroxetine (Young *et al.*, 2000).

There is also some weaker evidence suggesting that valproate monotherapy may be helpful in acute BP II depression. Monotherapy with valproate was found to be beneficial in reducing depressive symptoms in 63% of 19 patients with BP II in an open-label trial; interestingly, there were higher response rates (82%) in patients who had never previously received any medication treatment (Winsberg *et al.*, 2001). Although the small observational nature of this trial does not allow for any convincing inferences to be drawn, it does signal the possibility that depressed BP II patients might benefit more when treated initially with mood stabilisers.

Lamotrigine is increasingly recognised as a valuable medication in the treatment of bipolar depression (Thase, 2005). Two small, preliminary open-label studies initially found that the addition of lamotrigine significantly reduced depressive symptoms in samples of combined BP I and BP II patients who had inadequate responses to previous medications (Calabrese *et al.*, 1999; Suppes *et al.*, 1999). There have also been positive data from a double-blind RCT of 31 patients with refractory mood disorders, 14 of whom had BP II, comparing lamotrigine to gabapentin and placebo. Lamotrigine-treated patients showed significantly greater improvement over those treated with gabapentin or placebo (Frye *et al.*, 2000).

Some recent trials have explored the role of lamotrigine in combination with other mood stabilisers to augment acute treatment of bipolar depression. For instance, a preliminary 12-week double-blind RCT reported similar, significant improvements in depression in 20 BP I and BP II patients already on mood stabilisers, and who received either additional citalopram or lamotrigine (Schaffer *et al.*, 2006). Further, a study of 66 BP I and BP II patients with treatment-resistant depression showed more promise – as 24% of patients whose treatment was augmented with open-label lamotrigine recovered to a euthymic state, compared with 5% augmented with risperidone and 17% with inositol, though the differences were not statistically significant as the study was likely underpowered (Nierenberg *et al.*, 2006). Lamotrigine was also found to be of benefit as add-on therapy in the acute treatment of bipolar depression in an, as yet unpublished, 8-week double-blind, placebo-controlled study (van der Loos *et al.*, 2006) with 124 BP I or BP II patients. Similarly, preliminary data from a small, retrospective study of 21 relatively treatment-resistant patients with BP I or BP II conditions indicated that, when added to lithium, lamotrigine was effective in alleviating acute depressive symptoms in almost one-half of patients (Ghaemi *et al.*, 2006b). Although lamotrigine has not typically been associated with precipitating hypomania or mania, some recent data have suggested a possible increased risk of hypomania when it is used in combination therapy (Margolese *et al.*, 2003; Ghaemi *et al.*, 2006b; GlaxoSmithKline, 2006; van der Loos *et al.*, 2006). This issue requires further investigation.

Unfortunately, enthusiasm for lamotrigine monotherapy in the acute treatment of BP II depression is seriously undermined by the unpublished negative results of a large double-blind, placebo-controlled 8-week industry trial completed in 2005 of 220 patients randomised to either treatment with lamotrigine or placebo (GlaxoSmithKline, 2006). Patients treated with lamotrigine did not show significant improvement over those treated with placebo. It is also worth noting that adverse events were similar between groups, and there were no serious adverse events reported for lamotrigine (GlaxoSmithKline, 2006). At this point, available data suggest that lamotrigine should not be prescribed as monotherapy in acute BP II depression. Lamotrigine does, however, seem to be of value when used in combination, and it may also have an important therapeutic role in the long-term treatment of BP II (discussed below).

Studies of gabapentin and topiramate make some additional, albeit slender, contributions to the already too-thin evidence base for the acute treatment of BP II depression. Although the RCT with gabapentin mentioned above found that it was not significantly different from placebo as monotherapy, there are some retrospective data (Ghaemi *et al.*, 1998; Ghaemi and Goodwin, 2001) as well as a small, open-label trial (Young *et al.*, 1999) suggesting a potentially helpful adjunctive role in BP II depression. Gabapentin has also been noted to reduce symptoms of anxiety in depressed bipolar patients (Young *et al.*, 1999), and may be worth considering as an add-on when co-occurring anxiety complicates treatment. A study of 36 patients with BP I or BP II (n = 17) under randomised, single-blind conditions reported that topiramate had similar efficacy to bupropion in significantly reducing symptoms of depression when added to a mood stabiliser (McIntyre *et al.*, 2002).

Mood stabilisers in maintenance therapy

Natural history data indicate that patients with BP II tend to have a chronic course, dominated by fluctuating depressive symptoms, causing them to be sick during more than half of all follow-up weeks (Judd *et al.*, 2003, 2005). Despite being both disabling and distressing to patients, significant portions of their illness course may be missed, as their symptoms are frequently sub-syndromal, below the threshold for DSM–IV diagnoses of discrete mood episodes. This highlights the need for effective maintenance strategies, particularly ones that work in the depressive phase of the illness.

Further, reducing suicide-related morbidity and mortality is one of the most critical issues pertaining to maintenance treatment. Lithium alone has compelling data suggesting an anti-suicide effect in bipolar disorders. A meta-analysis of 33 studies reported a 13-fold decrease in annual reported rates of attempted or completed suicides during long-term lithium treatment (Baldessarini *et al.*, 2001). Similarly, a recent analysis of health plan data in the USA, of over 20 000 patients with BP I or BP II followed for an average of almost 3 years, found that the risk of death by suicide was 2.7 times greater during treatment with valproate compared to lithium (Goodwin *et al.*, 2003).

There are more data for lithium and anticonvulsants in maintenance therapy for BP II than there are for acute treatment. However, since mood stabilisers in BP II have been generally understudied, it remains to be seen whether they might indeed be better at long-term stabilisation and prevention of mood episodes than in treating them acutely. Given that lithium has been used since the 1940s, it is not surprising that it has been the most extensively studied maintenance treatment in bipolar disorder (Bauer and Mitchner, 2004). Small double-blind, placebo-controlled studies conducted in the late 1970s suggest that lithium is beneficial in reducing the frequency and severity of depressive episodes in patients with BP II (Fieve *et al.*, 1976; Quitkin *et al.*, 1978; Dunner *et al.*, 1982; Kane *et al.*, 1982; Yatham, 2004). More impressive data come from long-term observational studies showing substantial improvement with lithium treatment in over 300 patients with BP I or BP II (Tondo *et al.*, 1998, 2001; Baldessarini *et al.*, 1998; Baldessarini and Tondo, 2000). In one report, BP II patients showed a 98% reduction in hospitalisation rates during lithium treatment, as well as a decrease in the percentage of time spent ill and recurrence of mood episodes by 80% and 68%, respectively (Tondo *et al.*, 1998). Followed for an average of over 14 years, patients with BP II improved more than those with BP I from maintenance lithium treatment (Tondo *et al.*, 2001). There is evidence that lithium may take time to exert its positive prophylactic effect, with five patients with bipolar disorder treated for 2 years to prevent one mood relapse (Carney and Goodwin, 2005). Lithium was also shown to be of some benefit in a subgroup of patients with rapid cycling, which was five times more common among patients with BP II (Tondo *et al.*, 2001).

Although valproate is often considered more effective than lithium in the treatment of rapid-cycling bipolar disorder, a recent trial designed specifically to address this issue did not find a difference between the two (Calabrese *et al.*, 2005). Sixty patients with BP I or BP II who were stabilised on a combination of lithium and valproate were randomised to either maintenance monotherapy with lithium or valproate under double-blind conditions. Relapse rates for any mood episode were similar in both groups, with 56% treated with lithium relapsing compared with 50% treated with valproate (Calabrese *et al.*, 2005). It is worth noting that the 60 patients included in this maintenance portion of the study comprised only 24% of the 254 subjects initially enrolled in the acute open-label stabilisation phase, many of whom had refractory depression that did not respond sufficiently to the combination of lithium and valproate. These high attrition rates highlight the difficulties in effectively managing severe rapid-cycling bipolar disorder with recurrent depression. Whether patients with BP II fared better with lithium or valproate, or if their outcomes differed from those with BP I is not known as results have yet to be reported separately (Calabrese *et al.*, 2005). Previous observational data had also shown promise for valproate in rapid-cycling BP II (Jacobsen, 1993). For instance, a small open-label study of 33 patients with rapid-cycling BP II or cyclothymia treated with valproate reported marked or moderate improvement in 70% of those with BP II (Jacobsen, 1993).

There is evidence to suggest that lamotrigine may have an important role in the maintenance treatment of BP II, particularly for those with rapid-cycling. Although a large RCT of patients with rapid-cycling BP I or BP II failed to show a difference between lamotrigine and placebo on its primary outcome, time to additional therapy sub-group analyses of 52 patients with BP II on other important clinical measures were positive (Calabrese *et al.*, 2000). For instance, significantly more patients treated with lamotrigine (46%) remained stable without relapse over six months compared to placebo (18%). Small open-label studies also lend some additional support for lamotrigine as an adjunct in the long-term treatment of depression in BP II (Calabrese *et al.*, 1999; Suppes *et al.*, 1999). The

2006 UK National Institute for Health and Clinical Excellence (NICE) guidelines recommend the use of lamotrigine for long-term treatment of BP II patients with recurrent depressions (NICE, 2006). It also recommends combining lamotrigine with lithium or valproate in rapid-cycling BP II patients (NICE, 2006).

Carbamazepine may be of some use in maintenance treatment as well. In an analysis of 57 patients with BP II or Bipolar Disorder NOS followed for 2.5 years as part of a larger RCT, long-term prophylaxis with carbamazepine was shown to be equally efficacious to lithium, though with a slight trend favouring carbamazepine (Greil and Kleindienst, 1999; Kleindienst and Greil, 2000). However, patients with BP I showed significantly greater benefit from lithium, which contrasts with the findings from the observational studies of lithium above.

There are no data to support gabapentin or topiramate as monotherapies in the maintenance treatment of BP II, though preliminary findings from small open-label studies suggest that they may potentially be helpful on an add-on basis (Ghaemi et al., 1998; Ghaemi and Goodwin, 2001; McIntyre et al., 2005). In addition, a very recent double-blind, placebo-controlled RCT included 25 euthymic BP I or BP II patients treated with mood stabilisers who were randomised to receive either adjunctive gabapentin or placebo for one year. Although no patients in the study – whether treated with placebo or gabapentin – experienced measurable emerging manic or depressive symptoms, gabapentin was reported to be of some benefit based on significant changes in the Clinical Global Impressions scale, and fostered improved sleep compared to placebo (Vieta et al., 2006).

Very few studies have specifically addressed the prevalent issue of treating BP II patients possessing comorbid disorders. There are some promising data from small open-label studies that lamotrigine may be effective in treating BP II patients with co-occurring alcohol and substance abuse disorders (Brown et al., 2003; Rubio et al., 2006). An open-label study of lamotrigine used adjunctively in 25 patients with BP I or BP II and alcohol dependence (n = 7) reported significant improvement in mood, alcohol cravings and consumption (Rubio et al., 2006). Another small open-label study of BP I and BP II patients with cocaine dependence also reported a reduction in cocaine cravings along with a significant improvement in mood (Brown et al., 2003). Although valproate has double-blind, placebo-controlled data suggesting efficacy in reducing alcohol consumption in BP I patients with comorbid alcohol dependence, it has not been evaluated in patients with BP II for this indication (Brown, 2005). A placebo-controlled trial of patients with BP II and comorbid Borderline Personality Disorder found that valproate was helpful in significantly reducing aggression, irritability and interpersonal turmoil (Frankenburg and Zanarini, 2002).

Mood stabilisers form an important part of the overall pharmacological management of patients with BP II. However, they are only partial treatments, as very few patients can be completely treated with monotherapy. For instance, of the

500 patients with BP I, BP II or BP NOS in the study of prescription patterns mentioned at the beginning of the chapter, only about one-tenth (10.8%) were managed with mood stabilisers as monotherapy (Ghaemi *et al.*, 2006). Clearly, there are unmet therapeutic needs. How can these needs be addressed? There is growing acceptance that combination treatment, with rational polypharmacy, is inevitable in the effective management of bipolar disorder. Combinations of mood stabilisers with complementary activity offer a potentially viable approach, for which there is emerging, albeit scant, evidence (Calabrese *et al.*, 2005; Ghaemi *et al.*, 2006). Lamotrigine (which tends to stabilise mood from below and is useful in rapid-cycling BP II) and lithium (which has modest antidepressant effects acutely, and potentially reduces both hypomanic and depressive episodes) may be one such effective combination. The single long-term study to explore this strategy found that only 29% of patients given an open-label combination of lithium and lamotrigine maintained benefit at one year (Ghaemi *et al.*, 2006). Combining lithium with valproate is another alternative supported by some data. Mood stabilisation may also come from agents other than lithium and anti-convulsants, such as antidepressants (see Chapter 7) and antipsychotics (see Chapter 10), as well as psychosocial interventions (see Chapter 12).

In this chapter we have provided a sketch of the existing evidence for mood stabilisers in the treatment of BP II. Until data from large, well-designed controlled trials are available, firm evidence-based recommendations are impossible. We strongly recommend carefully taking into account the overall pattern of illness for each patient and paying particular attention to such issues as rapid cycling, mixed states and comorbid conditions in making decisions about treatment. Although the absence of compelling evidence certainly limits our endorsement of any single therapy, we should also be cautious not to dismiss potentially beneficial treatments prematurely – as is often noted in reviews, the absence of evidence should not be mistaken for evidence of absence. Numerous trials address-ing specific treatment issues in BP II, including the role of mood stabilisers, are now in progress. Readers are encouraged to keep abreast of these developments by searching the clinical trials register available online.

REFERENCES

Baldessarini, R. J. and Tondo, L. (2000). Does lithium therapy still work? Evidence of stable responses over three decades. *Archives of General Psychiatry*, **57**, 187–90.

Baldessarini, R. J., Tondo, L., Floris, G. and Hennen, J. (1998). Effects of rapid cycling on response to lithium maintenance treatment in 360 Bipolar I and II disorder patients. *Journal of Affective Disorders*, **155**, 1434–6.

Baldessarini, R. J., Tondo, L. and Hennen, J. (2001). Treating the suicidal patient with bipolar disorder: reducing suicide risk with lithium. *Annals of the New York Academy of Sciences*, **932**, 24–38.

Bauer, M. S. and Mitchner, L. (2004). What is a 'mood stabilizer'? An evidence-based response. *American Journal of Psychiatry*, **161**, 3–18.

Brown, E. S. (2005). Bipolar disorder and substance abuse. *Psychiatric Clinics of North America*, **28**, 415–25.

Brown, E. S., Nejtek, V. A., Perantie, D. C., Orsulak, P. J. and Bobadilla, L. (2003). Lamotrigine in patients with bipolar disorder and cocaine dependence. *Journal of Clinical Psychiatry*, **64**, 197–201.

Calabrese, J. R., Bowden, C. L., McElroy, S. L. *et al.* (1999). Spectrum of activity of lamotrigine in treatment-refractory bipolar disorder. *American Journal of Psychiatry*, **156**, 1019–23.

Calabrese, J. R., Shelton, M. D., Rapport, D. J. *et al.* (2005). A 20-month, double-blind, maintenance trial of lithium versus divalproex in rapid-cycling bipolar disorder. *American Journal of Psychiatry*, **162**, 2152–61.

Calabrese, J. R., Suppes, T., Bowden, C. L. *et al.* (2000). A double-blind, placebo-controlled, prophylaxis study of lamotrigine in rapid-cycling bipolar disorder. Lamictal 614 Study Group. *Journal of Clinical Psychiatry*, **61**, 841–50.

Carney, S. M. and Goodwin, G. M. (2005). Lithium – a continuing story in the treatment of bipolar disorder. *Acta Psychiatrica Scandinavica*, **111** (Suppl. 426), S7–12.

Dunner, D. L., Stallone, F. and Fieve, R. R. (1982). Prophylaxis with lithium carbonate: an update. *Archives of General Psychiatry*, **39**, 1344–5.

Fieve, R. R., Kumbaraci, T. and Dunner, D. L. (1976). Lithium prophylaxis of depression in Bipolar I, Bipolar II, and unipolar patients. *American Journal of Psychiatry*, **133**, 925–9.

Frankenburg, F. R. and Zanarini, M. C. (2002). Divalproex sodium treatment of women with Borderline Personality Disorder and Bipolar II: a double-blind placebo-controlled pilot study. *Journal of Clinical Psychiatry*, **63**, 442–6.

Frye, M. A., Ketter, T. A., Kimbrell, T. A. *et al.* (2000). A placebo-controlled study of lamotrigine and gabapentin monotherapy in refractory mood disorders. *Journal of Clinical Psychopharmacology*, **20**, 607–14.

Ghaemi, S. N. and Goodwin, F. K. (2001). Gabapentin treatment of the non-refractory bipolar spectrum: an open case series. *Journal of Affective Disorders*, **65**, 167–71.

Ghaemi, S. N., Katzow, J. J., Desai, S. P. and Goodwin, F. K. (1998). Gabapentin treatment of mood disorders: a preliminary study. *Journal of Clinical Psychiatry*, **59**, 426–9.

Ghaemi, S. N., Hsu, D. J., Thase, M. *et al.* (2006a). Pharmacological treatment patterns at study entry for the first 500 STEP-BD participants. *Psychiatric Services*, **57**, 660–5.

Ghaemi, S. N., Schrauwen, E., Klugman, J. *et al.* (2006b). Long-term lamotrigine plus lithium for bipolar disorder: one year outcome. *Journal of Psychiatric Practice*, **12**, 300–5.

GlaxoSmithKline (2006). A multicenter, double-blind, placebo-controlled, fixed-dose, eight-week evaluation of the efficacy and safety of lamotrigine in the treatment of major depression in patients with Type II bipolar disorder. http://ctr.gsk.co.uk.

Goodwin, F. K., Fireman, B., Simon, G. E. *et al.* (2003). Suicide risk in bipolar disorder during treatment with lithium and divalproex. *Journal of the American Medical Association*, **290**, 1467–73.

Greil, W. and Kleindienst, N. (1999). Lithium versus carbamazepine in the maintenance treatment of Bipolar II Disorder and Bipolar Disorder Not Otherwise Specified. *International Clinical Psychopharmacology*, **14**, 283–5.

Hadjipavlou, G. H. and Yatham, L. (2004). Bipolar II Disorder: an overview of recent developments. *Canadian Journal of Psychiatry*, **49**, 802–12.

Jacobsen, F. M. (1993). Low-dose valproate: a new treatment for cyclothymia, mild rapid-cycling disorders, and premenstrual syndrome. *Journal of Clinical Psychiatry*, **54**, 229–34.

Judd, L. L., Akiskal, H. S., Schettler, P. J. *et al.* (2003). A prospective investigation of the natural history of the long-term weekly symptomatic status of Bipolar II Disorder. *Archives of General Psychiatry*, **60**, 261–9.

Judd, L. L., Akiskal, H. S., Schettler, P. J. *et al.* (2005). Psychosocial disability in the course of Bipolar I and II Disorders. A prospective, comparative, longitudinal study. *Archives of General Psychiatry*, **62**, 1322–30.

Kane, J. M., Quitkin, F. M., Rifkin, A. *et al.* (1982). Lithium carbonate and imipramine in the prophylaxis of unipolar and Bipolar II illness: a prospective, placebo-controlled comparison. *Archives of General Psychiatry*, **39**, 1065–9.

Kleindienst, N. and Greil, W. (2000). Differential efficacy of lithium and carbamazepine in the prophylaxis of bipolar disorder: results of the MAP study. *Neuropsychobiology*, **42** (Suppl. 1), S2–10.

Malhi, G. S., Mitchell, P. B., Berk, M. and Goodwin, G. M. (2005). Mood stabilizers: a labile label. *Acta Psychiatrica Scandinavica*, **111** (Suppl. 426), S5–6.

Margolese, H. C., Beauclair, L., Szkrumelak, N. and Chouinard, G. (2003). Hypomania induced by adjunctive lamotrigine. *American Journal of Psychiatry*, **160**, 183–4.

McIntyre, R. S., Mancini, D. A., McCann, S. *et al.* (2002). Topiramate versus bupropion SR when added to mood stabilizer therapy for the depressive phase of bipolar disorder: a preliminary single-blind study. *Bipolar Disorders*, **4**, 207–13.

McIntyre, R. S., Riccardelli, R. and Binder, C. (2005). Open-label adjunctive topiramate in the treatment of unstable bipolar disorder. *Canadian Journal of Psychiatry*, **50**, 415–22.

National Institute for Health and Clinical Excellence (NICE) (2006). Bipolar disorder. *NICE clinical guideline 38*. http://www.nice.org.uk.

Nemeroff, C. B., Evans, D. L., Gyulai, L. *et al.* (2001). Double-blind, placebo-controlled comparison of imipramine and paroxetine in the treatment of bipolar depression. *American Journal of Psychiatry*, **158**, 906–12.

Nierenberg, A. A., Ostacher, M. J., Calabrese, J. R. *et al.* and STEP-BD Investigators (2006). Treatment-resistant bipolar depression: a STEP-BD equipoise randomized effectiveness trial of antidepressant augmentation with lamotrigine, inositol, or risperidone. *American Journal of Psychiatry*, **163**, 210–16.

Quitkin, F., Rifkin, A., Kane, J., Ramos-Lorenzi, J. R. and Klein, D. F. (1978). Prophylactic effect of lithium and imipramine in unipolar and Bipolar II patients: a preliminary report. *American Journal of Psychiatry*, **135**, 570–2.

Rubio, G., Lopez-Munoz, F. and Alamo, C. (2006). Effects of lamotrigine in patients with bipolar disorder and alcohol dependence. *Bipolar Disorders*, **8**, 289–93.

Schaffer, A., Zuker, P. and Levitt, A. (2006). Randomised, double-blind pilot trial comparing lamotrigine versus citalopram for the treatment of bipolar depression. *Journal of Affective Disorders*, **96**, 95–9.

Suppes, T., Brown, E. S., McElroy, S. L. *et al.* (1999). Lamotrigine for the treatment of bipolar disorder: a clinical case series. *Journal of Affective Disorders*, **53**, 95–8.

Thase, M. (2005). Bipolar depression: issues in diagnosis and treatment. *Harvard Review of Psychiatry*, **13**, 257–71.

Tondo, L., Baldessarini, R. J. and Floris, G. (2001). Long-term clinical effectiveness of lithium maintenance treatment in Types I and II bipolar disorders. *British Journal of Psychiatry*, **41** (Suppl. 178), S184–90.

Tondo, L., Baldessarini, R. J., Hennen, J. and Floris, G. (1998). Lithium maintenance treatment of depression and mania in Bipolar I and Bipolar II disorders. *American Journal of Psychiatry*, **155**, 638–45.

van der Loos, M., Nolen, W. A. and Vieta, E. (2006). Lamotrigine as add-on to lithium in bipolar depression. Paper presented at the fifth *European Stanley Conference on Bipolar Disorder*, Barcelona, 5–7 October.

Vieta, E., Sanchez-Moreno, J., Goikolea, J. M. *et al.* (2003). Adjunctive topiramate in Bipolar II Disorder. *World Journal of Biological Psychiatry*, **4**, 172–6.

Vieta, E., Goikolea, J. M., Martinez-Aran, A. *et al.* (2006). A double-blind, randomized, placebo-controlled, prophylaxis study of adjunctive gabapentin for bipolar disorder. *Journal of Clinical Psychiatry*, **67**, 473–7.

Winsberg, M. E., DeGolia, S. G., Strong, C. M. and Ketter, T. A. (2001). Divalproex therapy in medication-naïve and mood-stabilizer-naïve Bipolar II depression. *Journal of Affective Disorders*, **67**, 207–12.

Yatham, L. (2004). Diagnosis and management of patients with Bipolar II Disorder. *Journal of Clinical Psychiatry*, **66** (Suppl. 1), S13–17.

Yatham, L. N., Kennedy, S. H., O'Donovan, C. *et al.* (2005). Canadian Network for Mood and Anxiety Treatments (CANMAT) guidelines for the management of patients with bipolar disorder: Consensus and controversies. *Bipolar Disorders*, **7** (Suppl. 3), S5–69.

Young, L. T., Robb, J. C., Hasey, G. M. *et al.* (1999). Gabapentin as an adjunctive treatment in bipolar disorder. *Journal of Affective Disorders*, **55**, 73–7.

Young, L. T., Joffe, R. T. and Robb, J. C. (2000). Double-blind comparison of addition of a second mood stabilizer versus an antidepressant to an initial mood stabilizer for treatment of patients with bipolar depression. *American Journal of Psychiatry*, **157**, 124–6.

10

The use of atypical antipsychotic drugs in Bipolar II Disorder

David Fresno and Eduard Vieta

Introduction

The bipolar disorders are common, severe long-term conditions, with the World Health Organization reporting in 2001 that bipolar disorder was the fifth cause of 'life years lived with a disability' among young adults (WHO, 2001). Atypical antipsychotics are established as the main treatment for schizophrenia, but recently a growing number of trials have indicated that they may provide a therapeutic option for bipolar disorder, as both alternative and adjunctive treatments to traditional mood stabilisers (Vieta and Goikolea, 2005; Berk and Dodd, 2005). While they have been most commonly assessed as treatments for mania, there is increasing evidence of their efficacy and safety in the treatment of bipolar depression and as maintenance treatments of bipolar disorder.

The availability of atypical antipsychotics has brought important changes in the management of the bipolar disorders. Firstly, methodologically more rigorous trials have been developed in order to research their efficacy and safety as a treatment for the different bipolar phases. Secondly, the use of atypical antipsychotics in patients with schizophrenia has given short-term and long-term results suggesting that they provide a safer option than typical antipsychotics. Thirdly, it has been suggested that atypical antipsychotics, via neuronal plasticity determinant molecules, may relate to the therapeutic response process observed in drugs more commonly used as a treatment of affective disorders (Vieta, 2003). Fourthly, some atypical antipsychotics may have mood-stabilising properties (Yatham et al., 2005).

Special characteristics of Bipolar II Disorder

There are several special characteristics of Bipolar II (BP II) Disorder that have important clinical consequences. Although hypomanic episodes can occur in

Bipolar II Disorder. Modelling, Measuring and Managing, ed. Gordon Parker. Published by Cambridge University Press. © Cambridge University Press 2008.

Bipolar I (BP I) Disorder as well, it is a characteristic of BP II, and yet there are surprisingly few randomised trials focusing on how to treat hypomania. While hypomania can be considered as a phase preceding mania in BP I – and should be treated as such – this is not the model used in managing BP II (Vieta, 2007).

Bipolar depression is the most common phase of bipolar disorder (Judd *et al.*, 2002), and its management is a very real challenge (Hirschfeld, 2004). A NIMH study followed 146 patients over a mean of 13 years and found that bipolar patients were symptomatic for nearly half of their lives (i.e. 47%). They also found, consistent with previous studies (Vieta *et al.*, 1997), that BP II patients spent more time depressed than did BP I patients (50% vs 32% of their weeks). According to a naturalistic study carried out by Ghaemi *et al.* (2000) it took BP I patients nearly 6 years, and BP II patients nearly 12 years from first contact with the mental health system to achieve a correct diagnosis. This means that BP II patients, on average, spend double the time without a proper diagnosis and treatment (Ghaemi *et al.*, 2000).

As those with undiagnosed BP II are more likely to present for treatment for an episode of *depression*, antidepressant-induced 'switching' to hypomania is a possible and undesirable effect of being prescribed antidepressants (Altshuler *et al.*, 1995; Ghaemi *et al.*, 2003). Although some authors consider rapid cycling to be more frequent in BP II than in BP I patients (Kupka *et al.*, 2003), other experts find no difference (Dunner, 1979; Kuyler, 1988; Vieta *et al.*, 1997).

BP II patients are more frequently female (Vieta *et al.*, 1997); and may suffer from cognitive impairment as a result of their condition (Torrent *et al.*, 2006).

The use of atypical antipsychotics in Bipolar II Disorder

Monotherapy does not seem an adequate long-term option for managing the majority of patients with bipolar disorder. Current recommendations include combination therapy, particularly in patients with the treatment-refractory rapid-cycling variant (Muzina and Calabrese, 2005). Augmentation therapy with the atypical antipsychotics risperidone, olanzapine, quetiapine and ziprasidone has also been suggested to help control the depressive phase of bipolar disorder (Bowden, 2005), but results of randomised trials of atypical agents as add-on treatment to mood stabilisers for BP II patients are not available as yet.

Unexpectedly, there is very little literature about safety and efficacy of atypical antipsychotics in the treatment of BP II. The majority of studies investigating the pharmacotherapy of BP II have significant methodological limitations, as they comprise small samples and have involved observational or retrospective designs. Thus, the level of evidence is not high and therapeutic decisions must be made on a case-by-case basis. New trials with more adequate designs would be welcomed in order to develop effective treatment strategies for this subtype (Hadjipavlou *et al.*, 2004). The most widespread treatment guidelines for bipolar disorder are those of the American Psychiatric Association, the British Association for Psychopharmacology, the Expert Consensus Guideline Series and the Texas Medication Algorithm Project. These guides offer important data when a therapeutic decision is needed, but even when they discriminate between different possible phases of the disorder they do not offer specific information for BP II patients. The only exception is the Canadian Network for Mood and Anxiety Treatments (CANMAT) guidelines for the management of patients with bipolar disorder (Yatham *et al.*, 2005), which devote a section to BP II and which has been expanded in a recent update (Yatham *et al.*, 2006).

We now overview some specific studies.

Quetiapine

Quetiapine has recently become the first drug to be indicated by the US Federal Drug Authority (FDA) for monotherapy of bipolar depression, including BP II depression (El-Mallakh *et al.*, 2006). Although no specific controlled trial addressed the efficacy and safety of quetiapine monotherapy in BP II, there are two studies that included enough BP II depressed patients to enable analysis separate to those with BP I Disorder.

BOLDER (BipOLar DEpRession) studies I and II comprised two double-blind, randomised, placebo-controlled trials that investigated the efficacy and tolerability of quetiapine monotherapy for major depressive episodes in BP I and BP II patients (with 351 of the BOLDER I and II subjects having BP II Disorder). Combined results from both studies looking specifically at BP II patients have been reported recently (Suppes *et al.*, 2006). Efficacy was evaluated weekly using the Montgomery–Åsberg Depression Rating Scale (MADRS) and the Hamilton Rating Scale for Depression (HAMD). The MADRS scores were significantly lower from the first week in the quetiapine group. Adverse events reported were dry mouth, sedation and somnolence. Quetiapine may therefore be considered an effective and well-tolerated treatment for depressive episodes in BP II Disorder.

Quetiapine monotherapy's anxiolytic effects in BP II depression have also been analysed in the BOLDER I study, which examined scores on the Hamilton Rating Scale for Anxiety (HAMA) and some items from the MADRS and HAMD scales. Although the study was only positive for BP I depression, quetiapine improvement versus placebo was significant in several items, such as HAMA anxious mood, MADRS inner tension and HAMD psychic anxiety (Hirschfeld *et al.*, 2006).

Quetiapine has also been studied over a 12-month period as an add-on treatment for bipolar depression, and it showed promising results, although this was not a controlled trial, and it included both BP I and BP II patients (Milev *et al.*, 2006).

Quetiapine's potential tolerability issues include sedation, weight gain and, to a lesser extent, extrapyramidal symptoms.

Risperidone

There is evidence for risperidone as a safe and effective treatment for mania. In 2001, an open-label study of its effectiveness and tolerability in the hypomania associated with BP II was carried out with 44 DSM–IV-defined BP II patients. Their Young Mania Rating Scale (YMRS) scores were above 7, and they were followed-up for six months. The YMRS and Clinical Global Impression for Bipolar Disorder (CGI-BD) were used to measure efficacy, while treatment-emergent depression was rated with the Hamilton Depression Rating Scale (HDRS-17), and with the Udvalg for Kliniske Undersogelser (UKU) subscale used to estimate possible side-effects. Hypomanic patients received a mean 2.8 mg/day dose at endpoint. Thirty-four patients completed the trial. At the 6-month follow-up, 60% of the patients were asymptomatic according to the CGI. No differences were observed between risperidone as monotherapy, and as an adjunct to mood stabilisers. Risperidone was well tolerated by hypomanic BP II patients and seemed to be more protective against hypomanic than depressive relapses, but this was not a controlled trial (Vieta *et al.*, 2001). This is an important finding, as neuropsychological and outcome differences between risperidone and conventional antipsychotics in long-term treated patients have been studied. In these studies, those who received risperidone showed more cognitive flexibility and better occupational adaptation than did patients treated with conventional neuroleptics (Reinares *et al.*, 2000).

Finally, an observational study including BP I and BP II patients suggested that risperidone might have antidepressant properties (McIntyre *et al.*, 2004).

Potential tolerability issues with risperidone include mainly extrapyramidal symptoms, hyperprolactinaemia and weight gain.

Olanzapine

There are no published studies investigating the usefulness of olanzapine in samples of those with BP II Disorder only, so that only data on broader bipolar disorder samples can be considered.

In 2003 there was an 8-week, double-blind, randomised, placebo-controlled trial of 833 patients with bipolar depression – as quantified by a MADRS score of at least 20. They were divided into three groups: to receive placebo; olanzapine; or olanzapine plus fluoxetine. Olanzapine, but especially the olanzapine–fluoxetine combination, was associated with significantly improved MADRS scores compared with placebo ($P < 0.001$). Treatment-induced mania (YMRS score < 15 at baseline and at least 15 subsequently) was similar for the three arms of the trial (Tohen *et al.*, 2003). This combination is approved by the FDA for the treatment of bipolar depression, but all patients who joined this trial were diagnosed as having BP I.

A placebo-controlled study by Amsterdam and Shults (2005) randomly divided 34 bipolar patients with bipolar depression into four groups to receive, for up to 8 weeks, fluoxetine monotherapy 10–30 mg daily; olanzapine monotherapy 5–20 mg daily; combined therapy with fluoxetine 10–40 mg plus olanzapine 5–15 mg daily; or placebo. Several outcome measures were used: the 17-item HAMD, 17-item HAMD atypical symptom profile (HAMD 17-R), 28-item HAMD, MADRS and the YMRS. Results suggested that the combination of olanzapine–fluoxetine may be a safe initial treatment for major depressive episodes in a bipolar disorder, however an important caveat is the limited size of the study cohort. Also, length of treatment was just 8 weeks and, most important for this chapter, only two BP II patients were included.

Brown *et al.* (2006) compared olanzapine–fluoxetine combination (OFC) with lamotrigine. The OFC group showed greater improvement in depressive and manic symptoms, but more treatment-emergent adverse events, greater weight gain, and some elevated metabolic factors compared with those taking lamotrigine. Overall, treatment differences were modest. Again, only BP I patients were enrolled.

The principal tolerability concerns related to olanzapine treatment in general are weight gain and increased potential to develop the metabolic syndrome.

Other atypical antipsychotics

Conventional neuroleptics have traditionally been used as adjuncts to other medications in the treatment of some BP II patients, but there is little or no evidence of their efficacy. Aripiprazole has been approved in the USA for the treatment of mania and prevention of manic relapse. Further studies are ongoing in bipolar depression (García-Amador *et al.*, 2006), but its role in managing BP II Disorder is as yet unknown. None of the other antipsychotics, clozapine, ziprasidone or amisulpride, have been assessed in BP II Disorder.

Conclusions

Atypical antipsychotics now offer an option for the management of BP I, but limited trialling in relevant subjects means that their role in managing BP II remains to be studied.

The trials of atypical antipsychotics in mania have reported consistently positive results, as expected, but also a few trials in bipolar depression have been positive, probably due to their receptor activity profile (Brugue and Vieta, 2007). However, BP II has several special characteristics that make it necessary for separate studies to be undertaken for this subtype, especially when bipolar depression is particularly common in these patients.

There is very little literature, though, on the effects of atypical antipsychotics in BP II. There is controlled evidence of quetiapine monotherapy as an effective treatment for BP II depression, and of its anxiolytic effect in bipolar depression. And an open-label study suggests that risperidone is a well-tolerated and efficacious treatment of hypomania and that it might be protective against hypomanic episodes. Also, the olanzapine-fluoxetine combination is an option for major depressive episodes in bipolar disorder, but there is not enough evidence as to whether it might benefit BP II patients.

Thus there is a dearth of controlled studies in this area. No evidence is available with regards to theoretically attractive combinations with lithium, lamotrigine, or other antidepressants other than fluoxetine. Safety issues, including weight gain, metabolic syndrome, hyperprolactinaemia, extrapyramidal symptoms, akathisia, tardive dyskinesia and sedation are still a concern, particularly in the case of truly mild patients with good psychosocial functioning.

In conclusion, further research is needed in order to better understand the benefit–risk ratio of treating BP II with atypical antipsychotics.

Acknowledgements

Supported in part by the Red de Enfermedades Mentales (REM-TAP Network), Spain.

REFERENCES

Altshuler, L. L., Post, R. M., Leverich, G. S. *et al.* (1995). Antidepressant-induced mania and cycle acceleration: a controversy revisited. *American Journal of Psychiatry*, **152**, 1130–8.

Amsterdam, J. D. and Shults, J. (2005). Comparison of fluoxetine, olanzapine, and combined fluoxetine plus olanzapine initial therapy of Bipolar Type I and Type II major depression – lack of manic induction. *Journal of Affective Disorders*, **87**, 121–30.

Berk, M. and Dodd, S. (2005). Efficacy of atypical antipsychotics in bipolar disorder. *Drugs*, **65**, 257–69.

Bowden, C. L. (2005). Atypical antipsychotic augmentation of mood stabilizer therapy in bipolar disorder. *Journal of Clinical Psychiatry*, **66** (Suppl. 3), S12–19.

Brown, E. B., McElroy, S.L., Keck, P. E. Jr. *et al.* (2006). A seven-week, randomized, double-blind trial of olanzapine/fluoxetine combination versus lamotrigine in the treatment of Bipolar I depression. *Journal of Clinical Psychiatry*, **67**, 1025–33.

Brugue, E. and Vieta, E. (2007). Atypical antipsychotics in bipolar depression: neurobiological basis and clinical implications. *Progress in Neuropsychopharmacological and Biological Psychiatry*, **31**, 275–82.

Dunner, D. (1979). Rapid-cycling manic depressive illness. *Psychiatric Clinics of North America*, **2**, 461–7.

El-Mallakh, R., Weisler, R. H., Townsend, M. H. and Ginsberg, L. D. (2006). Bipolar II Disorder: current and future treatment options. *Annals of Clinical Psychiatry*, **18**, 259–66.

García-Amador, M., Pacchiarotti, I., Valenti, M. *et al.* (2006). Role of aripiprazole in treating mood disorders. *Expert Review of Neurotherapeutics*, **6**, 1777–83.

Ghaemi, S. N., Boiman, E. E. and Goodwin, F. K. (2000). Diagnosing bipolar disorder and the effect of antidepressants: a naturalistic study. *Journal of Clinical Psychiatry*, **61**, 804–8.

Ghaemi, N. S., Hsu, D. J., Soldani, F. and Goodwin, F. K. (2003). Antidepressants in bipolar disorder: the case for caution. *Bipolar Disorders*, **5**, 421–33.

Hadjipavlou, G., Mok, H. and Yatham, L. N. (2004). Pharmacotherapy of Bipolar II Disorder: a critical review of current evidence. *Bipolar Disorders*, **6**, 14–25.

Hirschfeld, R. M. A. (2004). Bipolar depression: the real challenge. *European Neuropsychopharmacology*, **14**, 83–8.

Hirschfeld, R. M., Weisler, R. H., Raines, S. R. and Macfadden, W. for the BOLDER Study Group (2006). Quetiapine in the treatment of anxiety in patients with Bipolar I or II depression: a secondary analysis from a randomized, double-blind, placebo-controlled study. *Journal of Clinical Psychiatry*, **67**, 355–62.

Judd, L. L., Akiskal, H. S., Schetter, P. J. *et al.* (2002). The long-term natural history of the weekly symptomatic status of Bipolar I Disorder. *Archives of General Psychiatry*, **59**, 530–7.

Kupka, R. W., Luckenbaugh, D. A., Post, R. M., Leverich, G. S. and Nolen, W. A. (2003). Rapid- and non-rapid-cycling bipolar disorder: A meta-analysis of clinical studies. *Journal of Clinical Psychiatry*, **64**, 1483–94.

Kuyler, P. L. (1988). Rapid-cycling Bipolar II illness in three closely related individuals. *American Journal of Psychiatry*, **145**, 114–15.

McIntyre, R. S., Mancini, D. A., Srinivasan, J. *et al.* (2004). The antidepressant effects of risperidone and olanzapine in bipolar disorder. *Canadian Journal of Clinical Pharmacology*, **11**, e218–26. Epub., October 4.

Milev, R., Abraham, G. and Zaheer, J. (2006). Add-on quetiapine for bipolar depression: a 12-month open-label trial. *Canadian Journal of Psychiatry*, **51**, 523–30.

Muzina, D. J. and Calabrese, J. R. (2005). Maintenance therapies in bipolar disorder: focus on randomised controlled trials. *Australian and New Zealand Journal of Psychiatry*, **39**, 652–61.

Reinares, M., Martinez-Aran, A., Colom, F. *et al.* (2000). Long-term effects of the treatment with risperidone versus conventional neuroleptics on the neuropsychological performance of euthymic bipolar patients. *Actas Españolas de Psiquiatría*, **28**, 231–8.

Suppes, T., Hirschfeld, R.M., Vieta, E. *et al.* (2006). Quetiapine monotherapy for depressive episodes in Bipolar II Disorder: combined results from two placebo-controlled studies. *Bipolar Disorders*, **8** (Suppl. 1), S34–5.

Tohen, M., Vieta, E., Calabrese, J. *et al.* (2003). Efficacy of olanzapine and olanzapine-fluoxetine combination in the treatment of Bipolar I depression. *Archives of General Psychiatry*, **60**, 1079–88.

Torrent, C., Martinez-Aran, A., Daban, C. *et al.* (2006). Cognitive impairment in Bipolar II Disorder. *British Journal of Psychiatry*, **189**, 254–9.

Vieta, E. (2003). Atypical antipsychotics in the treatment of mood disorders. *Current Opinion in Psychiatry*, **16**, 23–7.

Vieta, E. (2007). *Managing Bipolar Disorder in Clinical Practice*. London: Current Medicine Group.

Vieta, E. and Goikolea, J. M. (2005). Atypical antipsychotics: newer options for mania and maintenance therapy. *Bipolar Disorders*, **7** (Suppl. 2), S1–S13.

Vieta, E., Gastó, C., Otero, A., Nieto, E. and Vallejo, J. (1997). Differential features between Bipolar I and Bipolar II disorder. *Comprehensive Psychiatry*, **38**, 98–101.

Vieta, E., Gasto, C., Colom, F. *et al.* (2001). Role of risperidone in Bipolar II: an open six-month study. *Journal of Affective Disorders*, **67**, 213–19.

World Health Organization (2001). *World Health Report: Mental Health: New Understanding, New Hope*. Geneva: World Health Organization.

Yatham, L.N., Goldstein, J.M., Vieta, E. *et al.* (2005). Atypical antipsychotics in bipolar depression: potential mechanisms of action. *Journal of Clinical Psychiatry*, **66**, 40–8.

Yatham, L.N., Kennedy, S.H., O'Donovan, C. *et al.* (2006). Guidelines Group, CANMAT. Canadian Network for Mood and Anxiety Treatments guidelines for the management of patients with bipolar disorder: Update 2007. *Bipolar Disorders*, **8**, 721–39.

Yatham, L.N., Kennedy, S.H., O'Donovan, C. *et al.* (2005). CANMAT. Canadian Network for Mood and Anxiety Treatments guidelines for the management of patients with bipolar disorder: consensus and controversies. *Bipolar Disorders*, **7** (Suppl. 3), S5–69.

11

The role of fish oil in managing Bipolar II Disorder

Anne-Marie Rees and Gordon Parker

Introduction

As noted earlier (Chapter 5), an increase in Bipolar II Disorder (BP II) is suggested. Any prevalence increase could be artefactual, reflecting changes in attribution, definition, destigmatisation, help-seeking or other factors. Alternately, there may have been a real increase and numerous determinants have been proposed, including genetic factors, greater use of illicit drugs and many social and environmental factors. In relation to the last, there has been considerable interest in a dietary contribution, particularly involving omega-3 fatty acids.

What are omega-3 fatty acids?

Omega-3 (n-3) fatty acids are long-chain polyunsaturated fatty acids (PUFAs) found in various plant and marine life. The marine-based n-3 PUFAs primarily consist of eicosapentaenoic acid (EPA) and docosahexaenoic acid (DHA), and appear to be highly biologically active. In contrast, plant-based n-3 PUFAs, from flaxseed, walnuts and canola oil, are usually in the form of the parent n-3 PUFA, alpha-linolenic acid (ALA). Although dietary ALA can be endogenously converted to EPA and DHA (see the metabolic pathways in Figure 11.1), this process occurs inefficiently, with only 10–15% of ALA being metabolised in this way.

The history of n-3 PUFAs

In the last 150 years, rapid expansion in western populations has been associated with a change in diet, with n-3 PUFAs from fish, wild game and plants being replaced by saturated fats from domestic animals and omega-6 (n-6) PUFAs from common vegetable oils (corn, safflower and soybean) and other sources such as wheat germ. These changes have resulted in a large increase in the n-6/n-3 PUFA ratio in the general diet – from 1:1 to more than 10:1, which has led to a high

Bipolar II Disorder. Modelling, Measuring and Managing, ed. Gordon Parker. Published by Cambridge University Press. © Cambridge University Press 2008.

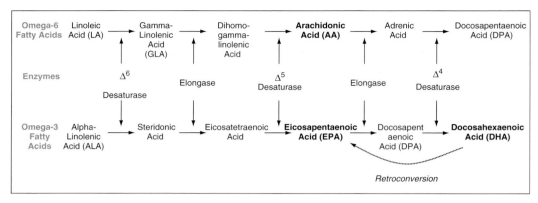

Figure 11.1. Metabolic pathway for polyunsaturated fatty acids.

proportion of the common *n*-6 PUFA, arachidonic acid (AA), as against EPA and DHA, in the cell membranes of most tissues; this leading, in turn, to a high proportion of pro-inflammatory eicosanoids. As shown in Figure 11.1, an increase in AA also affects the production of EPA and DHA, due to competition for metabolising enzymes.

Such dietary changes in fatty acid intake have been held to have numerous pathological consequences. These include links with cardiovascular disease, and compromised immune function and cognitive function, both in the infant and, later in life, in Alzheimer's disease. The sharp rises in rates of depression, bipolar disorder and other neurological disorders in the twentieth century may have been fuelled by the increased consumption of *n*-6-rich vegetable oils. Elevated levels of AA-derived inflammatory eicosanoids (e.g. prostaglandin E2) in patients with both unipolar and bipolar depression support this hypothesis (refer to Parker *et al.*, 2006 for further review of this area).

The use of fish oil for the treatment of psychiatric disorders is favoured by many patients, particularly those concerned about the side-effect profiles of psychotropic drugs. A naturally occurring dietary product is also appealing, and the notion that they are replenishing an element of their cells that has been depleted due to inadequate dietary intake appears intuitively acceptable to many patients.

Public health issues

Fish oil and its role in mood disorders is also a public health issue and research is already informing food policy. Certain foods, including infant formulas, are being fortified with *n*-3 PUFAs. The population needs nutritional advice with regard to *n*-3 PUFAs. This is starting to occur for particular conditions. For instance, the National Australian Heart Foundation has set guidelines about adequate fish intake per week in relation to preventing cardiac disease. Similar public health statements may need to be prepared regarding *n*-3 PUFA intake and mood disorders. Also food production methods, such as fish farming, need close monitoring and regulation to optimise *n*-3 PUFA content.

Research studies

Novel research into the role of fish oil as a treatment for mood disorders is being conducted internationally. We will review the literature published so far in the area of bipolar disorder. Unfortunately, most studies do not differentiate between Bipolar I Disorder (BP I) and BP II.

Epidemiological studies

Research has examined for links between seafood consumption and prevalence rates of bipolar disorder and schizophrenia. Links (Noaghuil and Hibbeln, 2003) were shown between greater seafood consumption and higher lifetime prevalence rates of BP I, BP II and bipolar spectrum disorder, with the strongest association being quantified for BP II ($r = -0.91$). The lack, however, of any association between seafood consumption and lifetime prevalence rates of schizophrenia was interpreted as reflecting specificity of the association to affective disorders. In a similar cross-national study (Hibbeln, 1998), a strong negative correlation ($r = -0.84$) was found between fish consumption and major depression.

Biological marker studies

One intrinsic advantage to this research domain is the capacity to pursue and quantify the proposed biological marker. PUFA levels can be measured in plasma, erythrocytes and adipose tissue using thin layer gas chromatography. Whole blood needs to be collected by venepuncture, however, finger prick techniques are becoming available.

Significant reductions in erythrocyte AA and DHA have been found in BP I subjects when compared with controls (Chiu *et al.*, 2003). No studies have yet been reported on PUFA levels for Bipolar II Disorder, however, several studies have reported reductions in *n*-3 PUFAs and an increase in the *n*-6:*n*-3 ratio for depressed compared with non-depressed subjects (Edwards *et al.*, 1998; Peet *et al.*, 1998; Maes *et al.*, 1999).

Treatment studies

Stoll *et al.* (1999b) undertook a 4-month double-blind, placebo-controlled trial of patients with bipolar disorder (BP I and BP II), with 14 receiving *n*-3 PUFA treatment (i.e. a total daily *n*-3 PUFA dosage of 6.2 g of EPA and 3.4 g of DHA) and 16 the (olive oil) placebo. As most were receiving a mood stabiliser, this was essentially an augmentation strategy, with the principal outcome measure being the duration of time before symptom exacerbation led to study exit. Those in the *n*-3 PUFA group reported greater symptom reduction and remained in remission for a significantly longer time. Consideration of the 'non-completors' of the 4-month study is of some interest. In the *n*-3 PUFA group, three of the 14 were 'non-completors' because of mania, hypomania, and worsening of a mixed state, respectively. In the placebo group, 10 of the 16 were 'non-completors', nine because of worsening depression, and one because of a 'continued mixed state'. Such indicative data were interpreted as demonstrating an antidepressant effect of *n*-3 PUFAs, while the authors noted that the baseline clinical state of their subjects disallowed any anti-manic effect of *n*-3 PUFAs to be evaluated. Thus, while this study is commonly viewed as demonstrating the benefits of *n*-3 PUFAs for bipolar disorder, it may also be that this study more demonstrated the antidepressant potential of *n*-3 PUFAs. Subsequently, Osher *et al.* (2005) reported an open-label study, with eight of 10 BP I patients (reporting depressive symptoms and/or being functionally impaired, and maintained on their pharmacotherapy) having a 50% or greater reduction in depression scores within one month.

A 4-month placebo-controlled randomised parallel group trial (Keck *et al.*, 2006) assessed the efficacy and safety of 6 g of EPA per day in 116 patients with acute bipolar (I, II or NOS) depression (including 59 patients with a rapid-cycling disorder). Subjects were receiving at least one mood stabiliser in addition to the trial medication. No differences were found in the depression or mania rating scale scores between the two groups. There were no significant differences in bleeding times between the groups, supporting *n*-3 PUFAs as a safe treatment. The authors commented, however, on the potential problem of using high doses of EPA as opposed to lower doses or EPA/DHA combinations.

One study (Chiu *et al.*, 2005), using a randomised placebo-controlled trial, has trialled treating acute mania with *n*-3 PUFAS. Fifteen patients were recruited and an *n*-3 PUFA product with an EPA:DHA ratio of 2:1 was used. The intervention was added to a fixed dose of sodium valproate (with lorazepam permitted for alleviating agitation or insomnia). Mean scores on the Young Mania Rating Scale decreased over the first 4 weeks but there was no statistically significant difference between the treatment and placebo groups. Numbers in this trial were small and the use of concomitant sodium valproate may have masked any anti-manic effects.

A pilot study by Marangell *et al.* (2006) reports a randomised double-blind placebo-controlled trial where 2 g of DHA per day or placebo were added to a psychosocial intervention for women with Bipolar Disorder (BP I = 9, BP II = 1). These women chose to discontinue standard pharmacological treatment while attempting to conceive. The DHA was well tolerated. While a non-significant result was reported, the very small cell numbers should be noted.

Another study (Frangou *et al.*, 2006) studied a synthetically manufactured product, ethyl-EPA (which contains 98% EPA). Patients with either BP I or BP II, and who were currently depressed, received either 1 g or 2 g of ethyl-EPA or placebo for 12 weeks in a randomised controlled trial. The intervention was added to usual treatment, required to have been unchanged for 8 weeks. Significant improvements in the Hamilton Depression Rating Scale scores were reported in the EPA groups compared to placebo. There was no difference between the 1 g or 2 g doses. There was no difference in scores on the Young Mania Rating Scale between the groups, and ethyl-EPA did not appear to precipitate polarity changes in people with bipolar disorder. Results for the BP I and BP II groups were not reported separately.

A 4-month placebo-controlled randomised parallel group trial (Keck *et al.*, 2002) assessed the efficacy and safety of 6 g of EPA per day in 59 patients with acute bipolar (I, II or NOS) depression. No differences were found in the depression or mania rating scale scores between the two groups. In the same study, 62 patients with rapid-cycling bipolar illness were similarly treated, with no significant differences found between treatment and placebo groups. There were no significant differences in bleeding times between the groups, supporting *n*-3 PUFAs as a safe treatment.

One study (Chiu *et al.*, 2005), using a randomised placebo-controlled trial, has looked at treating acute mania with *n*-3 PUFAS. Fifteen patients were recruited and an *n*-3 PUFA product with an EPA:DHA ratio of 2:1 was used. The intervention was added to a fixed dose of sodium valproate (with lorazepam permitted for alleviating agitation or insomnia). Mean scores on the Young Mania Rating Scale decreased over the first 4 weeks but there was no statistically significant difference between the treatment and placebo groups. Numbers in this trial were small and the use of concomitant sodium valproate may have masked any anti-manic effects.

Do n-3 PUFAs cause switching?

It is possible that N-3 PUFAs may cause switching from depression to hypomania. Switching is often reported as a marker of an effective antidepressant. Case reports of switching have included long-chain PUFAs (Kinrys, 2000). However, Stoll *et al.*

(2000) argued that hypomanic switching is rare with n-3 PUFAs and is mainly seen with the shorter-chain *n*-3 PUFA (alpha-linolenic acid), found in flaxseed oil.

In light of the above, more studies are needed to assess whether omega-3 has anti-manic or antidepressant mood-stabilising qualities. Most psychotropic drugs act differently across the bipolar spectrum (e.g. lithium and sodium valproate have stronger anti-manic compared with antidepressant effects), thus omega-3 (as for lamotrigine) may have greater mood-elevating effects.

Neuroscientific mechanisms

Several neurophysiological mechanisms have been proposed to explain the relationship between *n*-3 PUFAs and mood disorders. The two *n*-3 PUFAs, EPA and DHA, appear to decrease the production of inflammatory eicosanoids from AA via two mechanisms. Firstly, they compete with AA for incorporation into membrane phospholipids, decreasing both cellular and plasma AA levels. We know that DHA depletion in the brain leads to AA being upregulated, which increases the susceptibility to certain inflammatory diseases. Secondly, EPA competes with AA for the cyclo-oxygenase enzyme system, inhibiting the production of AA-derived pro-inflammatory eicosanoids (e.g. prostaglandins, leukotrienes and thromboxanes), with prostaglandin E2 and thromboxane B2 having been linked to bipolar disorder and depression. Docosahexaenoic acid and EPA also inhibit the release of pro-inflammatory cytokines, like interleukin-1 beta (IL-1β), interleukin-2 and interleukin-6, interferon-gamma and tumour necrosis factor (TNF)-α, which are dependent on eicosanoid release and also associated with bipolar disorder and depression (Logan, 2003).

These mechanisms are further supported by animal studies which suggest that AA turnover rates are reduced in rats fed lithium chloride. This is a highly specific effect, as turnover rates of DHA and palmitic acid are not affected. Similar effects are noted with long-term treatment of valproic acid and carbamazepine in animals, but no effect has been found with topiramate. This decrease in AA turnover corresponds to downregulating gene expression, and enzyme activity of cytosolic phospholipase A2 – an enzyme that selectively liberates AA but not DHA from phospholipids in the cell membrane. Lithium and carbamazepine also decrease brain protein level and activity of cyclooxygenase-2 (COX-2), as well as brain concentrations of prostaglandin E2, produced via cyclooxygenase-2 (Rapoport and Bosetti, 2002). Carbamazepine directly decreases eicosanoids. In essence, all three of these mood stabilisers decrease COX-2 and downregulate PGE2.

Further, *n*-3 PUFAs affect the brain-derived neurotrophic factor (BDNF) which encourages synaptic plasticity, provides neuroprotection and enhances neurotransmission. We know that BDNF and other neuroprotective factors are downregulated in bipolar disorder and upregulated by mood stabilisers such as lithium and the anticonvulsants. n-3 PUFAs also have anti-kindling properties making them a candidate for mood stabilisation. They also have direct effects on calcium channels (as in when verapamil and nimodipine are used as mood stabilisers). Also, they directly affect protein kinase C, as does sodium valproate (Stoll *et al.*, 1999a).

Another possible mechanism relates to the abundance of DHA in central nervous system membrane phospholipids, where it plays a vital role in maintaining membrane integrity and fluidity. By varying lipid concentrations in cell membranes, changes in fluidity can affect either the structure or function of proteins embedded in the membrane, including enzymes, receptors and ion channels, leading to changes in cellular signalling. As with the mood stabilisers lithium and sodium valproate, n-3 PUFAs suppress phosphatidylinositol-associated signal transduction mechanisms via changes in membrane fluidity.

The hypothesis that n-3 PUFAs can affect cell membrane fluidity is supported by a study using magnetic resonance imaging (Hirashima *et al.*, 2004). Twelve women with bipolar disorder received n-3 PUFAs for 4 weeks, and were contrasted with two non-treatment groups. T2 whole brain relaxation times were used to detect changes in membrane fluidity, measured at baseline and 4 weeks after treatment initiation. The bipolar subjects receiving n-3 PUFAs had significant decreases in T2 values, with a dose-dependent effect apparent when the bipolar treatment group was subdivided into high-dose (10 g n-3 PUFAs) and low-dose (2 g n-3 PUFAs) cohorts.

Another postulated more direct mechanism involves gene expression and the binding of fatty acids to specific nuclear receptors early in life, leading to genetic transcription (Sampath and Ntambi, 2004) and predisposing later in life to a range of diseases with DHA and EPA, such as Alzheimer's disease, cardiac disease, bipolar disorder and depression.

Potential treatment recommendations

Since research into n-3 PUFAs and bipolar disorder is still in its early stages, it is important that other evidence-based treatments are respected. It is unclear whether n-3 PUFAs work best by augmenting other treatments or as monotherapy. Also, the dose required and the amount of the different types of n-3 PUFAs (DHA and EPA) remains unresolved. Essentially, increasing dietary intake of n-3 PUFAs and decreasing the n-6:n-3 PUFA ratio is advisable for general wellbeing, and as a preventative strategy for mood disorders. Most research in this area has been into the prevention of cardiovascular disease. Approximately 300–500 mg per day of EPA and DHA are recommended for general wellbeing, which equates to about two fish oil capsules daily or two oily fish meals per week. Oily fish particularly high in *n*-3 PUFAs include swordfish and salmon, in particular, as well as tuna, mackerel, trout and anchovy. Local fishmongers are usually able to advise about the content of the local catch. To decrease *n*-6 PUFA intake, which is far too high in the Western diet, eating less processed food and increasing home cooking with monounsaturated fats such as olive oil should help.

For maintenance treatments, and to treat relapse in bipolar disorder, higher doses of *n*-3 PUFAs are likely to be required, via capsule intake, although more research is needed before dose recommendations can be made. The studies reported earlier suggest that adding fish oil to regular treatment at doses from 1–9 g *n*-3 PUFAs may be effective in preventing relapse in bipolar disorder, and that this treatment may be more effective in preventing bipolar depression than in preventing hypomania. Some researchers are arguing that EPA is the important active ingredient, despite DHA being much more abundant in the brain. Most fish oil capsule products available in Australia contain variable amounts of *n*-3 PUFAs, with the rest made up of *n*-6 PUFAs, monounsaturated and saturated fats. The proportion of DHA:EPA in the fish oil depends on the type of fish and location of catch, with southern hemisphere fish usually higher in DHA. Internationally, products are available with other ratios of *n*-3 PUFAs, including synthetic products which are almost pure EPA. It should be noted, however, that the short-chain omega-3 fatty acids, such as alpha-linoleic acid, which is found in flaxseed and linseed oil, have not been found effective in mood disorder management. Only small amounts are metabolised to the long-chain omega-3s and so it would be unwise to rely on this as the main source of omega-3.

Vegetarians may have to rely on short-chain omega-3, although eggs contain a reasonable amount of DHA, and micro-algae products are becoming available. There is a small amount of retroconversion of DHA to EPA (see Figure 11.1), but EPA intake in vegetarians is very limited.

Concerns relating to contamination of fish oil with mercury and other chemicals have received considerable press over the last few years. The amount of contamination, again, depends on the location of catch and the type of fish, while it appears that mercury contamination is a bigger problem in the northern hemisphere. Longer-living fish such as swordfish and shark are more likely to accumulate contaminants. Mercury poisoning has been associated with problems during pregnancy and therefore women in their reproductive years, and small children, should be cautioned about which fish they eat and in what quantities. Fish oil capsules that are approved by government regulatory bodies are checked for the level of contaminants, and therefore consumption of fish oil by this method should not be a problem.

Consuming very large amounts of polyunsaturated fats can increase oxidative stress, with potential tissue damage. The doses used for amelioration of mood disorders are unlikely to be a problem. However, ensuring a reasonable intake of antioxidants in one's diet is recommended. Antioxidants are high in foods containing vitamin C and E, or supplementation with these vitamins is an alternative.

Conclusions

Sufferers of BP II are usually much more debilitated by their depressive episodes than by their hypomanic episodes. For patients with mild bipolar illness, and who are concerned about side-effects of formal psychotropic drugs, a trial of high-dose fish oil as monotherapy may be warranted. In more severe illness, augmentation with fish oil may be a more advisable model. Research studies that focus on those with BP II should clarify these tentative recommendations over the next few years.

REFERENCES

Chiu, C. C., Huang, S. Y., Chen, C. C. and Su, K. P. (2005). Omega-3 fatty acids are more beneficial in the depressive phase than in the manic phase in patients with Bipolar I Disorder. (Letter to the Editor.) *Journal of Clinical Psychiatry*, **66**, 1613–14.

Chiu, C. C., Huang, S. Y., Su, K. P. *et al.* (2003). Polyunsaturated fatty acid deficit in patients with bipolar mania. *European Neuropsychopharmacology*, **13**, 99–103.

Edwards, R., Peet, M., Shay, J. and Horrobin, D. (1998). Omega-3 polyunsaturated fatty acid levels in the diet and in red blood cell membranes of depressed patients. *Journal of Affective Disorders*, **48**, 149–55.

Frangou, S., Lewis, M. and McCrone, P. (2006). Efficacy of ethyl-eicosapentaenoic acid in bipolar depression: randomised double-blind placebo-controlled study. *British Journal of Psychiatry*, **188**, 46–50.

Hibbeln, J. R. (1998). Fish consumption and major depression. *Lancet*, **351**, 1213.

Hirashima, F., Parow, A., Stoll, A. *et al.* (2004). Omega-3 fatty acid treatment and T2 whole brain relaxation times in bipolar disorder. *American Journal of Psychiatry*, **161**, 1922–4.

Keck, P. E. Jr, Freeman, M. P., McElroy, S. L. *et al.* (2002). A double-blind, placebo-controlled trial of eicosapentaenoic acid in rapid-cycling bipolar disorder. *Bipolar Disorders*, **4**, 26–7.

Keck, P. E. Jr, McElroy, S. L., Mintz, J. *et al.* (2006). Double-blind, placebo-controlled trials of ethyl-eicosapentaenoate in the treatment of bipolar depression and rapid-cycling bipolar disorder. *Biological Psychiatry*, **60**, 1020–2.

Kinrys, G. (2000). Are omega-3 fatty acids beneficial in depression but not mania? In reply. *Archives of General Psychiatry*, **57**, 716–17.

Logan, A. C. (2003). Neurobehavioural aspects of omega-3 fatty acids: possible mechanisms and therapeutic value in major depression. *Alternative Medicine Review*, **8**, 410–25.

Maes, M., Christophe, A., Delanghe, J. *et al.* (1999). Lowered omega-3 polyunsaturated fatty acids in serum phospholipids and cholesteryl esters of depressed patients. *Psychiatry Research*, **85**, 275–91.

Marangell, L. B., Suppes, T., Ketter, T. A. *et al.* (2006). Omega-3 fatty acids in bipolar disorder: clinical and research considerations. *Prostaglandins, Leukotrienes and Essential Fatty Acids*, **75**, 315–21.

Noaghuil, S. and Hibbeln, J. R. (2003). Cross-national comparisons of seafood consumption and rates of bipolar disorders. *American Journal of Psychiatry*, **160**, 2222–7.

Osher, Y., Bersudsky, Y. and Belmaker, R. H. (2005). Omega-3 eicosapentaenoic acid in bipolar depression: report of a small open-label study. *Journal of Clinical Psychiatry*, **66**, 726–9.

Parker, G., Gibson, N., Brotchie, H., Heruc, G., Rees A-M. and Hadzi-Pavlovic, D. (2006). Omega-3 fatty acids and mood disorders. *American Journal of Psychiatry*, **163**, 969–78.

Peet, M., Murphy, B., Shay, J. and Horrobin, D. (1998). Depletion of omega-3 fatty acid levels in red blood cell membranes of depressive patients. *Biological Psychiatry*, **43**, 315–19.

Rapoport, S. I. and Bosetti, F. (2002). Do lithium and the anticonvulsants target the brain arachidonic acid cascade in bipolar disorder? *Archives of General Psychiatry*, **59**, 592–6.

Sampath, H. and Ntambi, J. M. (2004). Polyunsaturated fatty acid regulation of gene expression. *Nutrition Review*, **62**, 333–9.

Stoll, A. L., Damico, K. E., Marangell, L. B. and Severus, W. E. (2000). Reply to Su, K-P., Shen W. W., Huang S-Y.: Are omega-3 fatty acids beneficial in depression but not mania? (letter). *Archives of General Psychiatry*, **57**, 716–17.

Stoll, A. L., Locke, L. B., Marangell, L. B. and Severus, W. E. (1999a). Omega-3 fatty acids and bipolar disorder: a review. *Prostaglandins, Leukotrienes and Essential Fatty Acids*, **60**, 329–37.

Stoll, A. L., Severus, W. E., Freeman, M. P. *et al.* (1999b). Omega-3 fatty acids in bipolar disorder: a preliminary double-blind, placebo-controlled trial. *Archives of General Psychiatry*, **56**, 407–12.

12

The role of psychological interventions in managing Bipolar II Disorder

Vijaya Manicavasagar

Introduction

The use of adjunctive psychological interventions represents an important new dimension to the treatment and management of bipolar disorder and especially Bipolar II Disorder (BP II). These interventions are gradually gaining in popularity amongst clinicians who wish to develop a comprehensive management plan once depressive or hypomanic episodes have been stabilised with medication. The impetus for this new emphasis has largely been driven by the recognition that individual differences in the severity, course and outcome of the disorder over time are not fully explained by biological factors and physical treatments alone. Furthermore, there has been increasing acceptance of stress-vulnerability models which highlight interactions between psychological, social and biological factors – which in turn play a significant role in the maintenance and recurrence of several serious psychiatric illnesses, including bipolar disorder and schizophrenia. Over the last decade, interest has also shifted to psychosocial factors which affect social and occupational functioning, treatment adherence and suicidality, and which are particularly amenable to psychological interventions (American Psychiatric Association, 2002).

Much has already been written about psychological interventions for unipolar depression and there is evidence to suggest that many of these strategies may also be useful in treating the depression that accompanies bipolar disorder. Thus, this chapter will primarily focus on addressing hypomanic symptoms and on managing the phasic nature of BP II.

Psychological interventions such as self-monitoring of symptoms and mood have usually been employed during the prodrome and/or the recovery phase of an episode (Perry *et al.*, 1999; Lam *et al.*, 2003). However, evidence is accruing to suggest that these strategies may also be beneficial as an adjunct to medication throughout the course of the illness (Glick *et al.*, 1994; Miklowitz *et al.*, 2003). At

Bipolar II Disorder. Modelling, Measuring and Managing, ed. Gordon Parker. Published by Cambridge University Press. © Cambridge University Press 2008.

the start of an episode, psychological approaches such as psychoeducation about the illness and mood charting can help to provide a rationale for treatment as well as empower patients to better manage their illness. Post-episode, a range of psychological strategies may be used to address psychosocial factors related to risk of relapse and concerns about the physical, psychological and behavioural consequences of the disorder. For some individuals, full symptomatic remission between episodes may be unrealistic and psychological interventions may be required to address sub-syndromal and persistent residual symptoms.

Clinicians should select and utilise relevant strategies from the range of psychotherapeutic approaches, depending on patient need. For example, if conflictual interactions amongst family members results in high stress levels, poor sleep patterns and disrupted work schedules (all of which contribute to relapse), then a combination of family therapy and behavioural strategies may form part of an effective intervention plan. If pessimistic thoughts and negative attributions, together with misinformation about the illness course, play a significant role in the onset of episodes of depression, then cognitive therapy and psychoeducational approaches may be relevant in developing a treatment plan. In this way a pluralistic rather than eclectic approach to treatment is recommended, where interventions are selected on the basis of the aetiology, psychosocial impact and coping strategies – based on information gathered during the assessment and case formulation stage of treatment.

As this is a relatively new area, there are few randomised controlled outcome studies on psychological interventions for bipolar disorder and none as yet examining whether such interventions are significantly different for Bipolar I Disorder (BP I) or BP II. For BP I – with its more severe and protracted 'highs' than BP II – it is likely that psychological interventions would be utilised much later in the episode, when symptoms have been controlled or markedly reduced by medication or other physical therapies. In contrast, psychological interventions are possibly of greater benefit to individuals with BP II, including during the highs, where such strategies may be used to directly dampen or control those symptoms.

Whilst the hypomanic episodes in BP II may not necessarily be as disabling as the manic episodes experienced in BP I, the depressive episodes can be just as severe and disabling (Parker, 2004; Mitchell *et al.*, 2004). Psychological interventions for BP II thus need to address both the highs and lows and psychosocial consequences of the phasic nature of the illness. Issues addressed by psychological approaches in the management of BP II include:

- strategies to improve treatment adherence (including understanding and accepting the diagnosis of BP II);
- strategies that facilitate the modification of problematic behaviours, irrational thoughts and emotional dysregulation during the acute stages of an episode;

- interventions that address comorbid conditions which can exacerbate the likelihood of relapse;
- reducing psychosocial factors related to relapse (such as family conflict, life stressors and maladaptive thinking styles);
- addressing physical, psychological and behavioural consequences of the disorder (including problems in interpersonal functioning, effects of stigma, isolation, poor self-esteem, hopelessness and demoralisation, difficulties in maintaining employment or fulfilling activities, and suicide risk); and
- strategies which address any wider problems in marital, parental, social and work relationships which result from the effects of the illness, including 'caregiver burden' (e.g. extending psychoeducation and psychological strategies to those in contact with or caring for the sufferer).

Long-term treatment and management of bipolar disorder is weighted towards prevention of future episodes and minimisation of adverse consequences during and after an episode. This is where the impact of families, friends and the wider social network can be particularly relevant.

Helping families, friends and colleagues understand and accept the disorder via education may lessen the burden of care, reduce stigma and reduce the risk of relapse. For example, participation in support or advocacy groups and in developing 'wellbeing plans' (described in Chapter 13) can engage carers, friends and others in the proactive management of the disorder. In turn, reciprocal positive interactions between the individual, their family and the wider social network through these strategies can facilitate effective management, reduce risk of relapse and minimise possible adverse psychosocial consequences after an episode.

Types of psychological interventions for BP II may vary depending on the stage of the illness at which treatment is sought. For example, at initial presentation, interventions may focus on education about the diagnosis, dealing with grief, and on issues related to medication compliance. At subsequent sessions, however, psychological interventions may need to focus on risk factors and early warning signs of relapse, strategies to manage acute symptoms, and on the psychosocial consequences following a depressive or hypomanic episode. The two case vignettes below illustrate presentations for BP II for which psychological approaches may vary.

Case vignette 1: first-episode BP II

Jason, a 17-year-old high-school student, was referred to a specialist mood disorders unit when his general practitioner, who suspected that he may be suffering from bipolar disorder, recommended a second opinion. For some time, his parents had noted Jason's intermittent episodes of 'moodiness', distractibility and irritability which were sometimes preceded by late nights socialising (and drinking) with friends, watching DVDs or playing computer games in his room. At those times, Jason would seem overly cheerful, talkative and expansive and entertain his friends and family with his ambitious career plans. Of late, however, these episodes were becoming more disturbing for the rest of the family. On some nights, Jason was awake the whole time and could be heard pacing about the house. His talkativeness had become overbearing as Jason monopolised the conversations at home and had begun to dominate his school class discussions with his opinions about the future. His teacher suggested to his parents that Jason needed an assessment from his general practitioner.

By the time Jason arrived at the specialist clinic, his family had accepted the provisional diagnosis of bipolar disorder given by their general practitioner, and had read about it on a website. When the psychiatrist at the clinic explained that Jason was suffering from BP II, his parents experienced a sense of relief tinged with sadness. They recalled that Jason's aunt had been institutionalised for several years because of 'manic depression' and contemplated a bleak future for their son. Jason, however, dismissed the diagnosis and did not see the need for any form of treatment. He enjoyed those periods when his thoughts seemed clearer, his mood was buoyant and he easily 'composed' songs for his band. It mattered little that he occasionally felt down (he reasoned that being in his final year of school was stressful enough without labelling it as 'depression' or 'bipolar disorder'). Besides, many of his friends reported that they too had periods when they felt gloomy.

A management plan developed for Jason comprised a mood stabiliser, together with psychological interventions to help him and his family understand the nature of BP II and how it differed from BP I (from which his aunt probably suffered). Jason especially needed to understand the role of medication and how to control some of his more flamboyant or inappropriate behaviours. Psychological interventions comprised psychoeducation about the disorder, advice on maintaining a healthy lifestyle, and mood-monitoring strategies that would enable Jason to detect when he was becoming over-stimulated. Of key concern in addressing this first episode was Jason's desire to preserve and encourage his periods of hypomania which he found especially enjoyable but which caused significant distress to his family.

First episode presentations of BP II – especially in young people – pose specific challenges to their therapists. Patients are frequently unwilling to accept the diagnosis, which then affects treatment compliance; they are likely to 'enjoy' or revel in their hypomanic episodes and are thus less likely to persist with medications or psychological interventions that dampen those emotional peaks; and finally, as the diagnosis is relatively novel and the illness has not yet impacted upon lifestyle, it may be perceived as a transient emotional state related to life events, stress, or social influences, rather than a disorder that requires active intervention. In summary, for the newly diagnosed patient, the key aspects of psychological intervention will include:

- education about the disorder,
- the use of mood graphs to monitor change,
- symptom management strategies, and
- instruction about lifestyle management.

Case vignette 2: sixth episode BP II

Narelle recalled that despite being a somewhat timid, socially awkward and anxious 15-year-old, there were hours or days when 'the world seemed friendlier', colours seemed brighter and sharper, and her confidence soared so that she found it much easier to voice her opinions and participate in her drama classes at school. When this 'magical time' ran its course, she often felt drained and irritable, which led to conflicts with her parents. Her mood plummeted to the extent that she found it difficult to motivate herself or keep up with her schoolwork and swimming which she usually enjoyed.

Now as a 36-year-old single mother of two young boys, Narelle had experienced six distinct 'episodes' over the last 10 years, each lasting 5–8 weeks, during which she felt as if she was 'on a high'. During each episode, she would feel less anxious, make plans to start new businesses, undergo a 'wardrobe makeover' (putting a strain on her already extended finances), and pursue different (and often highly inappropriate) relationships. Of particular concern to Narelle was that episodes were occurring more frequently and lasting longer.

She usually sought treatment after these episodes had run their course and she was experiencing a severe depressed mood, exacerbated by feelings of guilt and remorse for her behaviours when high. Her general practitioner, who had diagnosed depression but failed to detect her bipolar disorder, had intermittently prescribed antidepressants whenever Narelle plunged into a depressed state but the medications were relatively ineffective in halting the cycle of 'highs' and 'lows' now beginning to cause major disruptions to her life.

Her last episode had culminated in the break-up of a 3-year relationship because of her overspending and infidelity. Her general practitioner referred her to a psychiatrist who diagnosed BP II and prescribed both a mood stabiliser and an antidepressant. Narelle was also referred to a psychologist who helped her understand her diagnosis and its long-term management and engaged her and her ex-partner in counselling to examine whether they could retrieve their lost relationship.

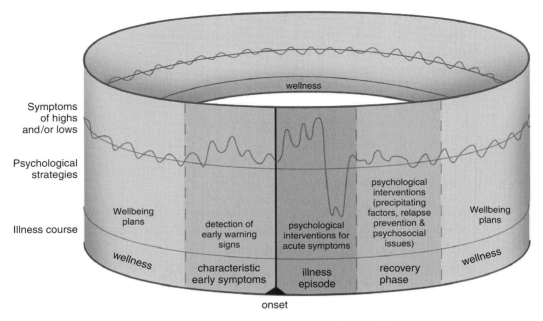

Figure 12.1. The role of psychological interventions in managing Bipolar II Disorder.

The legacy of several years of untreated or inappropriately treated BP II can result in considerable disruption to lifestyle. It is likely that the diagnosis of BP II will come as a relief to most who have suffered for some years and who have usually had to cope with the concomitant social and psychological consequences of their impaired judgement and impulsivity during episodes. The focus of psychological treatment in longstanding BP II is mainly to establish an acceptable medication regimen, recognise early warning signs, address possible precipitating factors, and learn how to overcome the psychosocial consequences of repeated episodes.

The cyclical and dynamic nature of bipolar disorder and its psychological management are represented in Figure 12.1, which illustrates the overlapping phases during which psychological interventions are to be employed. Wellbeing plans (described in Chapter 13) include several psychological strategies to stabilise mood and prevent relapse. Psychological strategies may also be used to detect and address early warning signs, manage hypomanic symptoms, examine risk factors or precipitants, prevent relapse, and address psychosocial issues associated with the illness.

Psychological interventions for bipolar disorder

Whilst medication is the mainstay of treatment, adjunctive psychological interventions can also play an important role in managing acute symptoms. Some of the more popular psychological interventions for bipolar disorder include psychoeducation, cognitive behaviour therapy (CBT), family focused therapy (FFT) and interpersonal and social rhythm therapy (IPSRT). These highly manualised therapies have been the focus of much of the psychological intervention research about bipolar disorder. They each share several psychological techniques including didactic education about bipolar disorder and medications used in its treatment, identification of risk factors and maladaptive lifestyle habits, as well as management of early warning signs and psychosocial problems. These interventions may also be used throughout different phases of the illness and in the development of Wellbeing Plans (see Chapter 13).

All psychological therapies, to a large extent, also rely on the development of an effective therapeutic alliance in order to effect change. Respect for the preferences and needs of the patient (despite the possibility that they may not be concordant with the preferences and needs of the therapist), the development of trust for the therapist, and an atmosphere of honesty and openness during treatment sessions are some of the crucial elements in dealing with bipolar disorder. The involvement of family members and other carers in treatment can pose significant challenges to the stability of the therapeutic alliance. However, given their impact on the course and outcome of the disorder, this aspect needs to be effectively managed rather than avoided.

Psychoeducation

Psychoeducation focuses on providing information to consumers about coping with a psychiatric illness while simultaneously dealing with their reactions to that information (Miklowitz, 2004). Information regarding bipolar disorder can focus on the nature of the disorder, medication, factors that affect mood swings and healthy lifestyle habits. It is equally important to recognise that not only can the symptoms themselves be problematic but that they can also cause impairments in various lifestyle areas. Table 12.1 describes the key randomised controlled outcome studies that have utilised psychoeducation as the main intervention for bipolar disorder.

Psychoeducation may be delivered in a structured or unstructured format to individuals, groups or families (Miklowitz *et al.*, 2003). Didactic instruction, role plays, experiential techniques, videos, web-based programs, and the provision of written materials can all be employed to enhance a greater understanding of the disorder, including its course over time, causes and precipitants, the medications used in treatment and management of the disorder, recognition of early warning signs and stress management techniques.

Possibly one of the most important aspects of psychoeducation about bipolar disorder is the cyclical nature of the disorder (Goodwin and Sachs, 2004).

Table 12.1. Randomised controlled trials for psychoeducation in the treatment of bipolar disorder.

Study	Sample characteristics and design	Outcome
Van Gent et al., 1988	34 participants randomly allocated to 4 sessions of psychoeducation or usual treatment; followed-up for 15 months	Participants in the psychoeducation group reported improvements in self-confidence, and in behavioural and social functioning
Van Gent and Zwart, 1991	35 participants randomly assigned to 5 sessions of psychoeducation or psychoeducation and psychotherapy; followed-up for 15 months	Both groups improved in psychosocial functioning, but the combination intervention group also improved on a measure of thinking and behaving
Van Gent and Zwart, 1993	26 partners of individuals with bipolar disorder randomly assigned to 5 group sessions of psychoeducation or control condition; monitored for 6 months	Partners in the psychoeducation condition demonstrated greater understanding of bipolar disorder than those in the control group
Colom et al., 2003	120 participants randomly assigned to either 20 sessions of group psychoeducation or to an unstructured support group; followed-up for 24 months	Intervention group had lower rates of relapse into mania and depression during treatment and at follow-up

Individuals and their families need to understand that episodes are likely to recur despite medication compliance, and that the recognition of early warning signs and the initiation of various preventative strategies may offset the likelihood of relapse.

Psychoeducation can also facilitate acceptance of the diagnosis, which is probably one of the most important components in its effective management. Better management is associated with greater acceptance and understanding of the illness. Open discussion of pertinent issues concerning bipolar disorder also serves to demystify and 'normalise' the illness as being no different from other types of chronic illnesses such as diabetes or inflammatory bowel disease, for example.

Cognitive behaviour therapy

The CBT model for the treatment of BP II focuses on both the depressive and hypomanic phases. Cognitive behaviour therapy is usually used to correct pre-existing dysfunctional thinking styles and maladaptive cognitive schemas which, once an episode has developed, interact with life events and behaviours to exacerbate symptoms and prolong the episode (Lam *et al.*, 2003). In patients whose dysfunctional thoughts are related to current mood state, CBT approaches may also be used to challenge and change these state-dependent cognitions. A recent study by Scott *et al.* (2006) has indicated that CBT may be more effective in the earlier stages of the illness (possibly before such maladaptive thinking styles become firmly entrenched) and among patients who are not experiencing frequent recurrences. A summary of some of the key randomised controlled outcome studies using CBT to treat bipolar disorder is provided in Table 12.2.

Addressing cognitive symptoms

Cognitive errors, including automatic thoughts, maladaptive assumptions and dysfunctional personal schemas, can be relevant to both the depressive and hypomanic phases of BP II. Commonly occurring negative thinking styles are 'mind-reading', overgeneralisation, black and white thinking and 'catastrophising'. Automatic thoughts in the depressive phase may focus on excessively pessimistic interpretations of events while those that occur during a hypomanic phase may be unrealistically optimistic or opportunistic. Depression is also associated with lowered self-esteem while hypomania is associated with grandiosity and increased self-confidence and optimism. Cognitive strategies include teaching individuals to identify and challenge their irrational thoughts by reframing them, checking the available evidence, looking for alternative explanations, and using Socratic questioning to refute irrational ideas.

Maladaptive assumptions drive the content of automatic thoughts in both depression and hypomania. For example, a person who is depressed may interpret being in a quiet, reserved social gathering with an automatic thought such as 'No one finds me worth talking to'. The resultant behavioural withdrawal may then reinforce the maladaptive assumption that 'When people ignore me at a social gathering, it means that I am worthless'. In a hypomanic state, the individual is likely to interpret the situation in a more personalised and positive light such as 'No one is as worth listening to as me' followed by behaviours that reflect that belief (e.g. speaking loudly, interrupting and intruding on others' conversations). Such behaviours may reinforce maladaptive beliefs such as 'I am an exceptional person' or 'Everyone only wants to listen to me'.

CBT instructs individuals in recognising irrational dysfunctional thoughts, to dispute the validity of such thoughts and substitute more appropriate and adaptive ones. In the above examples, challenging the logic of the initial self-statement and using 'cognitive experiments' may help to dispute the validity of such dysfunctional thoughts (see Table 12.3).

Table 12.2. Randomised controlled trials for cognitive behaviour therapy in the treatment of bipolar disorder.

Study	Sample characteristics and design	Outcome
Cochran, 1984	28 clients randomly assigned to standard clinical care alone or clinical care and 6 sessions of CBT techniques; followed-up for 12 months.	Clients receiving combination treatment had enhanced lithium adherence and fewer hospitalisations compared with the standard clinical care clients
Perry et al., 1999	69 participants randomly assigned to usual treatment, or usual treatment and 12 sessions of cognitive and behavioural techniques to identify early warning signs of relapse; followed-up for 18 months	Participants receiving combination treatment had fewer manic relapses, fewer days in hospital, longer time to relapse, and higher levels of social functioning and work performance in comparison with the control group
Scott et al., 2001	42 clients randomly allocated to waiting list control group or intervention group comprising 20 sessions of cognitive therapy; followed-up for 6 months post cognitive therapy	Those who received cognitive therapy significantly improved in levels of symptoms, global functioning and work and social adjustment compared with the clients on the waiting list
Lam et al., 2000	25 participants randomly allocated to 12–20 sessions of cognitive therapy and usual treatment or usual treatment alone (outpatient support); both treatments focused on relapse prevention; followed-up 6 months after therapy	Participants in the cognitive therapy group had significantly fewer bipolar relapses and total days in episode, and greater improvement in social adjustment and better coping strategies for bipolar prodromal symptoms compared with the control group. They also reported less hopelessness and better medication compliance
Lam et al., 2003	103 patients with Bipolar I randomly allocated to 14 sessions of cognitive therapy (and 2 booster sessions) plus usual treatment or usual treatment alone; monitored for 12 months	Cognitive therapy group had fewer bipolar episodes and numbers of admissions. They also had higher social functioning, fewer mood symptoms, less fluctuation in manic symptoms and better coping with manic prodromes
Ball et al., 2006	52 patients randomly allocated to cognitive therapy or usual treatment; followed up at 12 months	At follow-up patients allocated to cognitive therapy showed improvements in symptoms of mania, severity of illness status and a measure of overall improvement. However, these benefits were considerably less than those observed immediately after treatment
Scott et al., 2006	253 patients randomly assigned to usual treatment or usual treatment and up to 22 sessions of CBT. Assessed every 8 weeks for 18 months.	No significant differences between groups at 18 months in terms of recurrence rates. Adjunctive CBT more effective than usual treatment alone in those with fewer than 12 previous episodes

Table 12.3. Challenging and changing dysfunctional thoughts using 'cognitive experiments'.

Dysfunctional thought	Cognitive challenges	'Cognitive experiment'
'No one finds me worth talking to'	What evidence do I have that no one finds me worth talking to?	If someone responds to something I say it will probably mean that I am worth talking to
'No one is as worth listening to as me'	What evidence do I have that no one else is as worth listening to?	If people are in conversation with each other then others must also be worth listening to

More recently, 'emotive techniques' have been used to address negative cognitive schemas which are thought to be more difficult to access through direct methods such as simple cognitive challenges (Ball *et al.*, 2006). Emotive techniques include:

- acknowledging and validating the individual's initial experiences associated with the development of a particular cognitive schema,
- activating the emotional memories and any associated dysfunctional beliefs by arousing, for example, fear and shame in reaction to an imagined scene in the safety of the therapeutic situation, and
- activating healthy emotional resources in the patient such as anger at violation and sadness at loss as alternate responses to replace the individual's maladaptive emotional, social or behavioural responses.

Cognitive strategies may also be used to enhance therapy adherence, for example through challenging irrational and overly negative perceptions about medication, or they may be used to help change lifestyle factors that may be contributing to relapse. Cognitive behaviour therapies can also be used to address denial of the illness which usually occurs when people have been newly diagnosed, exploring their responses such as whether they actually have an illness, whether they require treatment, and whether they think they can cope with the illness.

Addressing behavioural symptoms

Managing behavioural symptoms in bipolar disorder includes identifying the triggers to hypomania such as medication non-compliance, sleep deprivation, overstimulation and the use of alcohol or drugs. Furthermore, behaviours associated with hypomania such as driving fast, socialising in 'noisy' environments, or risk-taking behaviours can further exacerbate overarousal and excitability. Activity scheduling can help to limit the number and extent of arousing or excitable activities that are likely to lead to problems.

Other behavioural symptoms may be associated with the depressive phase of the disorder. Again, it is important to focus on possible triggers to depressive episodes such as interpersonal stressors or events surrounding losses. Strategies to manage depressive symptoms may include graded exposure to tasks that will engender a sense of achievement on completion using rewards to motivate engagement in activities, periods of 'time out' where individuals can 'recharge their batteries', and goal-setting and problem-solving techniques.

Family focused therapy

High levels of interpersonal stress within families and other social environments are associated with higher rates of relapse and greater symptom severity for a number of psychiatric disorders including schizophrenia, unipolar depression and bipolar disorder (Miklowitz et al., 1988; O'Connell et al., 1991). Interpersonal stress within families, often referred to as 'Expressed Emotion' (EE), comprises high levels of hostility, criticism and overinvolvement/intrusiveness (Vaughn and Leff, 1976). High EE is often indicative of the level of stress within a family, particularly during the recovery period of the illness. High EE relatives are more likely to escalate negative verbal and non-verbal forms of interaction and to attribute problematic behaviours (such as irritability or impulsivity) to personal and controllable factors rather than uncontrollable factors associated with the illness.

There are several types of interventions which utilise the family to effect change and prevent relapse (see Table 12.4). One in particular that is gaining popularity in the treatment of bipolar disorder is family focused therapy (FFT) (Miklowitz, 2004).

Family focused therapy assumes that improving communication patterns and problem-solving capabilities within a family will encourage greater tolerance and acceptance of the illness which will, in turn, improve mood stability in the patient. Family focused therapy is a structured, time-limited form of intervention with five modules delivered over several months. The treatment modules comprise assessment of the family, education about bipolar disorder, training in communication-enhancement, problem-solving, and finally, strategies to address therapy termination (Miklowitz, 2004). The aims of therapy described by Miklowitz (2004) are to:

- understand the illness and recognise possible precipitants,
- help the family accept and plan for the likelihood that the illness will recur,
- understand and accept the role of medication,
- distinguish between illness-related and personality-related behaviours and mood states,
- learn to cope with the stressors that are likely to precipitate an episode, and
- improve the level of family functioning following an episode.

Table 12.4. Randomised controlled trials of family therapy for treatment of bipolar disorder.

Study	Sample characteristics and design	Outcome
Glick et al., 1994	19 inpatients randomly allocated to additional family therapy or usual inpatient care alone; followed-up at 18 months	Those patients allocated to additional family therapy showed significant improvements in social and work functioning and family attitudes compared with usual inpatient care alone
Clarkin et al., 1998	42 outpatients assigned to 11 months of standard treatment and 25 sessions of couples therapy	Of the participants who completed the treatments (n = 33), those who received couples therapy had higher levels of social adjustment and medication adherence than participants who received standard treatment
Miklowitz et al., 2000	101 patients receiving usual treatment randomly allocated to 21 sessions of FFT or case management; followed up for 12 months	Participants in the FFT interventions took longer to relapse and had lower symptom levels but benefits limited to depression not mania; high EE families benefited the most
Miklowitz et al., 2003	101 patients assigned to either 21 sessions of FFT or crisis management; followed-up for 2 years	Patients in the FFT intervention had fewer relapses, took longer to relapse, showed greater reductions in mood disorder symptoms and better medication adherence than patients in the crisis management group

Treatment may be commenced while the patient is being treated for the acute symptoms of the illness. During the assessment phase, the family is usually video-taped whilst engaging in a problem-solving discussion. Interactions are coded on dimensions such as criticism, guilt-induction, intrusiveness, self-disclosure, acceptance, acknowledgement and problem-solving (Miklowitz *et al.*, 1989; Simoneau *et al.*, 1998).

In the psychoeducation phase of the treatment, patients and families are encouraged to review the symptoms of the disorder (including prodromal features, resistance to the diagnosis and the issues of blame for the disorder); discuss possible genetic and predispositional factors; and develop an understanding of risk and protective factors in bipolar disorder and how they interact with biological vulnerability and stress. Patients are encouraged to track changes in mood, stress levels and medications using a mood chart, while family members are instructed in strategies to help the patient such as recognising and dealing with signs of relapse.

Communication enhancement training, utilising role-playing strategies, forms the third phase of the treatment, during which family members are instructed in expressing positive feelings, active listening, making positive requests for change, and expressing negative feelings. The fourth phase comprises problem-solving training while the last phase prepares the family for treatment termination. During the last phase, treatment goals and relapse prevention strategies are reviewed, medication adherence is stressed, and any other concerns are addressed. Follow-up arrangements are usually made during this termination phase including referral for other forms of therapy such as additional family or marital therapy if necessary.

Interpersonal and social rhythm therapy

Interpersonal and social rhythm therapy (IPSRT) asserts that exacerbations of bipolar disorder (both depression and hypomania) result from a combination of psychosocial and biological causes (Frank and Swartz, 2004). Based on the 'instability model' of Goodwin and Jamison (1990), IPSRT asserts that interpersonal stressors and disruptions in biological circadian rhythms play a key role in relapse and aims to help individuals identify and solve interpersonal problems and maintain daily regular biological rhythms such as:
- establishing good sleep habits,
- manipulation of exposure to sunlight and sleep-wake cycles,
- avoiding caffeine and other stimulants,
- engaging in regular exercise, and
- solving interpersonal problems and dealing with interpersonal stressors.

The model asserts that, in vulnerable individuals, disruptions to social 'zeit-bergers' or 'time-givers' (Aschoff, 1981) may give rise to affective disturbances.

Table 12.5. Randomised controlled trials for IPSRT in the treatment of bipolar disorder.

Study	Sample characteristics and design	Outcome
Frank *et al.*, 1999	82 participants allocated to IPSRT or to intensive clinical management; cross-over study where 50% of subjects cross over to the other treatment; followed-up at 2 years	IPSRT induces more stable social rhythms but no differences in time to remission and no differences in symptom reduction, suicide attempts, and total number of relapses
Frank *et al.*, 2005	175 inpatients and outpatients randomly allocated to IPSRT or intensive clinical management; monitored for 2 years	No differences in time to stabilisation of symptoms between the two treatments. However, patients in the IPSRT condition had longer times to relapse and higher regularity of social rhythms which was associated with reduced likelihood of relapse

The role of treatment is to restore these social and biological rhythms to reduce symptoms and prevent relapse. For example, disruptions to sleep patterns, by watching television late into the night and having to wake early, can result in biological perturbations which interact with genetic, temperament and life stresses to precipitate adverse mood states.

IPSRT helps patients develop regular and stable social rhythms such as going to bed at the same time each night, eating at set times during the day or engaging in regular and time-limited leisure activities. Patients are usually encouraged to monitor and record their baseline social rhythms, and work on establishing more optimal social rhythms. Prevention of relapse is encouraged by the maintenance of regular and stable social rhythms and the effective management of interpersonal stressors. There are few outcome studies on IPSRT and the two that are most frequently cited indicate that this treatment may be more effective as a strategy for relapse prevention rather than as a treatment during the acute phase of the disorder (see Table 12.5).

The administration of IPSRT is divided into four phases: the initial, intermediate, maintenance and termination phases of treatment, all of which utilise the components of psychoeducation, social rhythm therapy and interpersonal psychotherapy. The initial phase comprises a case formulation which defines the focus for treatment incorporating both the medical model of bipolar disorder and patient-specific interpersonal problem areas. Interpersonal issues that are usually the focus of attention include grief reactions associated with losses (including the loss of the 'healthy self'), interpersonal role disputes, role transitions and interpersonal deficits (Frank and Swartz, 2004).

'Unresolved grief' is the focus of treatment when a patient's current affective state is frequently associated with the death or loss of a significant attachment figure in their life. Treatment includes reviewing the relationship between the patient and the significant person, encouraging the expression of feelings for that person and supporting behavioural change such as forming new relationships and interests. 'Role transitions' involve major changes or transitions in life roles such as from being a daughter to becoming a wife, becoming a parent or becoming unemployed. As patients with bipolar disorder are particularly sensitive to change, the role of therapy is to help patients develop realistic expectations about their new role and to acquire skills in making this role transition. Becoming more emotionally stable can be the focus of treatment especially where there is apprehension or discomfort associated with this type of change. 'Role disputes' occur when there are significant problems in role expectations, communication patterns, and goals between patients and their families, partners and friends. Therapeutic strategies used to address role disputes can include role plays, communication skills and other techniques to facilitate role negotiation. 'Interpersonal deficits' usually occur when there is a long history of social isolation or unsuccessful relationships of an intimate and non-intimate nature usually as a result of the illness course. Therapy aims to help patients form and maintain new relationships including using the therapeutic relationship itself as a platform for learning.

The intermediate phase of treatment commences once the patient and therapist have agreed on an interpersonal area on which to focus. Only one interpersonal area is usually selected. Aims are to encourage adaptive 'social rhythms' and to resolve a specific interpersonal problem. The third phase of treatment involves the maintenance of adaptive social rhythms, resolving potential interpersonal difficulties before they cause significant distress, and maintaining mood stability. When appropriate, the fourth or termination phase of therapy is initiated.

As with other psychological interventions, IPSRT also involves the establishment of specific protocols for relapse prevention, monitoring symptoms and medication side-effects, monitoring drug and alcohol use, and the involvement of family members and significant others.

Although behavioural activation and positive social stimulation can be beneficial in the treatment and management of depression, the same level of activation may tip a susceptible individual into hypomania. Thus, the management of positive social stimulation may be yet another dimension that requires close monitoring. For example, a young person staying out late to socialise at a party at night may find the music, colours, conversation and social atmosphere highly stimulating to the extent that their sleep is significantly affected. A combination of further stimulation, fatigue and psychosocial stress the following day may be sufficient to trigger hypomanic symptoms in susceptible individuals.

Managing specific phases of the disorder

Detection and management of early warning signs

Because of the speed of onset of hypomanic episodes, regular use of psychological techniques such as self-monitoring and mood-charting are recommended for identifying prodromal symptoms. The detection and management of early warning signs also overlaps, to some extent, with Wellbeing Plans described in Chapter 13.

Early warning signs and triggers for relapse differ from individual to individual. Common triggers for relapse include high stress levels (or difficulties in coping) and medication discontinuation. The recognition and identification of these triggers is crucial for relapse prevention especially if such 'relapse signatures' (for example, insomnia, or starting to wear more colourful clothes) have been clearly established over several previous episodes of hypomania.

For individuals with longstanding bipolar disorder, self-monitoring usually involves focusing on two or three key symptoms which, in the past, may have been associated with relapse. Rating the intensity and/or frequency of such symptoms can help allay anxieties about minor symptom fluctuations and alert individuals and clinicians as to the likelihood of relapse. Common symptoms of relapse include:

- sleep disturbance such as requiring less sleep and not feeling tired,
- racing thoughts and speech,
- feeling 'high',
- increased 'driven' behaviours that are not checked by the need to eat or sleep,
- heightened anxiety levels, agitation, irritability and emotional intensity,
- feelings energised with new ideas or plans,
- spending more money than usual,
- increased sexual drive, flirtatiousness,
- reading extra symbolism into words and events, increased interest in religious/ spiritual ideas or themes,
- binge behaviours associated with eating, drug and alcohol use,
- arguments with family members or friends, and
- taking on more projects and working to the extreme.

Daily mood charting can also help to identify possible 'at risk' periods (such as overseas travel and the possibility of disruption to sleep routine, festive periods where social events may be clustered, or major lifestyle changes such as relocating to a different city or country) during which individuals are more likely to veer towards hypomania. Specific domains may include monitoring dysfunctional thoughts, levels of self-confidence, energy and creativity, level of social activity, sleep and speech patterns, and irritability, restlessness and concentration. Other domains (e.g. relevant to suicidal ideation), could include thoughts about death, and pessimism about their ability to function and achieve their goals.

One of the most frequently cited reasons for relapse in bipolar disorder is the premature cessation of medication. Reasons for stopping medication may include:

- side-effects ranging from a 'dulling' of the senses, loss of creativity, excessive weight gain, 'fuzzy-headedness' and sexual dysfunction,
- concerns about possible dangers of long-term use of medications such as lithium or SSRIs, including fears of becoming addicted and their effects in pregnancy,
- lack of understanding about the use of medication and possible 'misinformation' from family or friends which can result in individuals being reluctant to continue taking medication once their acute symptoms have significantly subsided, and
- lack of insight about the illness during hypomanic episodes during which medication is seen as unnecessary. If Wellbeing Plans have been developed, then this lack of insight may be obviated by the involvement of family members, friends and mental health professionals who may take limited responsibility for ensuring that medication is recommenced.

Education about the role of medication in reducing symptoms and preventing relapse can help patients and carers better manage the illness. Often family members experience anxiety about the need for long-term medication or may be hostile to the 'medicalisation' of a perceived personality characteristic or behavioural problem in the patient. Re-establishing circadian and social routines that may have been disrupted can also help to prevent relapse. This issue is discussed under Wellbeing Plans.

Psychological interventions for acute symptoms

Psychological interventions during the acute phase of the illness can involve techniques that – in conjunction with medication – help alleviate specific symptoms or mitigate the effects of such symptoms. The provision of information about these symptoms and their relationship to bipolar disorder can help engage patients and carers in the overall treatment plan comprising psychological strategies described in Tables 12.6 and 12.7.

There are also a number of key features which seem to emerge at the outset of an episode and which interact with symptom clusters and result in maladaptive behaviours. These features are firstly, a tendency to become hyper-stimulated or

Table 12.6. Psychological interventions for acute symptoms during hypomanic episodes.

Symptoms	Possible psychological interventions
High energy levels	Gradual exposure to activities such as mindful meditation, relaxation training and guided imagery. Strategies to regulate biological and social rhythms may be employed including ensuring regular mealtimes, engaging in a regular exercise routine, and reducing over-stimulation from social activities. Despite sleep difficulties, individuals may need to be encouraged to attempt to go to sleep at a regular bedtime using a combination of relaxation exercises and guided imagery
Excessively positive or hedonistic mood	Use of cognitive strategies to challenge overly positive and unrealistic thoughts, the use of 'cognitive experiments' whereby individuals are encouraged to test the veracity of their over-optimistic cognitions
Irritability and anger	Strategies that help patients to 'slow down' in reacting to stressors such as counting to 100 before saying or doing anything, use of cognitive strategies to challenge thoughts associated with irritability. Education and communication training for patients and carers to improve interactions within families
Inappropriate behaviours	Behavioural contracts may be developed with carers to help prevent inappropriate behaviours, such as restricting access to finances, car keys and alcohol when patients are hypomanic. Patients are encouraged to discuss their plans with carers before engaging in new activities
Upsetting mystical experiences	Use of cognitive therapy and cognitive experiments to challenge thoughts and emotions associated with mystical experiences

overexcited (and difficulties in self-regulation of arousal) and secondly, high levels of impulsivity (or difficulties in delaying gratification) (see Table 12.8). Such features can exacerbate the symptoms of bipolar disorder and contribute to their intensity and frequency and may need to be addressed through psychoeducation, CBT, FFT and IPSRT.

In addition, comorbidity with other psychiatric disorders and conditions is common in bipolar disorder. The most frequently reported comorbid conditions include alcohol and substance abuse, anxiety disorders and Clusters B (antisocial, borderline, histrionic and narcissistic) and C (avoidant, dependent and obsessive-compulsive) personality disorders. Significant alcohol or drug use will compromise most treatment plans and it may be advisable to address this comorbid condition first despite the primacy of the bipolar disorder. Comorbidity is associated with a poorer course over time, more frequent relapses, poor medication adherence and higher rates of suicidality.

Table 12.7. Psychological interventions for acute symptoms during the depressed phase.

Symptoms	Possible psychological interventions
Lowered energy levels	Gradual exposure to simple tasks and pleasurable activities, and monitoring energy levels
Excessively pessimistic mood	Use of cognitive strategies to challenge negative thoughts and the use of 'cognitive experiments' whereby individuals are encouraged to test the veracity of their pessimistic cognitions
Irritability and anger	Strategies that help patients to 'slow down' in reacting to stressors such as counting to 100 before saying or doing anything, use of cognitive strategies to challenge thoughts associated with irritability. Education and communication training for patients and carers to improve interactions within families
Cessation of usual activities	Setting realistic goals, engaging in activities, monitoring progress, and the use of self-reward, encouragement by friends and carers to engage in activities

Table 12.8. Maladaptive behaviours associated with the escalation of hypomanic symptoms.

Symptoms	Escalation of arousal	Difficulties in controlling impulsivity	Behaviours
High energy levels	Feeling increasingly wired and 'hyper'	Inability to slow down	Escalation of social activities, driving oneself to the limit at work, not sleeping, disorganised thinking, not completing tasks
Positive or hedonistic mood	Over-confidence and over-optimism, increased sexual arousal	Grandiose and unrealistic ideas	Initiation of complex or unrealistic plans, saying and doing outrageous things, spending more money, sexual promiscuity
Irritability	Escalation into anger or rage	Impatience and intolerance	Arguments, interpersonal problems, restlessness

Addressing precipitating factors, and relapse prevention

The course of bipolar disorder tends to be highly variable and depends upon type of treatment, treatment adherence, level of education about the disorder, comorbidity and several other factors. Most people with the disorder suffer many episodes over their lifetime and relapses are common even for those taking mood-stabilising medications.

Sub-syndromal and prodromal symptoms of bipolar disorder can develop in a few days and herald the onset of an acute episode of hypomania. However, many suffer from persistent low-grade symptoms (with a fluctuating course) that do not conform to the pattern of discrete episodes of mania or depression separated by symptom-free periods. Psychosocial factors related to relapse include:

- High levels of 'expressed emotion' (EE) amongst family members towards the sufferer which may result from misattributions about the illness. High EE may be lowered by psychoeducation and family focused therapy.
- Low levels of social support, which may be addressed by CBT if maladaptive thinking styles are a problem. Interpersonal and social rhythm therapy (IPSRT) and social skills training may also be used to address chronic interpersonal difficulties.
- Adverse life events are a general risk factor for a number of psychiatric illnesses. In bipolar disorder, life events, particularly those of an interpersonal nature or those that involve loss events, are associated with high rates of relapse. Cognitive behaviour therapy and IPSRT may be used to address dysfunctional thinking styles and grief associated with certain types of life events.
- Personality factors such as high levels of neuroticism, impulsivity and interpersonal sensitivity seem to be related to a poorer outcome in bipolar disorder. Anxiety-reduction strategies, learning to delay gratification, and cognitive and behavioural techniques that address sensitivity to perceived losses and abandonment are all helpful in preventing relapse.

Psychological interventions also need to include helping individuals develop and sustain optimal social environments, maintain healthy lifestyles, improve self-esteem and self-confidence, and regain a 'sense of self'. Personality factors that affect the course and outcome of the disorder may need to be addressed separately with more intensive and/or long-term interventions.

Psychosocial issues associated with the illness

Grandiosity, heightened activity levels, distractibility, impulsiveness and poor judgement, as well as low mood, low energy levels, impatience, irritability and hopelessness affect the sufferer as well as the people around them. Both hypomanic and depressive symptoms significantly impact upon wider social networks.

People with bipolar disorder may also be at risk of significant personal and social impairments in functioning (e.g. deficient interpersonal relationships, poor ability to problem-solve, lack of specialised work skills) which are independent of their mood swing episodes. Such impairments may reflect the wider impact of suffering from a serious psychiatric illness (e.g. alienating friends and close attachments over time).

Several types of psychological interventions including CBT, FFT, goal-setting, problem-solving techniques and communication skills training may be used to

Table 12.9. Psychological strategies used to address medication non-compliance.

Cognitive 'dulling', fuzzy-headedness and loss of creativity	Discuss with prescribing physician the possibility of changing medication or dosage
Weight gain	Embark on exercise programme and/or modify diet; use of reinforcement schedules to maintain motivation and reward weight loss
Sexual dysfunction	Discuss with prescribing physician and/or partner the cost/benefits of changing medication or dosage
Fears of long-term effects	Discuss with prescribing physician concerns regarding addiction, effects on pregnancy and breastfeeding; challenging irrational thoughts about medication
Lack of insight during hypomanic episodes	Enlist the help of significant others to ensure that medication is not discontinued; use of Wellbeing Plans

address psychosocial issues associated with the illness. If appropriate, individuals may also be encouraged to participate in sports and support groups or engage in consumer advocacy activities which may help build social networks and improve self-esteem.

Other issues

Facilitating medication continuation

Despite the proven necessity of medication management for bipolar disorder, many individuals choose to discontinue their medication regimen. The reasons for stopping medication have been described earlier in this chapter and can be addressed using a number of psychological strategies (see Table 12.9).

Treatment compliance

In order to ensure commitment, a 'compliance contract' may be developed. Such contracts may be time limited so that patients are encouraged to adhere to treatment for a specified period of time regardless of their level of motivation. Compliance contracts may also include support people whose role it is to remind or help facilitate treatment adherence (e.g. ensuring that the patient does not run out of medication, driving patients to appointments). In adolescents with bipolar disorder, management of the illness can pose significant challenges, especially when medication needs to be taken regularly and over-stimulation is to be avoided. Parents may need to find a careful balance between becoming over-involved or, alternatively, neglectful of their adolescent's treatment regimen. Education through a variety of modalities can help young people and their families better understand and manage the illness and prevent relapse.

Suicide prevention

Evidence suggests that patients with BP II are at greater risk of suicide than those with BP I (Rihmer and Kiss, 2002). Symptoms of bipolar disorder can include severe depressive lows and reckless highs which engender, alternatively, feelings of hopelessness, helplessness and impulsive destructiveness (Newman, 2004). The recurrent nature of episodes results in serious disruptions to life course including terminations of interpersonal relationships, academic, financial and vocational goals, and loss of social standing in the community. In addition, frequent comorbidity with drug and alcohol abuse can exacerbate impulsive and risk-taking behaviours – all of which increase the likelihood of harm.

Suicide risk needs to be continually assessed and monitored. Level of intention or commitment, plans and opportunities for suicide, as well as reasons for suicide provide important information from which a suicide prevention plan may be developed.

Thoughts associated with feelings of helplessness and hopelessness, and maladaptive cognitive schemas about the self can be addressed by cognitive therapy. Irrational thoughts about suicide as a 'way out' or as a method to alleviate perceived family burden can also be challenged by a combination of problem-solving skills, family therapy and reattributional techniques.

If patients are expressing suicidal ideas, the frequency of therapy sessions may be increased, emergency phone numbers provided, and family members enlisted to help monitor worrying behaviours. Psychological techniques that have been employed have also included exercises that help patients focus on meaningful aspects of their lives such as close relationships, personal goals, achievements and 'unfinished business'. Other strategies include empowering patients to recognise and deal with prodromal symptoms so that depressive or hypomanic episodes are not inevitable, addressing 'habitual' suicidal ideation, ensuring that medication is being adhered to at the correct frequency and dose, helping patients overcome feelings of shame, stigma and isolation, and making an 'anti-suicide contract' which allows patients and therapists to collaborate against suicidal ideation and intention.

It is important to realise, however, that the risk of suicide remains one of the key issues in the treatment of bipolar disorder and ultimately it is a combination of therapeutic interventions, self-monitoring by patients and medication adherence that will prevent the likelihood of completed suicide.

Conclusions

Although there is no definitive evidence to recommend any one psychological therapy over another, the results of several randomised controlled trials suggest that specific psychological interventions such as mood charting or challenging irrational thoughts about medication can be extremely helpful. Delivering psychological interventions in a flexible format according to patient need is reflected in our pluralistic approach to treatment. This can only be achieved by thorough assessment and case formulation.

There is every reason to be optimistic about the treatment and management of BP II as the range and scope of reputable and reliable psychological interventions steadily increases. Whilst medication plays a crucial role in symptom management, psychological interventions empower individuals to deal with the myriad psychosocial problems that afflict the sufferer and affect their carers throughout the illness. In addition, psychological interventions are crucial to ensure treatment compliance, facilitate recovery, prevent suicide, and ultimately to help patients with BP II to live full and satisfying lives.

REFERENCES

American Psychiatric Association (2002). Practice Guidelines for the Treatment of Patients with Bipolar Disorder (revision). *American Journal of Psychiatry*, **159** (Suppl. 4), S1–50.

Aschoff, J. (1981). *Handbook of Behavioural Neurobiology. Vol. 4. Biological Rhythms*. New York: Plenum Press.

Ball, J., Mitchell, P., Corry, J., Skillecorn, A. M. S. and Malhi, G. S. (2006). A randomised controlled trial of cognitive therapy for bipolar disorder: focus on long-term change. *Journal of Clinical Psychiatry*, **67**, 277–86.

Clarkin, J. F., Carpenter, D., Hull, J., Wilner, P. and Glick, I. (1998). Effects of psychoeducation for married patients with bipolar disorder and their spouses. *Psychiatric Services*, **49**, 531–3.

Cochran, S. (1984). Preventing medication non-compliance in the outpatient treatment of bipolar affective disorder. *Journal of Consulting and Clinical Psychology*, **52**, 873–8.

Colom, F., Vieta, E., Martinez-Aran, A. *et al.* (2003). A randomized trial on the efficacy of group psychoeducation in the prophylaxis of recurrences in bipolar patients whose disease is in remission. *Archives of General Psychiatry*, **60**, 402–7.

Frank, E., Kupfer, D. J., Thase, M. E. *et al.* (2005). Two-year outcomes for interpersonal and social rhythm therapy in individuals with bipolar disorder. *Archives of General Psychiatry*, **62**, 996–1003.

Frank, E. and Swartz, H. (2004). Interpersonal and social rhythm. In *Psychological Treatment of Bipolar Disorder*, ed. S. L. Johnson and R. L. Leahy. New York: The Guilford Press.

Frank, E., Swartz, H., Mallinger, A. *et al.* (1999). Adjunctive psychotherapy for bipolar disorder: effects of changing treatment modality. *Journal of Abnormal Psychology*, **108**, 579–87.

Glick, I. D., Burti, L., Okonogi, K. and Sacks, M. (1994). Effectiveness in psychiatric care: psychoeducational outcome for patients with major affective disorder and their families. *British Journal of Psychiatry*, **164**, 104–6.

Goodwin, F. K. and Jamison, K. R. (1990). *Manic-Depressive Illness*. New York: Oxford University Press.

Goodwin, G. and Sachs, G. (2004). *Fast Facts – Bipolar Disorder*. Oxford: Health Press Limited.

Lam, D. H., Bright, J., Jones, S. *et al.* (2000). Cognitive therapy for bipolar illness: a pilot study of relapse prevention. *Cognitive Therapy and Research*, **24**, 503–20.

Lam, D., Watkins, E., Hayward, P. *et al.* (2003). A randomised controlled study of cognitive therapy of relapse prevention for bipolar affective disorder: outcome of the first year. *Archives of General Psychiatry*, **60**, 145–52.

Miklowitz, D. J. (2004). Family therapy. In *Psychological Treatment of Bipolar Disorder*, ed. S. L. Johnson and R. L. Leahy. New York: The Guilford Press.

Miklowitz, D. J., Goldstein, M. J., Nuechterlein, K. H., Snyder, K. S. and Mintz, J. (1988). Family factors and the course of bipolar affective disorder. *Archives of General Psychiatry*, **45**, 225–31.

Miklowitz, D. J., Goldstein, M. J., Doane, J. A. *et al.* (1989). Is expressed emotion an index of a transactional process? I. Parents' affective style. *Family Process*, **28**, 153–67.

Miklowitz, D. J., Simoneau, T., George, E. *et al.* (2000). Family focused treatment of bipolar disorder: one-year effects of a psychoeducational program in conjunction with pharmaco-therapy. *Biological Psychiatry*, **48**, 582–92.

Miklowitz, D. J, George, E. L., Richards, J. A., Simoneau, T. L. and Suddath, R. L. (2003). A randomised study of family-focused psychoeducation and pharmacotherapy in the out-patient management of bipolar disorder. *Archives of General Psychiatry*, **60**, 904–12.

Mitchell, P. B., Malhi, G. and Ball, J. R. (2004). Major advances in bipolar disorder. *Medical Journal of Australia*, **181**, 207–10.

Newman, C. F. (2004). Suicidality. In *Psychological Treatment of Bipolar Disorder*, ed. S. L. Johnson and R. L. Leahy. New York: Guilford Press.

O'Connell, R. A., Mayo, J. A., Flatow, L., Cuthbertson, B. and O'Brien, B. E. (1991). Outcome of bipolar disorder on long-term treatment with lithium. *British Journal of Psychiatry*, **159**, 123–9.

Parker, G. (2004). Highlighting Bipolar II Disorder. *Canadian Journal of Psychiatry*, **49**, 791–3.

Perry, A., Tarrier, N., Morriss, R., McCarthy, E. and Limb, K. (1999). Randomised controlled trial of efficacy of teaching patients with bipolar disorder to identify early symptoms of relapse and obtain treatment. *British Medical Journal*, **318**, 149–53.

Rihmer, Z. and Kiss, K. (2002). Bipolar disorders and suicide behaviour. *Bipolar Disorder*, **4**, 21–5.

Scott, J., Garland, A. and Moorhead, S. (2001). A pilot study of cognitive therapy in bipolar disorders. *Psychological Medicine*, **31**, 459–67.

Scott, J., Paykel, E., Morriss, R., Bentall, R. *et al.* (2006). Cognitive-behaviour therapy for bipolar disorder. *British Journal of Psychiatry*, **188**, 313–20.

Simoneau, T. L., Miklowitz, D. J. and Saleem, R. (1998). Expressed emotion and interactional patterns in the families of bipolar patients. *Journal of Abnormal Psychology*, **107**, 497–507.

Van Gent, E. and Zwart, F. (1991). Psychoeducation of partners of bipolar manic patients. *Journal of Affective Disorders*, **21**, 15–18.

Van Gent, E. and Zwart, F. (1993). Ultra-short versus short group therapy in addition to lithium. *Patient Education and Counselling*, **21**, 135–41.

Van Gent, E., Vida, S. and Zwart, F. (1988). Group therapy in addition to lithium in patients with bipolar disorders. *Acta Psychiatrica Belgica*, **88**, 405–18.

Vaughn, C. E. and Leff, J. P. (1976). The influence of family and social factors on the course of psychiatric illness: a comparison of schizophrenic and depressed neurotic patients. *British Journal of Psychiatry*, **129**, 125–37.

13

The role of wellbeing plans in managing Bipolar II Disorder

Margo Orum

Introduction

In recent years, the treatment of bipolar disorder has increasingly recognised the central importance of helping people to identify their early warning signs and episode triggers, and to develop strategies aimed at preventing or minimising future episodes. The axiom 'knowledge is power' holds true for those with bipolar disorder who wish to manage their illness well. The 'knowledge' part of the axiom refers to the need to develop a fine-tuned awareness of one's own early warning signs and triggers, as well as becoming well informed about the medical, physical and psychological aspects of the illness in general. Gathering a large body of information about one's 'enemy' in this way is how one gains 'power' over this illness – the power to recognise a potential risk, and to know how to act swiftly to neutralise it.

In recent research (Russell and Browne, 2005), in which 100 people with bipolar disorder were interviewed about how they had remained well for long stretches, *all* participants indicated they had developed some kind of plan or strategy to remain well. Many had remained well for more than 10 or even 20 years. The plans these people developed to stay well were highly personalised and surprisingly diverse in the needs addressed and the solutions adopted. The most used strategies included a commitment to getting adequate sleep, being aware of warning signs and triggers, keeping stress to a manageable level, taking appropriate medication, and making use of compassionate social and professional supports. Some people had made major lifestyle changes, while others stayed well with only very minor adjustments.

Crucially, perhaps, most of the participants appeared to have a strong sense of ownership in relation to their strategies. They were not merely 'following doctor's orders' but, rather, appeared to have assumed responsibility for the overall management of their illness, which included accepting the diagnosis, taking

Bipolar II Disorder. Modelling, Measuring and Managing, ed. Gordon Parker. Published by Cambridge University Press. © Cambridge University Press 2008.

medication and seeking appropriate help. In particular, they were prepared to remain mindful about the presence of the illness in their lives so that they could act decisively when early warning signs appeared, yet at most other times they were able to keep it sufficiently out of mind to enjoy life (Russell, 2005).

The knack of achieving balance between a healthy approach to self-monitoring and an unhealthy preoccupation with early warning signs is a difficult art to learn. Indeed, finessing a comfortable level of mindfulness about the illness is something that can take months or even years of practice. It is here proposed that in order to learn the art of maintaining a healthy balance, the person with bipolar disorder must eventually become willing to take on the responsibility for, or stewardship of his/her own 'wellbeing plan' – namely, a set of strategies developed with the unique needs and interests of the individual in mind, aimed at helping him/her achieve a healthy and satisfying lifestyle, and usually developed collaboratively with health professionals, family and/or friends. This proposed wellbeing plan is a component of a three-pronged approach to recovery which incorporates (a) medication, (b) education and (c) wellbeing plans.

The term 'wellbeing plan' as used here involves more than simply a plan for avoiding symptoms or keeping an illness in check. Rather, it seeks to raise the level of response to a higher level. It aims first to inform, keep safe and to protect from the risk of episodes. Secondly, when the time is right, it seeks to remind, inspire and challenge the individual to take measured steps towards adding value to his/her life, thus creating a more interesting and fulfilling existence. Thirdly, it works toward a more robust sense of self, which can then act as a protection against further episodes, buffering against depression and diluting the impulse to escape into hypomanias.

Clearly, individual differences in resilience, self-esteem and vulnerability (not only in the person with bipolar disorder, but also in the members of his/her support team – including the health professional) will have a significant impact on the degree of difficulty that might ensue in collaborating on such a plan.

This chapter seeks to distil the best elements of what has been learned so far about how people have managed to remain well despite the presence of this illness, by drawing on the experience both of people with bipolar disorder, and the professionals treating it. It further seeks to open discussion about how one might go about developing a wellbeing plan, and what the likely differences might be in motivation for wellbeing plans as a result of differences in the experiences of those with Bipolar II Disorder (BP II) as opposed to those with Bipolar I Disorder (BP I).

At this point I might add that 21 years ago I had my first episode of BP I and have been managing it successfully for the past 14 years, following a conscious decision to beat the illness. The manner of my management has been similar to the strategies described above. The main components have been a willingness to stick with medication and to seek professional help from psychiatrists and psychologists as needed; to remain mindful of stress levels and sleep quality; to accept the need for self-monitoring and to continually strive to raise my general level of self-awareness (assisted by psychotherapy and mindfulness meditation practice); and finally, to make it all worthwhile, by moving into a career I found stimulating and congruent with my interests (psychology).

Differences in BP II versus BP I in motivation to develop wellbeing plans

One of the main differences between a diagnosis of BP I and BP II is that those with BP I have experienced psychosis, while those with BP II have not.

When individuals with BP I look back on their psychotic experience and see they have been demonstrably 'crazy' – in their own eyes as well as the eyes of friends, family or workmates – then the idea of avoiding another episode can often be readily, even heartily, embraced. The bulk of their memories of psychotic thoughts and behaviours do not fit with their usual view of reality or their sense of self. Thus, ironically, the extreme nature of this experience tends to help them accept that their reality was indeed different during that time, and this may in turn help them find the motivation to develop and act on a plan (initially, at least).

For those with BP II, however, the appeal of committing to strategies to remain episode free may not be so self-evident, especially after a hypomanic episode. Even in the face of strong evidence from family and friends that the hypomanic episode caused damage to relationships, finances or career path, it can be difficult for both the person (and the professional treating them) to know just where the boundary might lie between ordinary emotional reactions and hypomanic magnification of emotions.

Part of the reason for this is that for the person with BP II, it can be difficult to recognise, on looking back, the degree to which they were 'not themselves'. Whether they were mainly euphoric during hypomania, or irritable/angry, their memories of the time nonetheless tend to remain indistinguishable from their 'everyday' thoughts and motivations. Unlike the chaotic thoughts and confusion of psychosis, thoughts during hypomania connect almost seamlessly with deeply held personal beliefs and motivations, so that in a gut sense the person may feel convinced there is a good 'reason' for the excesses in their behaviour, and thus resist the idea they were hypomanic. Sometimes those 'reasons' for emotional excess may be quite legitimate. And yet it may also be true that their behaviour went beyond their ordinary range because their responses were magnified by hypomania. It is very important that both these parallel truths be acknowledged by the clinician or support person. Doing so will also help the person 'under the microscope' to move towards acceptance of the fact they were hypomanic (if indeed true). The clinician who dismisses the relevance of thoughts or ideas simply because they appeared to typify hypomania will lose credibility for unnecessarily negating experience that was, for the patient, highly meaningful.

Similarly, when a person is depressed (but not to a psychotic degree), their negatively based emotions – fears and concerns – are magnified by the depression, and yet they may still be firmly set in the person's real life issues. Again, it is important to recognise that there are parallel truths in operation. One truth is that the content and context of the person's negative thoughts are consonant with their inner concerns, and the other is that the implications drawn by the person are magnified by depressive thinking.

Indeed, many people who experience BP II tend to have more depressive episodes than hypomanias, and in general appear to spend much more time depressed than do those with BP I. Those who have only the odd mild episode of hypomania punctuating long bouts of demoralising depressive doldrums are highly unlikely to welcome the notion of avoiding hypomanias. The chief desire for these people in terms of motivation for a wellbeing plan, is to rid themselves of the depressions. Thus the only way they are likely to countenance steering clear of the hypomanias would be if, in sacrificing them, they were better able to achieve a balanced 'middle way' whereby mood swings in both directions were less likely.

To summarise, people with BP II (as well as some with BP I) may feel conflicted about the need to develop strategies to remain well or, specifically, a wellbeing plan, for any of the following reasons:
- they had not perceived themselves as being all that 'different' when hypomanic
- they felt fantastic and enjoyed the extra creativity or productivity of hypomania
- they felt either intense euphoria or, alternatively, deep distress in relation to some of their life concerns during hypomania or depression, and thus the notion of a plan to remain well is suspect because it appears to discount or relegate those emotions to nothing more than symptoms of an 'episode'.
- they do not want to lose the hypomanias because they had been, for them, such welcome holidays from depression.

One of the objections raised regarding strategising about what to do when early warning signs appear, is the notion that this may be a doomed enterprise – doomed because the target time for action is a time of reduced insight and control for the person with bipolar disorder, and thus a time when adherence to the plan can be very easily thwarted. For example, a person who has willingly and painstakingly drafted up a plan when well may very likely sweep it aside as irrelevant when hypomanic, or alternatively lose faith in it along with any motivation to follow it, when depressed. A good plan needs to foresee these problems and include a 'plan B' set of options and alternatives (see the plan format in Box 13.4.)

Finally, whether a person has BP II or BP I, there is a strong chance they will feel some level of ambivalence about drawing up a plan to remain well. As mentioned above, those with BP II may have more ambivalence as a group, because of the nature of their experiences. However, at the level of the individual, it is basic psychological logic that anyone compelled by ill health to live by new restrictions will naturally feel ambivalent.

Finding motivation for a wellbeing plan

A wellbeing plan need not be in any particular format. Essentially, it could be anything from a private decision by an individual to adopt a certain strategy designed to better control his/her illness, to a formal document drawn up by the individual in close consultation with family, friends, workmates and/or health professionals.

As more is understood about the importance of engaging in such collaborative planning, it is now increasingly common for clinicians of all types to at least instigate, and preferably, become involved in helping their patients to formulate a workable set of strategies for recovery and maintenance of wellness. What is offered here as a wellbeing plan is suggested as an optimal component in assisting recovery from bipolar disorder – a plan that will not only help people to return to wellness, but encourage them towards lifestyle practices that will maintain well-ness, and also boost self-efficacy and resilience.

The primary consideration as to how a wellbeing plan should be formulated, and by whom, needs to be driven by the question: what will work best for the individual involved? It is suggested that the clinician's main duty, at minimum, should be to supply the individual with appropriate information and psychoeducation (includ-ing lists of books, videos and websites) to inform the making of such a plan.

In order to be motivated to work on developing a wellbeing plan, an individual needs to be given a chance to explore his or her feelings about the diagnosis, and to feel confident that the plan will serve his or her particular interests and circum-stances, and reflect his or her preferences, in both the short and long term. It needs to achieve this while also being guided by current wisdom about risk factors and triggers. The presence or absence of relationships at home or at work, and the quality of them, are another critical consideration. Who can be relied upon and who is best avoided when ill? The individual needs to gain a sense of ownership over the decisions that went into formulating the plan, as well as the strategies outlined in it. In other words, people are unlikely to be motivated to work on, or stick to, a wellbeing plan unless it feels real, do-able, and like something that will serve their unique needs.

Some people are overly cautious and safety conscious, while others brush away the need for any kind of concessions to the presence of bipolar disorder in their

> **Box 13.1. Checklist before embarking on a wellbeing plan**
>
> **Costs of the illness**
>
> Explore your *negative* thoughts and feelings about having this illness. How does it *negatively* affect:
> - your sense of self (the kind of person you believe yourself to be)
> - your life (e.g. future career, study, living situation, lifestyle)
> - your relationships (with partners, family, friends, workmates, etc.)
>
> **Benefits of the illness**
>
> Explore any *positive* thoughts and feelings you may have had about your experiences with this illness. Are there ways it has *positively* affected:
> - your sense of self (the kind of person you believe yourself to be)
> - your life (e.g. future career, study, living situation, lifestyle)
> - your relationships (with partners, family, friends, workmates, etc.)
>
> **Imagine life with fewer episodes (i.e. with successful management)**
>
> If you were able to learn to manage this illness so that you could last several years at a time without episodes (as many do), what difference would this make to:
> - your sense of self (the kind of person you believe yourself to be)
> - your life (e.g. future career, study, living situation, lifestyle)
> - your relationships (with friends, family, workmates, life partners, etc.)

life. Helping those with each of these personality styles to flesh out a workable plan that speaks to their sense of self while also guiding them in the direction of maintaining good psychological health is something of an art.

Box 13.1 suggests a format for encouraging the patient to explore his or her own beliefs, feelings and concerns about both the *negative* and *positive* experiences and implications of the illness. This approach is influenced by the motivational interviewing technique developed by Miller and Rollnick (1991), whereby the clinician prompts the patient to express *both* sides of any ambivalences in him/herself (in this case, about the diagnosis, and thus also, the proposed need for a wellbeing plan). The basic tenet here is that people are always persuaded more surely by their own deliberations than by those of others. When there is ambivalence (a very common state), presenting one side of the argument only will add fuel to the other side. All too often in therapy the clinician falls into a trap of arguing strongly in favour of 'good management' practices, which leaves the patient with a strong inclination to give voice to the unvoiced side of the ambivalence – thus talking him/herself further into a position of opposing what has been proposed.

It may seem obvious, given the amount of disruption caused to self and others by bipolar disorder, that anyone would want to be rid of it. However, because hypomania can be a wonderful feeling and a time of great creativity, the desire to re-experience it can (perhaps sometimes unconsciously) sabotage more conscious efforts to remain well. Recognising and expressing one's own subversive feelings through being encouraged to express both sides helps the patient to put all his or her conscious motivational 'cards on the table' and thus to more accurately weigh up the personal pros and cons of managing the illness.

The instructions to then imagine a life more free of the illness, and to scan the same three things (sense of self, work/life/study plans, relationships) in each case intends to prompt a vivid scenario of the possible life improvements that could be experienced from learning to manage the illness well. People completing this exercise in my workshops have commented that, for the first time, they lost some of their fear and sense of helplessness about the illness, and felt inspired that they could indeed imagine a much more hopeful future by becoming more proactive in keeping episodes at bay.

Ideally, work on formulating a wellbeing plan takes place during a period of wellness, and most often it follows on from diagnosis and/or an episode. It can be best to sketch out initial ideas soon after an episode, and to save more detailed work on a plan for a time when the individual is reasonably well and regaining confidence. A little space after an episode helps to allow distortions to interpretations (influenced by hypomanic or depressive thinking) to fade.

Involving others

As mentioned earlier, the person who has bipolar disorder needs to be the main 'voice' driving the wellbeing plan. The clinician may or may not be directly involved in helping to draw up the plan, depending on the patient's preference. Either way, the clinician should prepare the ground for a plan; supply relevant information and psychoeducation about BP II; help the patient work through, or at least address, possible ambivalence that might sabotage a plan; and examine any relationship difficulties that might need to be taken into account.

In most cases, where possible, the involvement of helpful family members or friends is desirable, especially those who may well be involved if episodes break through in future. The patient should choose those he or she trusts most, and preferably those who are in daily (or almost daily) contact so that they have the opportunity to notice very early warning signs. This may be somewhat difficult if the patient lives alone or if the closest family or friends live at some distance. However, the experience of others has shown that phone or email contact can sometimes serve quite effectively as early warning detection – mostly in conjunction with regular professional help, or additional arrangements with a trusted neighbour or workmate to phone relatives if they have concerns. Such arrangements *must* be the choice of the patient, though (and be warranted by past experience), or else they become more like surveillance than a safety net.

A plan can also include an intention to join a support group or a community group when the person is able, to develop some regular contacts. Sarah Russell's (2005) book, which features dozens of first-hand accounts, illustrates a wide variety of ways that people have chosen to involve others in their successful strategies to remain well. Interestingly, few of those people chose to join mental health support groups, preferring instead to join community groups such as sporting clubs, book clubs, music groups and so on. Formal bipolar support groups seem to be of optimum help when a person first receives a diagnosis and is still struggling to come to terms with the diagnosis and is learning about the illness and how to manage it. The person might aim to move on to interest-based community groups as they become able, in order to gain confidence and a sense of integration back into the general community.

Making a wellbeing plan

Let us review the key elements that should be addressed in collaboratively making a wellbeing plan by following an example. In this case, three people have gathered to make a wellbeing plan: the person who has BP II ('David'), his sister 'Louise' with whom he shares a flat while they are both at university, and a treating clinician, such as a psychiatrist or psychologist.

As a general rule, the patient should always be given the first opportunity to speak at each step in the process, followed by the support team members. If there happen to be any misconceptions voiced about the illness and its implications, the clinician needs to sensitively correct those, and can also add in any further suggestions (preferably in the form of a range of options) for the team to consider.

Debrief past efforts by others to help

It is useful to start with a debriefing of what others did in the past that worked, and what did not, in the lead up to, during, and immediately after, the episode/s. Some example questions to David might be:

- How were your family/friends involved in helping (if at all) in this (or past) episode/s?
- What was most difficult for you about the way they acted/spoke at the time?

- What did they do/say that helped you the most?
- Do you see their input at the time differently now that you are somewhat recovered?
- What did you do yourself that helped/did not help?

Questions to Louise might be:

- What was most difficult for you when David was ill?
- What did you do or say that you believed helped/did not help? (Ask David to comment on her responses.)

The discussions that flow from these questions (albeit often emotional) provide an excellent opportunity to address and sometimes correct communication difficulties, hurts or resentments that may have arisen between family members due to the stress of the illness, either in the current or previous episode/s. For example, David might not have fully realised how much his excessive spending had distressed his parents until Louise spoke of it during the debriefing. Similarly, it might not have been until the debriefing that Louise came to understand at a deeper level that David had indeed been 'ill' and subject to distorted thinking, rather than acting out some personal vengeance or intentionally being difficult.

Identify early warning signs

David is asked to identify any possible early warning signs in his thoughts or behaviour leading up to the time when he began to show clear signs of an episode. After David has exhausted his ideas, Louise can be asked to add her observations, and the clinician also can add comments. This discussion reveals that in his recent episode of *hypomania* (which occurred in early spring), David had been sleeping two hours less for several nights, and yet still felt slightly buoyant, with increasing energy, and had been spending more than usual for some days before other, more obvious, signs appeared. This happened in a week where he had attended several 21st birthday parties, had been drinking heavily, and getting only patchy sleep. Looking back further, to his previous episodes of *depression*, David was able to remember that in the early stages he had found returning phone calls difficult, and that he did not want to go to lunch to socialise with others at work. One of his previous depressions was after a relationship break-up, and another was in winter, at a time when he felt overloaded at work, and deeply disappointed about a low grade on an assignment at university. Finally, David might be asked to check through a list of other people's early warning signs (see Box 13.2), in case any of those might also apply to him.

Identify risk factors and triggers

Again, David should be given first opportunity to nominate those situations that have appeared to trigger his mood to escalate either up or down, before

Box 13.2. Early warning signs

Some common early (and not so early) warning signs for hypomania (and mania)

- Not sleeping (the most commonly experienced sign)
- Agitation, irritability, emotional intensity, anger, aggression
- Energised with ideas, plans, motivation for schemes
- Intense expression laden with implied extra meaning
- Inability to concentrate
- Rapid thoughts and speech
- Spending money more than usual
- Increased sexual drive, flirtatiousness
- Increasing incidence of paranoid thoughts
- Losing track of time
- Reading extra symbolism into words, events, patterns, seeing 'codes'
- Increased use of telephone or writing – making contact with many people
- Insistent and persuasive
- Erratic thinking, speech, behaviour
- Increases in, or binges in, alcohol and/or drugs, e.g. cannabis
- Arguments with friends or family
- Increased 'driven' activity without stopping to eat, drink or sleep
- Increased interest in religious/spiritual ideas or themes
- Taking on more work, working to extremes in hours or projects
- Grandiose plans or claims

Some common early warning signs for depression

- Change in sleep patterns – insomnia, or excessive sleeping
- Fatigue
- Staying up late to watch TV
- Increased irritability
- Loss of concentration
- Lack of motivation
- Withdrawal – avoiding social contact, not answering the phone, cancelling social activities
- Change in eating habits – loss of appetite, or overeating
- Reduced libido
- Increased anxiety and feelings of worthlessness
- Loss of interest in leisure activities and hobbies
- Listening to sad/nostalgic music
- Taking sick days
- Procrastinating and putting off responsibilities
- Bursting into tears for no apparent reason
- Thoughts of suicide

> **Box 13.3. High-risk activities and possible triggers**
>
> - Taking cannabis and other drugs
> - Excessive stress at work and/or home
> - Getting too little sleep (hypomania), or too much (depression)
> - Stressed metabolism (with irregular energy/sleeping/eating patterns)
> - Excessive alcohol
> - Suddenly stopping prescribed drugs without consulting psychiatrist
> - Excessive caffeine rich drinks late in the day (that can disrupt sleep)
> - Doing intense emotional/spiritual workshops (gentle growth is fine)
> - Being in any intense, accelerated learning environment where there is challenge to old beliefs or sudden change to foundational beliefs
> - Acting on impulses, if they arise from possible hypomania
> - Flying overseas where different time zones may disrupt sleep-wake rhythms

his sister and the clinician contribute their suggestions. A list of common risk factors and triggers such as those shown in Box 13.3 can then be consulted for further possible matches to David's experience. Some early warning signs can be seen as risk factors as well, because they herald the possibility of an episode, and thus continued engagement in those behaviours constitutes risk. Working from David's story so far, some initial potential triggers for hypomania might be:

- a string of nights of drinking and not much sleep
- perhaps the intensive social stimulation of parties
- sleeping fewer hours and still feeling energised
- spending more than usual
- vulnerability to hypomania in early spring.

For depressive episodes, his initial list would be:

- overloaded with work
- losses and disappointment
- break-up with romantic partners
- reluctance to socialise
- reluctance to return phone calls
- vulnerability to depression in winter.

From the list of known risk factors and triggers supplied by his clinician, David also adds to his plan:

- a commitment to avoid illicit recreational drugs
- a commitment to be mindful of the need for preventive safety action when he travels overseas next year with friends.

Box 13.4. Wellbeing plan   **Date:**_____

Plan A

We, _____

   Person A (who has bipolar disorder) and

_____

Person B (who has been entrusted by Person A to note early warning signs)
agree to work as a team as shown below, in a bid to minimise or stop future episodes of
bipolar disorder invading our lives. I/we also commit to continually seek out wellbeing
attitudes and activities that will keep bipolar at bay, and boost enjoyment and quality of
life in the long term.

   Early warning signs, triggers and risk factors that we agree warrant action are:

. . . .

. . . .

   If Person A begins to notice any of those above he/she agrees to take action such as:

. . . .

. . . .

   If Person B begins to notice any of those above he/she agrees to take action such as:

. . . .

. . . .

Plan B

If, due to the illness, Person A refuses to act as agreed above, he/she acknowledges the
following actions may then become necessary:

. . . .

. . . .

   Strategies that I will commit to in order to prioritise my continuing wellbeing are:

. . . .

. . . .

Specify how the feedback will be delivered

David nominated his sister Louise to be the family member he would prefer to
provide him with feedback if she (or other family members) notices early warning
signs. Louise has agreed to this arrangement, and they have settled on the wording
that David finds least irritating. David will tell Louise whenever his private
monitoring has picked up some very early warning signs, and invite her to help
him monitor things further, until he gets them back into control. Getting the form
of the feedback to a comfortable level for the person with bipolar disorder is
crucial to the workability of the plan. Box 13.4 shows a sample plan format.

Acknowledge how difficult it is to receive feedback

David and Louise need to be aware that no matter how good the relationship between them, nor how tactfully she might give feedback, it will nonetheless be *very* hard for David to hear it. He is likely to feel stripped of his dignity and, especially, his credibility as an equal, when she first tells him she is noticing signs. Particularly difficult is the fact that if he denies that there is anything wrong, this can all too easily sound like the lack of insight that typifies the early stages of hypomania. Thus he must be prepared to *consider the possibility* that the signs may be present, even when he feels strongly that Louise is mistaken, or making much about nothing. He needs to be able to content himself with the fact that time and his continued wellness will show that either he was right (she was mistaken), or that he successfully acted upon the signs. He must learn to live with that level of ambiguity.

Intervene at the earliest possible moment

If David can muster the willingness to act upon Louise's feedback by taking the agreed safety precautions, just in case, he is well on his way to managing the illness well. Similarly, his own self-monitoring may pick up some early signs, to which he needs to respond with similar open-mindedness. Catching signs at a very early stage generally means that safety precautions are quite minimal and do-able. Sometimes all that is required is an acceptance of the possibility, and a willingness to become more watchful in self-monitoring for a short time. These early interventions cannot be seen by others, but may be the most powerful in terms of their ability to prevent episodes. A personal example is provided in Box 13.5.

Specify what safety measures will be taken, and by whom

When early warning signs appear, David agrees to consider reducing his work pressure, perhaps take a day off, cancel stressful appointments, or take extra contingency medication, as arranged with his psychiatrist. If he has not been sleeping well, he may take a sleeping tablet, or get some exercise to help him sleep. If he has been forgetting medication, he will ask Louise to help him remember for the next week or so. As a basic precaution when he travels overseas, he will take a day off work before and after the trip to avoid overload stress and give him time to adjust.

Take into account the strengths and weaknesses of close relationships

David structured the feedback to come through Louise in order to avoid adding stress to his relationship with his mother. He had become angry and defensive when ill with his mother, in particular, due to her style of relating to him when ill. He would not mind his father's involvement, but believed Louise was more

> **Box 13.5. Author's examples of very early prevention**
>
> One Sunday morning years ago I awoke at 6 am feeling sparkly and energised. It was such a lovely morning I was about to get up straight away and start digging in my garden to make a new flower bed. Then a monitoring thought popped up: "Hang on, I don't usually get up at 6 am on a Sunday morning." As I considered it further, I realised that the sparkly urge to tag along on the magic carpet joy-ride felt very like the first seductive tentacles of hypomania. I had a decision to make. I could tempt fate by accepting the joy-ride, or I could refuse to be seduced. I chose the latter. With a quick promise to myself that I could still do the gardening a couple of hours later, I rolled over, turned my back on hypomania's lure, and amazingly, went back to sleep. When I woke again, the magic carpet sparkles had all dissolved. Quite often, I believe, it can be that simple.
>
> I use a similar approach to downgrade the credibility of the 'can't do' messages that depressive thinking sometimes presents to me. On days when my confidence dips low I can feel very stressed at the thought of all my usual activities. I have learned to accept that some days are like this, and to remind myself that these feelings need not – and usually do not – last beyond that day. Depression is not always this easy to sidestep for those who are more prone to it, but the strategy of refusing to take its bleak messages seriously works much more powerfully when they first appear, than after it has taken hold.

perceptive and able to accurately pick up early warning signs. Furthermore, he and Louise live together, have a fairly equitable relationship, and during the last episode she was less 'in his face' than others. Some people drafting their own management plans have written in a simple declaration like 'our strengths are that we care about each other, even if we sometimes get angry – and we agree to make a special effort not to let anger get in the way of this important task of catching signs early'.

Include a commitment to quality-of-life activities

The importance of quality of life as an integral component of wellbeing plans will be addressed further in the next section. David's quality of life commitments, however, were to take up tai chi, to avoid heavy drinking and keep a more regular sleeping pattern, and to say 'no' to overtime when he felt pressured at work. He decided to start playing his guitar again (after a long break), because his guitar had always provided a good way to relax and relieve stress.

Don't aim too low for too long – aim for stages of recovery

Sometimes people make the mistake of aiming too low, for too long – and this becomes, in effect, the antithesis of a wellbeing strategy, because over time it is almost inevitable that they will become depressed again. A depressing life begets depression, and depression in turn begets a depressing life. It is well known that depression is sparked by loss, and there are many real and imagined threats of loss when it comes to bipolar disorder – loss of self-confidence, loss of hope, loss of relationships with family, friends and lovers, loss of future expectations, loss of ability to work in one's former chosen field, loss of reputation, loss of identity. Therefore a strategy that enshrines a strict or overly cautious approach to recovery may also enshrine loss as the prevailing state of that person's life. This is why it is important for a wellbeing plan to flag the idea that things can improve, that further stages of recovery can be attained, and that the individual can work his or her way back to a life that feels meaningful and satisfying, albeit with some concessions made towards managing the illness. David's plan foreshadowed these issues simply with an intention to review his plan's contents in a year's time, to consider what had worked and what had not, and to reflect on any new information or different needs he might then have. It would be likely, if things went well, that his revision would include a partial phasing out or reformulating of Louise's support role.

The plan needs to fit the person

David, in the example given above, illustrates just one way that a wellbeing plan might develop. Obviously, individual differences in patients and their families/ friends in terms of their self-esteem and communication abilities will make an enormous impact on the ease or difficulty of drafting a plan. Where communication is seriously compromised between the patient and family support team, it is best to suggest the family work through this in therapy, as serious communication difficulties are bound to compromise not only the making of the plan, but also the family's ability to act on it appropriately. Some patients may be better off drafting up a plan by themselves or with their professional helpers, and only then showing it to their family with a request as to the ways they believe their family could help them most.

Benefits of collaborating on making a wellbeing plan

The main benefit of making a wellbeing plan in the manner described is that the patient is motivated to take over the responsibility or stewardship of a set of strategies for keeping him or herself well, usually with the assistance of appropriate others. This gives the patient a voice in how he or she will be treated when ill, and because the patient has been central to formulating and personally selecting the set of strategies, it is much more likely that he or she will remain committed to making them work.

Furthermore, from the vantage point of 'wellness', the patient can decide how he or she wants to be treated when ill. Obviously this helps to reduce any lingering sense of helplessness in relation to the illness, and restores a sense of control and mastery.

Even if things don't go exactly to plan at crunch time, the experience of having collaborated on a plan is likely to have some helpful moderating effects, one being that family and friends have permission to act, and this relieves them of some of the burdens of decision-making. In addition, in the process of collaborating, the patient and family may learn much about the strengths and weaknesses of their usual style of communicating, and thus some lasting improvements in mutual cooperation and understanding can sometimes be achieved.

Summary of key secrets for optimum management of bipolar disorder

A willingness to:

- accept that one has the illness
- take medication as a preventative safety net
- identify and be vigilant of one's own early warning signs
- learn about the nature of bipolar disorder, especially high-risk activities
- manage your particular stressors and potential triggers at work and play
- keep regular patterns of eating, exercise, sleep and relaxation
- make use of counselling to come to terms with bipolar disorder
- formulate a wellbeing plan and work through issues which may be fuelling stress and triggering depression
- work on relationship issues to ensure/improve cooperation with family or friends in detecting early warning signs
- allow trusted others to mention warning signs, and be willing to manage one's own aggravation when they do
- alternatively, if family/friends are themselves problematic stressors, find ways to avoid/nullify those stressors
- take a preventative self-management approach overall to become adept at avoiding episodes
- cultivate mindfulness so that self-monitoring happens naturally in response to potential triggers.

Quality of life matters

The commitment to manage bipolar disorder via a wellbeing plan is essentially a commitment to personal growth. Although wellbeing and personal growth are desirable for all people, those with bipolar disorder have more at stake, and thus a more urgent need to cultivate self-mastery, personal insight and resourcefulness.

Recently there has been a surge of interest in mindfulness techniques as a means of stress reduction, attaining greater insight and managing depression (Kabat-Zinn, 1990; Segal *et al.*, 2002). Mindfulness is an invaluable personal skill for a population of people who have a need to become adept at observing themselves. The practise of mindfulness also helps with sleeping well, staying calm, managing stress and achieving the detachment to monitor one's thoughts and emotions without undue judgement.

A great many people with BP II are highly creative, and often more so when hypomanic. This sometimes leads them to believe they can only be creative when they are hypomanic, and thus to court hypomanias, even when 'highs' are destructive in other areas, such as maintaining relationships. A wellbeing plan can address this potential problem by incorporating the commitment to foster creativity in everyday life, rather than assuming it can only happen during hypomania. Hopefully, everyday life will then become too precious to risk a hypomania, and the result is a vastly improved quality of life overall.

In much of the current literature aimed at helping people understand and manage bipolar disorder (e.g. the excellent book by Miklowitz, 2002), early warning signs, triggers and risk factors stand alongside strategies to remain well. It is here proposed that replacing the more benign 'strategies to remain well' with a more dynamic, overarching, lifestyle-enriching wellbeing plan might serve to galvanise the interest and dedication of the person in a way that has not as yet been expressly operationalised in the more traditional management plan approach.

Before going further it may be useful to define what is meant here by the word 'recovery'. A hard line definition invokes the notion of a total (and presumed lifelong) absence of episodes and symptoms – but this definition cannot be applied until one is on one's deathbed, and has long been rejected as unhelpful. And recovery can never be a return to the person's pre-illness level of functioning (it is impossible to leap backwards upstream in the river of experience to resume a sense of self untrammelled by the illness). A more empowering and reasonable definition might hold that recovery is achieved when coping with the illness no longer occupies centre stage in a person's psyche and no longer limits lifestyle choices to a debilitating degree. One way or another, the experience of bipolar disorder leaves a mark on a person's identity. So perhaps sustainable recovery is best seen as a commitment to learn the lessons of life that spring from having to manage the illness, to follow one's dreams despite, or because of the illness, and to accumulate skills and mastery that assist in achieving longer stretches between episodes; and dealing more efficiently and skilfully with the episodes that do break through, with a personal minimum of down-time. With commitment like this driving the wellbeing plan, personal growth becomes almost inevitable over time.

With its sights set purposefully on positive outcomes, and with an emphasis on collaborative formulation, the wellbeing plan is proposed as a kind of paradigm shift in treatment approach. At the outset of treatment the wellbeing plan can enshrine the premise of meaning and lifestyle as ultimate and necessary considerations underpinning sustainable recovery, with the first-order principles of medication and education forming a springboard from which the 'lifestyle treatment' can be launched. The assumptions inherent in such a plan are that the individual with bipolar disorder has every reason to hope for better outcomes in future – just as much, in fact, as someone without the illness (given similar underlying personality characteristics).

The positive psychology movement describes three main roads to happiness, or wellbeing: seeking out *pleasurable* activities; being fully *engaged* in activities that are interesting and absorbing, and seeking deeper *meaning* in life, chiefly through a sense of contribution (Seligman, 2002). The wellbeing plan described here encompasses each of these strategies. A prudent wellbeing plan would factor in a commitment to a staged recovery, which includes an initial recuperation stage, mastering basic management skills, and later when the person is able, a commitment to searching out paths back to a lifestyle that is pleasurable, engaging and meaningful. These positive goals are likely to have strong appeal for most patients, and would provide a powerful incentive for patients to adhere to their wellbeing plan.

To recap, the bottom line is that wellbeing plans must reflect the preferences and personal style of the people for whom they are intended. They should be responsive to current needs, and foreshadow future ones. They can – and should – be flexible, not set in stone. They can be simple or complicated, and developed alone, but preferably with professionals, family/friends, or a combination. Ideally they incorporate lessons from the past, identify early warning signs and triggers, set out a plan of action for minimising or preventing future episodes, and include carefully articulated quality-of-life commitments – so that remaining well becomes a viable long-term prospect.

REFERENCES

Kabat-Zinn, J. (1990). *Full Catastrophe Living: Using the Wisdom of your Body and Mind to Face Stress, Pain and Illness.* New York: Delta.

Miklowitz, D. J. (2002). *The Bipolar Disorder Survival Guide: What You and your Family need to Know.* London: Guilford Press.

Miller, W. R. and Rollnick, S. (1991). *Motivational Interviewing: Preparing People to change Addictive Behavior.* New York: Guilford Press.

Russell, S. (2005). *A Lifelong Journey: Staying well with Manic Depression/Bipolar Disorder.* Melbourne: Michelle Anderson Publishing.

Russell, S. J. and Browne, J. L. (2005). Staying well with bipolar disorder. *Australian and New Zealand Journal of Psychiatry*, **39**, 187–93.

Segal, Z. V., Williams, J. M. G. and Teasdale, J. D. (2002). *Mindfulness-based Cognitive Therapy for Depression.* New York: Guilford Press.

Seligman, M. E. P. (2002). *Authentic Happiness.* New York: Free Press.

14

Survival strategies for managing and prospering with Bipolar II Disorder

Meg Smith

Introduction

The psychiatrist looks at me. I am pleading for antidepressants. I stumble, inarticulate, over why I think I am now depressed enough to warrant the magic pills. The words don't come out of my mouth. There is a loud roar. I wake out of the nightmare to the sound of the first plane of the day thundering over the bedroom. I stumble into the bathroom, decide I can't face a shower and head off to the kitchen to grab some coffee to wake me up and get me into the land of the living.

There is something horribly familiar about this scenario. It is the recurring cycle of sliding into depression, trying to decide if this one is a 'normal' depression or if it will continue as weeks of a bleak, grey existence – or if it is just the fear that the usual stresses of life will precipitate a depressive episode.

The early episodes of Bipolar II Disorder (BP II) are dominated by depressive bouts, with a few nice periods of high activity, creativity and elation to spice things up. But eventually, the periods of depression drive most of us to seek help. Life stresses, getting older, medical crises and too much risk-taking lengthen and deepen the depressions until, finally, it is hard to ignore that there is something badly wrong.

So – the diagnosis has been made and the treatment has been prescribed. Now what? Perhaps the most important thing about surviving bipolar disorder is accepting the knowledge that there is a biochemical disorder in the first place, and that you have to be careful and take care of yourself. BP II is not new to most individuals by that time: what is new is that the mood swings can be recognised and that there is a choice in relation to what to do about them.

Given that most people with BP II will have, on average, 10–15 years of undiagnosed mood swings, it can take some time to accept the fact that what you thought was your personality can be more accurately described as a biochemical vulnerability which has the potential to 'swing' the individual into periods of

Bipolar II Disorder. Modelling, Measuring and Managing, ed. Gordon Parker. Published by Cambridge University Press. © Cambridge University Press 2008.

illness that can have a devastating effect on relationships, employment, financial stability and self-concept.

Living with bipolar disorder has been variously described. Some say it can be like living on the edge of a precipice: most of the time it might be possible to deny that the edge is there, but then an event happens which can be a brutal reminder that an episode can happen quickly and catastrophically. Others say it is like riding a canoe along a river: there are wonderful vistas and generally smooth gliding through the rapids, waterfalls and sandbanks. But most people living with bipolar disorder are familiar with the periods when life is on hold, when there is a painful recuperation from living too high and too fast. Surviving bipolar disorder is a skilful mix of dodging the rapids and learning where the problems are likely to be.

The first 15 years – developing the 'bipolar personality'

The course of bipolar disorder varies from person to person but there are some commonalities shared by everyone. For example, there is commonly a time lag between onset of symptoms and eventual diagnosis and access to appropriate medication and treatment. For most people, the path to diagnosis and effective treatment is a long one. Because the early symptoms are often depressive, and antidepressant drugs have been around since the late 1950s, this has generally meant treatment by general practitioners, often mistakenly, for 'depression'. Then come the subsequent problems resulting from antidepressant use: mixed states, hypomania and sleeplessness. Some people who have experienced poor management of their medication give up attempting to obtain treatment and try to accept that the mood states are part of their personality – rather than risk the side-effects and complications caused by many medications.

Effective treatment brings its own problems – for many people this can mean having to 'unlearn' a range of adaptive strategies that were developed to cope with depressive or hypomanic symptoms, or having to recognise personality characteristics as contributors to a mood cycle. Depressive symptoms may have been interpreted as shyness or lack of social skills, and hypomania viewed as self-confidence and motivation.

One of the first people I met who had BP II was a successful psychotherapist. Successful, however, for only part of the year. Spring and summer brought wonderful creative ideas, and he organised seminars, networked amongst his colleagues, wrote many papers and was very busy on a number of committees. During autumn and winter, he vanished into his unit. During some spring creative sessions, his behaviour was regarded as somewhat unorthodox and avant garde by his professional colleagues, and he acquired a reputation for pushing the limits in psychotherapy. He was neither diagnosed nor effectively treated until his late forties. What would his life have been had the diagnosis and treatment been available to him earlier? Would he have been as successful financially as his well-known brother? Would he have had a stable emotional relationship, a centred and judicious life, instead of a sadly premature death?

People develop their own strategies for understanding what is happening to them. Blaming others for the 'breakdowns' is one tactic. For example, deciding that a previous decision to be in a relationship, or job, or project, must have been wrong, and that moving into something different will solve the problem. People with bipolar disorder have very interesting and varied lives as a result of such strategies. Diagnosis means taking a long hard look at your life to date and deciding what is 'you' (and your personality) and what is the consequence of your mood disorder.

Dissociation and alternative identities

One of the most striking ways in which people living with bipolar disorder explain their mood swings to themselves is by the development of different identities or personalities that fit the constellation of moods. Developing a new personality can be a way of leaving behind the trauma and pain of a period of depression – particularly when one's mood starts to lift. The development of such personalities is not necessarily pathological. Many successful people have developed stage or professional or creative identities that are at odds with the personae in other parts of their lives. Alternate identities can be useful as a way of confining thoughts, perceptions and behaviours to one area of your life.

Everyone has roles in life, but usually you are aware of the roles and the set of behaviours that go along with them. Bipolar disorder blurs the boundaries between roles so, while you might usually wear a suit to work and watch your language with your superiors, during a hypomanic period it can seem quite reasonable to wear a holiday shirt and become more familiar with your boss. At best, you acquire an interesting reputation – at worst you lose your job!

One survival strategy is to know where the boundaries are and be very firm about not crossing them when you feel like it. One of the positive things about bipolar disorder is that the moods can be very elastic – it is possible to hold onto a set of behaviours for short periods of time. So an effective approach is to decide what is important and what you need to do to retain your reputation. The work identity might mean a particular set of clothes and a particular set of tasks. If you want to hold on to the job, don't get creative with that role.

Best of all for the individual is to decide *ahead of an episode* what is important to them and put in place what needs to happen to preserve that part of their life.

A time to decide, a time to defer

Hypomania is wonderful for deciding that great life changes must be made. Unfortunately, hypomania also goes along with poor judgement, general inability to weigh up the consequences, and feelings that things are wonderful when they are in reality often far from wonderful. Most of us learn the hard way that decisions made during periods of hypomania are not always the best decisions.

Individuals need to recognise the time of year that they are more likely to be hypomanic, or the constellation of symptoms that signals hypomania, and put off any major decisions. If it really is a major decision, a few more days or weeks are not going to make much of a difference. Hypomania can be very useful for engendering creative ideas, and generating an archive of wonderful schemes and projects – but wait until the hypomania has subsided before acting on those great ideas. If the idea is any good, it needs a period of stability to come to fruition.

Choices and dilemmas: living a life more ordinary

Does treating bipolar disorder douse the magic of the mood swings? Psychotic manic episodes which result in hospital treatment and months of restabilisation present a different dilemma from the milder highs of Bipolar II Disorder. People generally seek treatment when something is uncomfortable or needs to change – so the depressive phase is more likely to bring people into the consultant's office than the hypomanic phase. Given the choice of removing the depressive symptoms by eliminating the hypomanic phase, some people will opt for the life and the personality they know, and decide not to take medication.

Newer medications may make this choice easier. In his book *Listening to Prozac*, Peter Kramer introduced the idea that the SSRI antidepressants could subtly modify personality. This is an intriguing notion. The SSRI antidepressants do seem to have the ability to subtly remove some of the more unpleasant symptoms of depression. I remember being amazed when a few days of paroxetine eliminated the anxiety I felt about making phone calls. I don't think I had even registered that the anxiety was part of the depressive phase. I would not have sought help for this particular symptom because it simply seemed to be part of my reticent personality. But faced with the evidence that medication helped this particular symptom I started to look at other parts of my 'personality' that were probably aspects of mood disorder rather than of the real me.

Perhaps the essential difference between Bipolar I Disorder (BP I) and BP II is the size of the steps that people will take to modify the symptoms. BP I has such huge consequences that heavy medication seems quite justifiable to prevent future disasters. But for those with BP II it is a hard call to make the decision to knock out those mild hypomanic periods that, after all, seem to be very productive and pleasant and creative. I can be persuaded to take a drug that regulates my sleep patterns and, incidentally, returns my mood to normal. But I probably won't be persuaded to take an antipsychotic drug that has unpleasant and immediate or ongoing side-effects.

Seasons and life changes

Some bipolar disorders have a seasonal predilection – creative, hypomanic swings in spring and summer; low mood and withdrawal in winter. These commonly feel part of the normal rhythm of life and – most of the time – that is fine. But stress at particular times can escalate mood or deepen depression, so it is worth being aware of the at-risk times. People with bipolar disorder take longer to recover from stress – so a number of stresses close together during an at-risk period can result in a full-blown manic episode. Being aware of potential stressors, monitoring sleep patterns, and ensuring there is adequate time to recover from stressful events, can make it easier to reduce their impact on the individual's life.

Alcohol and other recreational drugs

Drugs that only need to be taken once or for a short time to bring about a change in mood or intellectual functioning or perception have, of course, been around for thousands of years. Many young people experiencing a mood disorder learn very quickly that alcohol, at least in the short term, has some benefits. Alcohol can provide a short period of euphoria so, for people in the depressive phase of a bipolar disorder, the enjoyment of alcohol at the end of a gloomy day is commonly anticipated with eagerness. Unfortunately, of course, over-indulgence in alcohol can make the next day's gloom even darker, so a dependence on alcohol, in order to experience at least some hours of light relief in the evening, can very easily develop.

Thus, it is not surprising that many researchers have found that comorbid substance abuse is common in people living with bipolar disorders, with research studies estimating that between one in five and one in two people with bipolar disorder also have a substance abuse problem.

From a survival point of view, management of substance use is a key factor in staying well. Whether the substance is alcohol, nicotine, marijuana, cocaine, ecstasy or amphetamines, there is now significant evidence that some recreational drugs make episodes of mood disorder worse and prevent the learning of social and emotional skills. Drug use can also cause other medical problems which can make medication management of the mood disorder that much more difficult.

This is not to say that people living with bipolar disorder should not use *any* recreational drugs. But there do seem to be some indications that people with such mood disorders may be more easily addicted to some drugs (Bratfos and Haug, 1968), and that mood disorders, in some cases, can be secondary to recreational drug use (Shobe and Brion, 1971). New drugs and new combinations of drugs appearing on the social scene will always complicate life for people with bipolar disorder.

There may be some substances that people with bipolar disorders should avoid. Cold and flu medications and other 'over the counter' drugs may not necessarily include warnings about the particular sensitivities that people with bipolar disorder may experience. Illicit drugs have the added problem that dosage and contamination vary enormously from batch to batch so it can be impossible to determine a 'safe dose'. Cocaine, and methamphetamine in particular, have caused a rise in psychotic episodes in Australia, and it can take weeks or months for a drug-induced psychotic episode to be brought under control. Drugs such as these can switch a period of elation into a complicated psychotic episode that is difficult to treat and manage.

Most people with a bipolar disorder which has been untreated will have tried non-prescription drugs in an attempt to alleviate the symptoms. These are commonly used to help the sufferer get to sleep, to help cut down on the amount of stimulation, to assist with waking up in the morning, to boost concentration, and to offset the effects of prescribed medication. A frank and open discussion about drug use and medication is essential to challenge assumptions and to educate people about drugs – including illicit, recreational, and 'over the counter drugs' – as well as prescribed drugs.

Some of the reasons for drug use given by people living with bipolar disorder are sensible but some may be based on misinformation, peer pressure or anecdotal experiences. In many cases there are probably better alternatives available via carefully working out the effects of current drugs and developing ideas to get similar effects from other sources with less harmful consequences. Sleep-inducing drugs are a case in point. A tricyclic antidepressant in the bathroom cupboard that, from previous experience, induced drowsiness, might not be the best drug in the early stages of a hypomanic episode. A drug such as olanzapine or clonazepam that can reduce early hypomanic symptoms, and also has the effect of inducing sleep, may be a much better choice.

Eating, exercising and body shape

Ernst Kretschmer noted that people with manic depressive illness were more likely to have a pyknic body type – in essence, short and stocky, and with a tendency to flab and fat. While the idea of body type and its relationship to mental illness and other characteristics such as, say, criminality, is no longer fashionable or supported by any real evidence, the effect of severe or moderate periods of mood disorder, and the drugs used to treat the disorder, can have a big influence on body shape and weight. The combination of medications which cause weight gain, the lack of motivation to exercise during depressive periods and the disturbances in carbohydrate metabolism from many medications can result in a body type that is overweight, full bellied and flabby. A few weeks in hospital on the old phenothiazine tranquillisers could result in a huge gain in weight. Or poor hospital treatment programmes with large meals, no exercise and much sitting around drowsily in the day room could result in the same effect.

Many people living with bipolar disorder report that an episode of mood illness caused a rapid gain or loss in weight. Such rapid weight changes can leave the person feeling powerless to take over control again. So, weight control has to be an important discussion at the beginning of any treatment.

Weight gain is multifactorial – so the remedy must be multifactorial, with several issues noted:

(i)   *Medication effects.* Medication plans should include a discussion about weight gain, particularly if drugs which are known to cause weight gain in a significant number of individuals (such as olanzapine) are being prescribed.

(ii)   *Thirst.* Dry mouth is common with some medications. Lithium alters kidney function and thirst is a common side-effect of lithium treatment. For those who use soft drinks to relieve the thirst, weight gain is a common consequence. So some commonsense guidelines about managing dry mouth and thirst (e.g. by drinking water) are required.

(iii)   *Eating patterns as a consequence of mood disorder.* Common problems in eating patterns for people living with mood disorder include:
  • not feeling like eating in the morning – and therefore skipping breakfast, or using coffee and/or nicotine to overcome an early morning depressive slump
  • having better appetite later in the day – and so eating larger meals at night – often with alcohol.
Over time, such patterns of eating can result in significant weight gain.

(iv)   *Biochemical changes in mood disorder.* Craving carbohydrates is a common biochemical symptom experienced by those with bipolar disorder. Any mood improvement induced by snack foods and pastries is usually transient – the consequent weight gain is less so.

Women and BP II Disorder

The rates for BP II are higher for women. Mood changes following events such as childbirth, abortion and miscarriage may bring women into treatment or encourage them to seek help. Women with bipolar disorder have a much higher risk of experiencing depression, both during pregnancy and following childbirth (and, most commonly, in the first 4 weeks postnatally).

Some women with BP II report moderate to severe premenstrual symptoms. It has long been known that women are more likely to be admitted to psychiatric hospitals during the premenstrual phase. While most women cope with the fluctuations in hormone levels following ovulation, a few women appear to be vulnerable to changes in hormone levels and experience significant mood problems.

Whatever the reason for the higher rates of bipolar disorder and depression reported for women, it should be recognised that women have specific needs when it comes to treatment. Hormonal treatments (whether used for birth control, menopausal symptoms or control of heavy menstrual bleeding) may also affect mood and should be taken into account when discussing treatments with those with bipolar disorders. Drugs used to treat bipolar disorder and which are metabolised in the liver may also affect the reliability of contraceptive pills.

Surviving suicidal thoughts

People with BP II are more vulnerable to suicidal thoughts and more liable to act on them. The first experience of depressive illness can also bring with it suicidal thoughts. Because the depression may appear to be a reactive depression to circumstances at the time, and/or not serious enough to warrant admission to hospital, the seriousness of suicidal ideation can easily be overlooked. Most people who have survived an episode of suicidal thinking learn from the experience and can subsequently recognise that the patterns of thinking are part of the illness. They develop strategies to stop themselves acting on the thoughts and can take quick action to get onto medication to prevent such thoughts.

Tragically, many suicides of young people may be because the first suicidal thoughts are believed and acted upon. Or people are too ashamed or frightened of the thoughts to talk about them to others and to seek help. Many with BP II are high functioning and highly achieving people who are bewildered and confused by suicidal ideation.

Some antidepressant medications are recognised as elevating mood but not reducing suicidal ideation so, as the depression lifts, the individual regains the energy to carry out suicidal or self-harm behaviours. Some of the tricyclic antidepressant drugs prescribed in the 1970s became lethal in combination with a prescription for an anti-anxiety drug.

Some key points in surviving suicidal thoughts

Individuals should be encouraged to talk about the specifics of the thoughts – and then work out what strategies can be put in place to keep safe.

Periods of suicidal thinking often do not last long or can be sporadic – so work out when the worst times are and what can be done to stay safe.

Common strategies nominated as helpful by those with bipolar disorder include:

- being with other people
- keeping harmful objects out of reach
- countering the suicidal thoughts with positive thoughts
- thinking of why you need to survive, and deciding to survive.

And finally ...

Perhaps the real key to surviving and prospering despite BP II is for the individual to decide for themself the upper and lower limits of mood, and what the duration of extreme moods is going to be. Clipping off the tops and bottoms of mood swings can mean that they retain creativity and energy – but without the devastation of the lows, or the chaos and confusion of periods of hypomania. Potentially, we who have bipolar disorder have the greatest probability of creativity, energy, enterprise and sensitivity during our periods of depressive reflection and high energy.

REFERENCES

Bratfos, O. and Haug, J. O. (1968). The course of manic–depressive psychosis. A follow-up investigation of 215 patients. *Acta Psychiatrica Scandinavica*, **44**, 89–112.

Shobe, F. O. and Brion, P. (1971). Long-term prognosis in manic-depressive illness: a follow-up investigation of 111 patients. *Archives of General Psychiatry*, **24**, 334–7.

15

A clinical model for managing Bipolar II Disorder

Gordon Parker

Introduction

As stated earlier in several sections of this book, we currently lack an evidence base for knowing how best to manage Bipolar II Disorder (BP II). We can presume, however, that three modalities (i.e. psychotropic drugs, information and education, wellbeing plans) that have been demonstrated as effective and beneficial for the management of Bipolar I Disorder (BP I) have similar broad relevance. The roles and effectiveness of specific drug classes (i.e. antidepressants, antipsychotics and mood stabilisers) remain unclear, however, and as noted in many of the earlier chapters, it may be erroneous to extrapolate decision rules for psychotropic drugs from guidelines derived for managing BP I Disorder. In the absence of randomised controlled studies, we are left with either opinion or clinical observation – a strategy risking idiosyncratic views. In this chapter, my personal approaches are detailed to lay down a template for consideration. To address concerns about any idiosyncrasies, the views of a number of internationally respected experts are provided as commentaries – either in relation to the template or their independent management observations. As Ghaemi (Chapter 26), quoting Peirce, so percipiently notes, 'Scientific truth is not the purview of any individual but rather flows from the consensus of the community of investigators: we are all in this together'.

Providing a diagnosis and introducing a management plan

While the impact of receiving a diagnosis of bipolar disorder can range from relief to profound distress, most people appreciate a firm diagnosis, particularly if they have had their mood swings misconstrued, misdiagnosed or minimised by others. Family and friends may not have suspected a categorical mood disorder. Health professionals may have merely informed the individual that they have 'depression'

Bipolar II Disorder. Modelling, Measuring and Managing, ed. Gordon Parker. Published by Cambridge University Press. © Cambridge University Press 2008.

or 'clinical depression', or provided alternate and incorrect diagnoses such as 'borderline personality' or 'attention deficit hyperactivity disorder'. A 'new' diagnosis of BP II requires some processing by the individual.

If diagnostic confidence is not strong, it is reasonable for the clinician to state why they are not certain – and the steps that might be needed for clarification. Ideally, the patient will allow a relative to sit in on the diagnostic briefing following history taking – or at a subsequent interview – for a number of reasons. Firstly, to identify any markers of bipolar disorder not detailed by the patient, or to corroborate or clarify diagnostic nuances. Secondly, for the family to be made aware of the diagnosis – and, in particular, allow clarification or challenges to be openly discussed. Thirdly, to assist with 'locking' the patient into a management plan. If a diagnosis is given to the patient only, it is not uncommon for family members to reject any such diagnosis, causing bewilderment in the patient about whether to side with the family or with the clinician. Allowing the family to be present when diagnosis and management options are discussed reduces the chance of disjunction, and promotes family members' involvement and support over time.

There is wisdom in emphasising to the patient that BP II is not the same as 'manic depressive illness', and (my personal view despite some opposing studies) that BP II rarely worsens to a BP I (or psychotic) condition. I tend to suggest to individuals that they have the milder form of bipolar disorder and try to take the edge off the diagnostic impact and their apprehension by suggesting that the 'milder type' is the one 'that the British comedian Stephen Fry has described as 'bipolar lite''. I do emphasise, however, that while the 'highs' are usually not too disabling and may even be associated with greater productivity and superior performance, they can – in addition to presaging a depressive fall – have some mood-specific deleterious effects. I give examples of disinhibition that individuals can relate to theoretically or practically ('Having a tattoo that you really don't want') and which generally evince a wry smile, or I focus on signal behaviours ('Hitting the credit card'; 'Drinking too much alcohol'; 'Driving too fast') that have been identified or alluded to by the patient. Reference to potentially more shameful disinhibited behaviours (e.g. going to prostitutes, taking a job in a strip club) are best avoided as examples. Even if personally relevant, any such detailing may 'spook' the patient and reify the mortification that they attach to such normally uncharacteristic behaviours, which can then increase any shame that they associate with their illness.

I suggest to the patient that most people enjoy their highs, and that they are genuinely likely to be more creative and productive up to a certain level, but go on to note that the risk carried by significant highs (above and beyond events driven by the high at that time) is the subsequent depression – and it is the depression that puts the argument for treatment. Many individuals are concerned that medication will take away the pleasure or creativity they experience when high, or cause them to feel that they are no longer 'themselves'. Such issues are either raised by patients early after diagnosis, or are not articulated but influence ongoing ambivalence about taking medication and continuing with professional help.

The lever, then, to encourage the patient to accept treatment is generally the severity of the depression associated with BP II, and which – as detailed in Chapter 4 – is (overall) as severe and impairing as the depression experienced by those with BP I depression.

It is worth emphasising that the condition will not compromise any of their aspirations or plans in life – including work, marriage, parenthood. There are few exceptions to this working rule. For example, I remain unsure whether a person with BP II should continue as an airline pilot, even if the condition is well controlled. Such rare exceptions should not challenge the need to make such a positive statement.

Management plans should be pluralistic, involving a mix of medication and 'well-being' plans, with the components considered below, first in relation to medication.

Medication strategies

Mood stabilisation is clearly a primary objective but not easy to achieve for three principal reasons. First, as detailed elsewhere, we lack an evidence base to inform us whether those mood stabilisers used for managing BP I are efficacious for managing BP II. Secondly, we lack the capacity to clearly predict which medication options are most likely to be beneficial. It is therefore wise to forewarn patients that, while their condition can be brought under control, it is difficult for the clinician to estimate whether they will achieve benefit with the first drug trialled or with subsequent drugs – or even with combinations that may need to be trialled over months and sometimes years. While this is disappointing news for most, it preempts later disappointment and is generally wiser than suggesting rapid improvement and control. It also builds to the third issue and one that underlies the management paradigm – 'quick fix' drug strategies for BP II are rare, and this is an ongoing condition that needs to be 'managed' rather than viewed as able to be 'cured'.

Drug management will be considered in relation to the three commonest scenarios: mood stabilisation, managing episodes of 'bipolar depression' and managing 'break-through' highs.

Mood stabilisation

There appears to be little doubt that orthodox mood stabilisers (e.g. lithium, valproate) are beneficial for many patients with BP II. Further, and as discussed in Chapter 9, many clinicians and researchers judge lamotrigine as beneficial; in some regions of the world, it is the first medication trialled by many clinicians. However, all mood stabilisers have a risk of side effects, some quite serious, and while the argument to commence mood stabilisation with one of these drugs appears relatively straightforward (and is the approach adopted by most clinicians), their cost: benefit can be problematic.

In light of such concerns it is my practice to first trial an SSRI. As noted in Chapters 7 and 8, while the SSRIs (as for all effective antidepressants) can result in individuals reporting manic or hypomanic 'switching' and increased mood swing cycling, I suggest that such risks are far lower than generally viewed. Further, our SSRI 'proof of concept' study (Chapter 8) was consistent with our clinical observations over the last decade in suggesting that some 40–50% of patients with BP II report effective mood stabilising (albeit more distinctly for depressive episodes) with an SSRI. However, about one half of those who report such clear mood stabilising benefits to me describe a progressive 'poop out' effect after some months or years. If an SSRI (or venlafaxine monotherapy) fails, I then move to a formal mood stabiliser but argue that it is worth trialling an SSRI initially as the cost: benefit ratio is generally superior, largely in terms of fewer significant side effects (and thus better patient adherence). If those drugs cause increased switching or cycling, a lower dose is trialled before necessarily rejecting the strategy and moving to a formal mood stabiliser.

I also recommend that BP II patients trial fish oil (omega-3 fatty acid) supplementation in combination with other medication. Again there are no data for its use in those with BP II, but studies of those with bipolar disorder (see Chapter 11) suggest some limited support. In those trials where it has been reported to be efficacious, fish oil supplementation tended to be of greater benefit for the depressed phase than for highs, a finding also observed by us clinically. Further, our observations suggest that only 5–10% of those with BP II report distinct improvement with fish oil, with 'improvement' being either reduced cycle frequency or intensity, or the individual being able to lower their dose of mood stabiliser or antidepressant medication. While there appears to be a low overall benefit, fish oil supplementation has high acceptability by those with mood disorders. In essence, while many patients are concerned about taking psychotropic drugs for short or for extended periods (often reflecting concerns about becoming 'dependent' on such drugs), they view fish oil as a 'natural' strategy. Even if only beneficial for a small percentage, trialling appears warranted in light of side-effects being rare and acceptability high.

While most of the atypical antipsychotic drugs have been demonstrated in controlled trials as efficacious mood stabilisers for those with BP I, there are limited data in relation to their application in BP II, as reviewed principally in Chapter 10. My personal view is not to use them as mood stabilisers in light of the risk of long-term side effects, unless the patient has failed several formal mood stabilisers.

Bipolar depression

Most BP II patients will present with an episode of depression as the immediate management focus, with subsequent break-through episodes of depression common and concerning. While all treatment guidelines for managing BP I recommend commencing a depressed patient on a mood stabiliser before initiating an antidepressant, as noted in several sections of this book it is likely that the risk of 'switching' is not as high as previously judged. My personal practice is to immediately commence an antidepressant drug. If the patient has not previously received any antidepressant, I first trial an SSRI (thereby seeking to relieve the depression and then, during maintenance, to examine its impact as a mood stabiliser). If minimal or no improvement occurs after one week, I augment the SSRI with low dose olanzapine (1.25 – 5 mg nocte). If the patient is going to respond to this regime, our data indicate that improvement will occur in one week or less, so I seek to cease the olanzapine in the week following recovery to avoid the risk of side effects. If this regime fails, or is successful but the patient's depression returns after ceasing olanzapine, I regard the SSRI as having too narrow a spectrum of action as a maintenance antidepressant for that patient, and taper and cease the SSRI. I then trial venlafaxine, using a similar regime (i.e. initially as monotherapy; if unsuccessful, then adding low-dose olanzapine for one week, and then, if the patient's depression has resolved, ceasing the latter one week later). If this approach fails, a similar process involving a tricyclic antidepressant and sometimes an MAOI (i.e. alone and then augmented briefly) is trialled.

Our Clinic model is based on the following logic. Firstly, that antidepressants vary in terms of the 'spread' or 'spectrum' of their actions. For example, the 'narrow-spectrum' SSRIs principally affect the serotonergic system; dual action drugs (such as venlafaxine) have both noradrenergic and serotonergic actions; while the TCAs and MAOIs are broad-action drugs (affecting serotonergic, noradrenergic and dopaminergic systems). As BP II depression is most commonly melancholic depression, broader-spectrum antidepressants are generally more effective (overall) than narrow-spectrum strategies. Secondly, I personally view the atypical antipsychotic drug olanzapine as being distinctly more efficacious than other atypical antipsychotic drugs in augmenting antidepressant drugs (i.e. broadening the spectrum of impact), possibly as a reflection of its impact on multiple (dopaminergic, serotonergic, adrenergic, histaminergic and muscarinic) receptors. In further support, we have had patients respond well to olanzapine augmentation having failed augmentation with other atypical antipsychotic drugs, and have reported both a series of case studies examining its augmentation propensity (Parker and Malhi, 2001), and a 'proof of concept' study (Parker *et al.*, 2005) suggesting that olanzapine augmentation of an antidepressant drug is associated with either greater efficacy and/or more rapid onset of action effects than use of an antidepressant drug alone. In the latter paper, we noted a phenomenon previously described in relation to lithium augmentation of antidepressant medication – that the addition of olanzapine after the antidepressant has been prescribed for a few days appears to be associated with a more distinct and rapid remission effect than their co-prescription, and it may be that there is a need for the antidepressant to first sensitise the serotonin receptor.

Some 40–60% of those with melancholic depression (both unipolar and BP II depressed individuals) will report rapid remission in 1–7 days after adding low-dose olanzapine. In one study (Parker, 2002), we showed that olanzapine was associated with an immediate impact on sleep and anxiety levels and a slower impact (over days) on mood improvement, suggesting that the antidepressant effect is not merely due to anxiolytic or sedative effects. We view such a strategy as akin to ECT in terms of the treatment logic. As ECT is commonly ceased once remission has occurred, we similarly argue that there should be no need for olanzapine to be continued once remission has occurred and that it should be redundant if the maintenance antidepressant and/or mood stabiliser is 'intrinsically' efficacious. If the latter criterion is not met, we argue for changing that regime rather than continuing the olanzapine augmentation. We also seek to cease the olanzapine rapidly as a consequence of the high prevalence of weight gain and other concerning side effects experienced by many receiving this drug over longer periods. If the patient appears to require an ongoing antipsychotic for augmentation (which is generally rare in BP II), we generally use an alternate atypical antipsychotic with fewer long-term side effects.

It is important to note that a significant percentage of depressed patients will experience a 'high' following olanzapine augmentation (including unipolar patients who have never reported a high or antidepressant-induced switching). Usually it is mild and transient and does not require any specific treatment. It is easily missed. The patient who thanks the clinician for the rapid benefit ('It's a miracle Doc') can invoke clinician satisfaction or relief – but should also invite review as to whether the patient has had their mood 'switch'.

The logic to the model just detailed is worthy of restating. It assumes that (i) a narrow-spectrum antidepressant drug may work and – as it is likely to have fewer side-effects – is therefore an appropriate initial strategy, (ii) if such an antidepressant drug fails, the move should be to introduce progressively more broad-spectrum antidepressants, which, while likely to be more effective, risk more troubling side effects, (iii) olanzapine (and, less commonly, other atypical antipsychotics and lithium) effectively broaden the spectrum of action of the base antidepressant and may effect a 'jump lead to the battery' phenomenon in inducing remission, but that (iv) any such augmentor should be able to be ceased and antidepressant monotherapy maintained if *that* antidepressant is sufficiently broad spectrum in its action to maintain remission – if an antidepressant is required for maintenance. Unfortunately, the intrinsic propensity of any antidepressant class to provide maintenance can rarely be estimated prospectively.

If antidepressant monotherapy does not induce remission or fails to maintain adequate mood stabilisation, I then trial the addition of a formal mood stabiliser. If initiated and the patient becomes euthymic, the next consideration is generally whether to continue the two drugs (i.e. mood stabiliser and the antidepressant) or to taper and cease the antidepressant. The ideal objective of maintaining the patient on a mood stabiliser alone appears to be successful in only a minority (say, one-third). Another one-third of patients appear to benefit from a combination of mood stabiliser and antidepressant drugs, but here the clinician needs to watch for periods when the antidepressant drug may be causing more switching or, more commonly for the broader action antidepressants, new or more frequent 'mixed states'. Such changes (either detected from the patient's mood chart or from their symptom report) may require lowering the dose of the antidepressant, ceasing it, or trialling an alternate antidepressant (usually a narrower spectrum antidepressant).

Bipolar 'highs' or hypomania

In comparison to the manic episodes of BP I – and where there are distinct behavioural changes, risks of collateral damage at work and with family, and/or hospitalisation, and where medication is generally required, BP II hypomanic episodes do not always necessitate medication changes. For those not receiving any medication, drug choice will more be determined by the severity and impact of depressive episodes than by the highs. For those who are taking medication, distinctive hypomanic episodes or break-through highs argue the need for medication readjustments and/or adjustments to wellbeing plans. The clinician should not necessarily seek to eradicate the mild highs (when life is enjoyable and efficiency is also high) for those many individuals who can handle them. An informed patient is often the best judge – a corroborative witness (e.g. family member) the next most useful.

Non-drug management components

If a patient with BP II is to be managed successfully, the following components are as important as medication strategies. Firstly, education. Secondly, mood charting.

Thirdly, the development of a wellbeing plan. All three components are subsumed by an operating principle. When an individual is informed that they have bipolar disorder it has a major impact, threatening their image, their identity and the way in which they see themselves in the world and their own future. It can be akin to an adolescent being told that they have Type I diabetes or another major chronic medical illness. After impact and 'why me' phases, most individuals feel controlled by their illness. Such a feeling of loss of control or mastery settles over time as the individual comes to terms with the numerous challenges, so that after years (rarely months) the individual feels more that *they* control *it* rather than feeling that *it* controls *them*. We believe that a key objective to managing bipolar disorder, one principally addressed by education, is to reduce that interval. The move is from 'I am a Bipolar sufferer' to 'I am me and I have bipolar disorder. I am not defined by my condition'.

While medication is almost invariably necessary to control bipolar disorder it is rarely sufficient. While medication may be primary, it has downside risks. Firstly, drugs are usually prescribed within an innately hierarchical system, where the doctor holds the expertise, and writes prescriptions and recommends certain drugs one above another. The patient predictably is a recipient of a process that is not easily able to be assimilated. This is not to criticise such system nuances but more to consider their impact. Over the months or the years, the hierarchical system can reinforce the patient's natural concern about their need to take medication, activating perceptions that the medication may be changing their true self or that they may be overly dependent on it. Essentially, the patient lacks 'ownership'.

Strategies that involve a patient in their own management therefore have the capacity to build to a more reciprocal and collaborative management model linking the clinician and the patient. Such a model allows that the clinician will have more expertise in certain areas (e.g. medication choice) and the patient in other areas (e.g. non-drug strategies that 'work for me'). In addition, educational components, mood charting and wellbeing plans have their own advantages, now detailed.

Education

With so much excellent information available, presumably every clinician (whatever their professional background) provides their patient with some education about the nature and nuances of BP II. In addition, there are general sources of education that can be recommended. While there have been many books written about bipolar disorder, including academic texts such as Goodwin and Jamison's *Manic-Depressive Illness*, and personal accounts such as Kay Jamison's *An Unquiet Mind*, textbooks and autobiographies tend to focus on BP I. Encouraging a patient with BP II Disorder to read the autobiography of an individual with BP I can be disconcerting and inappropriate, heightening concerns that they might develop psychotic episodes and be hospitalised. This makes the treating health professional even more relevant as a source of appropriate and less confronting information.

In addition to the patient receiving education, it is also important that relevant relatives or friends involve themselves in aspects of that educational programme or in independent educational activities, ideally with the agreement and support of the patient. Carer groups, when well managed, can be a superb source of general education, practical wisdom and support.

Patients, relatives and those in the general community now increasingly turn to the web to receive education about medical and psychiatric conditions. There are many excellent websites providing information about BP I, but few that provide education on BP II. The risk of encouraging a patient with BP II to go to a more generic website is, again, to have the patient disconcerted, and even receive misleading information if it is weighted to BP I management. In regard to this, the Black Dog Institute's website (blackdoginstitute.org.au) has a modular educational programme that articulates differences between BP I and BP II, considers the common management ingredients and draws attention to specific nuances in relation to BP II. Research studies looking at the effectiveness of delivering information about the management of depression via this mode have found it to be both beneficial and appreciated by patients and consumers. 'E-health' strategies for bipolar disorder will clearly develop further and rapidly over the next few years, and will benefit from research evaluation.

Mood charting

Mood charting is not new. Virginia Woolf had her mood swings charted by her husband for over 40 years. Charting has a number of advantages to both the patient and to the clinician. An ideal mood chart should allow the patient to chart – at the end of each day – the extent to which their mood was 'high' and/or 'low' and to rate the severity of each swing extreme. In addition, it should note medication or medication changes, whether there were any particular triggers (e.g. alcohol, drugs, overseas travel, break-up of a relationship) and the level of impairment across that particular day. A representative mood chart is available on our website (blackdoginstitute.org.au) but frequently patients will feel even more empowered if they develop their own, and some show great imagination in creating a computer-based system. One patient decided that one of her key perturbing symptoms was feeling 'scratchy' – in essence a 'mixed state'. In addition to charting 'highs', 'lows' and intensity of 'scratchiness', she also rated her pleasure in life and anxiety levels, but also built in an 'ennui' pole.

At the finish of our 9-month trial of SSRI antidepressants as mood stabilisers (see Chapter 8), we provided our subjects with a number of educational 'take aways' and a copy of their study mood chart. Invariably they rated the 9-month record of their daily mood swings as the most important piece of material, and most felt encouraged to continue to chart their moods subsequently.

For the clinician, the patient's ongoing mood chart is also invaluable. Most clinicians record information reflecting either the functioning of the patient at the time of their visit or some 'product moment' of the interval between visits. This misses the richness of the potentially available interval information. For most patients with BP II it takes months or years to find the ideal medication, combination medication or overall management programme. A mood chart over that extended period provides the clinician with a permanent record of differing interventions, enabling judgement of whether 'tweaks' or substantive management changes were associated with changes observed by the patient and recorded in the mood chart.

Wellbeing plans

As detailed in Chapter 13, the development of such a plan can be of fundamental importance to so many with BP II. It locks the patient into a more collaborative endeavour, gives them greater 'ownership' of their condition, promotes self-management and advances the process whereby the patient feels that they are able to control it rather than be controlled by their bipolar disorder. Importantly, the information that is generated to produce a successful wellbeing plan is often new information to the clinician or outside the clinician's general list of management strategies. For example, most clinicians view certain self-help strategies (e.g. exercise) as, at best, possibly effective at times or of no relevance, even fatuous. However, many individuals with BP II will identify exercise (or some other self-help strategy) as of fundamental importance to them at some time during the course of their disorder. When asked later in their 'journey' (see Wigney et al., 2007) to nominate factors contributing to their successful self-management, these strategies are generally nominated ahead of medication or ahead of the mental health professional. Professionals should not find such information galling. Just as most people who have survived a cancer nominate their coping style rather than their surgeon, it is a rather back-handed compliment that medical competence is taken as a given and that the professional will easily determine the right medication for their condition. Also, while some people merely wish to lie back and have the cancer cut out or the problem go away, most people who cope well wish to contribute to their own improvement. The contributions that work for the individual patient can rarely be predicted by the clinician. It is often outside the clinician's purview. Thus, there is often little commonality between the information derived at clinical assessment and the development of a wellbeing plan.

It is problematic to know when best, following diagnosis, is the optimal time to develop a wellbeing plan, and whether it should be a task undertaken by the managing clinician or by another health professional. My own approach is to encourage the patient to start mood charting immediately after a diagnosis is made, and to focus on implementing initial medication strategies, reflecting the fact that most patients usually present at a time when they are significantly depressed. It seems appropriate to start to develop a wellbeing plan when the individual is functioning reasonably and this usually requires their depression to be under sufficient control. While many clinicians successfully combine clinical management and the development of a wellbeing plan, I generally choose to refer patients to a psychologist, who will understand the nuances involved in developing such a plan and, when identifying a particular problem area, be competent in implementing appropriate psychological strategies.

Psychotherapy

For an extended period, we tended to overly weight the contribution of medication to the management of bipolar disorder. In the last decade or more there has been an increasing appreciation of the role of the psychotherapies in assisting those with bipolar disorder, whether BP I or BP II, as detailed in Chapter 12. The majority of studies of adding a psychotherapy to pharmacotherapy show a range of benefits to those with bipolar disorder.

Initial concerns that psychotherapy did little more than improve adherence to medication were allayed by a number of studies showing that psychotherapy had additional benefits. It is a feature now of many guidelines to recommend a psychotherapy as a mandatory component to a management package, whether it be for bipolar or for a unipolar depressive disorder. However, it is worth considering why any particular psychotherapy might add value rather than necessarily accept such findings at face value.

The psychotherapies have many constituent ingredients, both specific and non-specific. Specific components mandate a target or goal to be addressed. This could represent dealing with bipolar disorder itself – perhaps in assisting the patient to accommodate to the conditions, or nuances related to the disorder and its consequences. Such issues may be addressed by psychotherapy but are as likely to be addressed by the development of a wellbeing plan with a particular patient. Additionally, though, there will be individuals with bipolar disorder who have independent issues that are not resolved by the strategies detailed above and who would benefit from a psychotherapeutic approach. However, and as many patients with bipolar disorder are fortunate in responding well to medication, it strikes me that a psychotherapy should not be mandated as a 'necessary' component.

As noted, psychotherapy also has non-specific ingredients. Ideally, an empathic and understanding therapist providing the patient with an opportunity to detail their world and receive understanding, support and cogent counselling. Such components are not unique to psychotherapy and should be elements of a pluralistic approach by the mental health professional. As many professionals have focused on the prescription of psychotropic medications and moved away from spending time with the patient, a case for psychotherapy emerges – addressing that therapeutic vacuum. While there are patients who are well served by independent professionals who focus separately on medication, and on interpersonal and psychotherapeutic issues, there are also therapists who offer a pluralistic approach. As Kay Jamison (1995) wrote in *An Unquiet Mind*: 'Lithium ... diminishes my depression ... gentles me out ... But, ineffably, psychotherapy heals'. Further: 'The debt I owe my psychiatrist is beyond description . . . all the . . . things he didn't say that kept me alive . . . all the compassion and warmth . . . and his granite belief that mine was a life worth saving . . . Most difficult to put into words, but in many ways, the essence of everything.'

Thus, some of the studies that have shown the benefit of including a psychotherapy in conjunction with pharmacotherapy may not have demonstrated any distinct benefit from psychotherapy per se but more the benefit from a pluralistic approach. To the extent that the last is true, then it raises certain ways of proceeding. Firstly, it is unlikely that psychotherapy is necessary for all patients with BP II. Thus, rather than regard a psychotherapy as a necessary component to be mandated in a therapeutic package, there is wisdom in considering whether there are definable problems that might be best addressed by a psychotherapeutic approach. If so, the issue is whether they are likely to be appropriately dealt with by a pluralistic management plan or require an added-on therapy. This can be resolved, generally, by putting the option to the patient and respecting their priorities.

Conclusions

This chapter argues for a pluralistic approach which prioritises medication, education, mood charting and the development of a wellbeing plan, ideally involving the patient's family and weighting a strong self-management component. The aims are to ensure greater control of the mood swings and to allow the patient to move to a stage where, while recognising that they have BP II, they are not defined by the condition and feel that they can control it. Some specific nuances in regard to medication strategies reflect a personal approach and this will now be counterbalanced by the viewpoints of others with experience in managing BP II.

REFERENCES

Jamison, K. (1995). *An Unquiet Mind: A Memoir of Moods and Madness*. New York: Alfred A. Knopf.

Parker, G. (2002). Olanzapine augmentation in the treatment of melancholia: the trajectory of improvement in rapid responders. *Journal of Clinical Psychopharmacology*, **17**, 87–9.

Parker, G. and Malhi, G. (2001). Are atypical antidepressant drugs also atypical antidepressants? *Australian and New Zealand Journal of Psychiatry*, **35**, 677–83.

Parker, G., Brotchie, H. and Parker, K. (2005). Is combination olanzapine and antidepressant medication associated with a more rapid response trajectory than antidepressant alone? *American Journal of Psychiatry*, **162**, 796–8.

Wigney, T., Eyers, K. and Parker, G. (2007). *Journeys with the Black Dog. Inspirational Stories of Bringing Depression to Heel*. Sydney: Allen & Unwin.

16

Management commentary

Terence A. Ketter and Po W. Wang

Introduction

As noted by Parker, management of Bipolar II Disorder is challenging for several reasons, including the scarcity of controlled data to inform evidence-based care. Such limited data mean that clinicians commonly extrapolate information regarding BP I and/or (unipolar) major depressive disorder, and view BP II as an intermediate category. Such an approach has strengths and limitations. One notable limitation is that it may underemphasise the heterogeneity of BP II, a condition with substantial inter-patient variability.

Thus, some patients with BP II may have an illness more like major depressive disorder: relatively infrequent recurrent pure (with minimal mixed features) depressive episodes, rare hypomanias, and – with antidepressants – they experience relief of depression without treatment-emergent affective switch (TEAS) into hypomania or accelerating episodes. Antidepressants may be considered foundational treatments for this presentation. In academic centres with specialty clinics, such patients are more likely referred to major depressive disorder clinics, where clinicians may view antidepressants as the treatment of choice for this type of BP II.

However, other patients with BP II may have an illness more akin to BP I. These patients experience relatively frequent recurrent depressive episodes that include mixed features (in some instances with concurrent depression and hypomania, i.e. dysphoric hypomania), common hypomanias and, in some instances, rapid cycling. Antidepressants give inadequate relief of their depression and can confer TEAS, and/or cycle acceleration. For these patients, mood stabilisers or atypical antipsychotics – not antidepressants – may be considered foundational treatments. In academic centres, such patients are more likely referred to bipolar disorder clinics, where clinicians may view antidepressants as potentially problematic for this type of BP II.

Clinicians in the community, compared to providers in subspecialty depression or bipolar disorder clinics, arguably face greater challenges related to the full

Bipolar II Disorder. Modelling, Measuring and Managing, ed. Gordon Parker. Published by Cambridge University Press. © Cambridge University Press 2008.

spectrum of clinical heterogeneity in patients with BP II. They need to administer individually tailored treatments, carefully balancing the relative risks and benefits of intervening with antidepressants.

Parker observes that, as a consequence of the scarcity of controlled data regarding BP II, we turn to either opinion or clinical observation – approaches that risk idiosyncratic views. This chapter provides a synthesis of the scarce controlled data combined with personal observations.

Providing a diagnosis and introducing a management plan

The approach to diagnosis described by Parker is sound. Certain aspects benefit from additional emphasis. Involvement of a family member or significant other is not only ideal, but is arguably mandatory for the accurate diagnosis of BP II. The DSM–IV criteria for a hypomanic episode tacitly suggests that a collateral objective information source is required, as the change in mood and function during hypomania needs to be objectively evident (American Psychiatric Association, 2000). Hypomanic episodes which, by definition, are not severe, may be viewed by the patient as not abnormal or problematic, while they are more sensitive to reporting clinically relevant depression or anhedonia. Hypomanic episodes may, in fact, be seen as times of 'enhanced' health. Furthermore, as patients commonly present with depression, state-dependent memory effects may impair their ability to recall features of prior hypomanic episodes. Thus, a lack of collateral information may result in a misdiagnosis of major depression or Bipolar Disorder Not Otherwise Specified (NOS), rather than the appropriate BP II diagnosis.

Similarly, lack of collateral information may result in a misdiagnosis of BP II in a patient who actually has BP I. This risk is perhaps greatest where episodes of mood elevation have not involved psychosis or hospitalisation (which makes the diagnosis of a syndromal manic or mixed episode more straightforward), but have involved an indeterminate (moderate versus severe) degree of interpersonal or occupational dysfunction. One limitation of the DSM–IV distinction between hypomanic and manic or mixed episodes is the lack of an operationalised approach to quantifying the degree of dysfunction, and attributing causality of such dysfunction to mood elevation episodes. It can be challenging to quantify whether dysfunction is 'severe' (as required for manic and mixed episodes) or merely 'mild to moderate' (as required for hypomanic episodes). Although histories of bankruptcy, incarceration, multiple relationship failures or multiple employment terminations indicate severe dysfunction, the degree to which such problems relate to episodes of mood elevation as opposed to episodes of depression, comorbid Axis I and Axis II psychiatric disorders, comorbid medical disorders, or environmental factors, can vary widely. In patients, denial and other factors may lead to underestimating the degree or relationship of dysfunction to episodes of mood elevation. Observers can provide crucial additional information to aid in assessing these factors.

When even collateral information yields an indeterminate assessment, a convention of 'rounding-upwards', from major depressive disorder to Bipolar Disorder NOS, from Bipolar Disorder NOS to BP II, and from BP II to BP I, may be a worthwhile approach. Such 'erring on the side of bipolarity' would be expected to decrease the risk of iatrogenic illness otherwise exacerbated by administration of unopposed (in the absence of anti-manic counterbalance), or inadequately opposed, antidepressant therapy. Additionally, this appreciation of bipolarity over unipolar depression focuses patients' attention towards monitoring the frequent associations between hypomanic and depressive episodes, so countering their tendency to long for the return of the periods of productive hypomania, and their ensuing neglect of the risk of the subsequent depression.

The use of a structured assessment instrument such as the Mood Disorders Questionnaire (MDQ) (Hirschfeld *et al.*, 2000), modified to include input from both the patient and an observer, can more rigorously assess for a history of symptoms of mood elevation, and also serve as an educational tool to inform clients and significant others of crucial symptoms that can herald a mood elevation.

Some patients are focused on obtaining a definitive categorical diagnosis of either bipolar disorder or major depressive disorder, and are distressed by any ambiguity. In instances where the patient's diagnosis appears to be at the boundary of a category, a dimensional approach emphasising commonalities across categories may prove useful. For example, mood stabilisers may yield benefit in those patients with frequently recurring major depressive disorder who have subthreshold mood elevation symptoms on the MDQ, and antidepressant resistance.

Care must be taken in helping patients assess the significance of having BP II. In some respects (less disabling mood elevation, lower risk of problems with antidepressants), BP II might be considered less severe than BP I. However, in other respects, such as depressive illness burden and consequent risk of suicidal acts, BP II may be considered equally or even more severe. An alternative to considering BP II as 'bipolar lite' is to focus on the benefits of client awareness of mood fluctuations (via, for example, mood charting) and on the currently available and emerging therapeutic options available for optimising functional outcomes. A balanced assessment can be formed by individualising patients' expectations based on prognostic factors such as age of onset, comorbid psychiatric and medical disorders, and the presence or absence of treatment resistance, psychosis, rapid cycling or TEAS. Advising patients to avoid trivialising the disorder (leading to non-adherence) or catastrophising it (leading to diminished life goals and expectations) can also help promote an appropriate assessment. Many patients can expect that a reasonable lifestyle (e.g. avoiding sleep deprivation and excessive alcohol), plus medical and psychological efforts, will allow minimal symptoms and normal function. However, in spite of such efforts, some patients will experience a more difficult course, with frequently recurrent or chronic episodes. In such instances, characterised by inadequate efficacy or tolerability with multiple medications, the contribution of psychosocial interventions becomes even more crucial.

As suggested by Parker, a desire to relieve and prevent depressive episodes is a key commonality for clinicians and patients from the outset. Over time, however, clinicians may be able to enhance patients' appreciation of the need to control symptoms of mood elevation so as to minimise the risk of triggering depression, and other problems more directly related to mood elevation (irritability, impulsivity), that can compromise longer-term interpersonal or occupational function.

Medication strategies

Parker provides a persuasive argument that mood stabilisation is a primary objective for patients with BP II, but it may not be easy to achieve. Although the evidence base to inform therapeutics is limited, it is encouraging for patients that therapeutic data are steadily expanding. Thus, there are controlled data supporting (in rank order): the use of quetiapine in acute BP II depression (Calabrese *et al.*, 2005; Thase *et al.*, 2006); lamotrigine maintenance in rapid-cycling BP II (Calabrese *et al.*, 2000); lithium in acute BP II depression (Goodwin *et al.*, 1972; Baron *et al.*, 1975), and for maintenance treatment (Dunner *et al.*, 1976; Fieve *et al.*, 1976; Quitkin *et al.*, 1978; Tondo *et al.*, 1997, 1998); and the use of antidepressants in acute BP II depression (Himmelhoch *et al.*, 1991; Amsterdam, 1998; Amsterdam *et al.*, 1998, 2004; Amsterdam and Garcia-Espana, 2000; Amsterdam and Brunswick, 2003). Next, we consider medication approaches from the perspectives of achieving mood stabilisation, treating episodes of acute BP II depression, and managing 'break-through' mood elevation.

Mood stabilisation

Clinicians commonly commence pharmacotherapy with the medication having the fewest adverse effects that adequately addresses the patient's particular psychiatric disorder. This approach assumes that efficacy is generally equivalent for the therapeutic options. Thus, antidepressants might be considered foundational agents for some patients with BP II, in view of their generally favourable adverse effect profiles. However, mood stabilisers or atypical antipsychotics may be foundational agents for patients with psychosis, concurrent hypomania (dysphoric hypomania), rapid cycling or antidepressant TEAS.

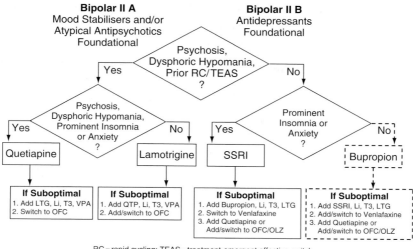

Figure 16.1. Proposed treatment scheme for acute Bipolar II depression.

Figure 16.1 maps an approach which defines a BP II 'A' sub-group with an illness more akin to a BP I disorder. Such patients crucially require interventions to stabilise mood from 'Above baseline' (i.e. addressing hypomania and dysphoric hypomania). For this sub-group, mood stabilisers and/or atypical antipsychotics could prove to be foundational treatments (Bipolar II **A**, Figure 16.1 – left). Such a group might also include patients with psychotic depressive episodes, as such episodes crucially require antipsychotics. However, a different sub-group, Bipolar II 'B', might have an illness more like unipolar major depressive disorder, primarily requiring interventions to stabilise mood from 'Below baseline' (i.e. addressing depression). For this group antidepressants could be foundational agents (Bipolar II **B**, Figure 16.1 – right).

This approach takes into account the possibility that, for Bipolar II A patients, the risk:benefit analysis does not favour antidepressants as these agents may exacerbate their illness (going against the Hippocratic maxim of 'first do no harm'), or may fail to provide expedient benefits for their illness (going against the contemporary clinical practice of trying to relieve symptoms as quickly as possible). In the absence of an adequate evidence base for the treatment of BP II Disorder, Figure 16.1 provides a schema for determining whether to rely more upon evidence regarding BP I, or psychotic unipolar major depressive disorder (in patients with Bipolar II A); or upon data regarding non-psychotic unipolar major depressive disorder (in patients with Bipolar II B).

Thus, for those with Bipolar II B, the approach described by Parker – or variants (Figure 16.1 – right) may best address the desire for minimal risk of adverse effects and expedient relief of acute depression. However, for those with Bipolar II A, other approaches (Figure 16.1 – left) may provide a more favourable risk:benefit ratio. To give an example: the generally favourable tolerability profile of lamotrigine is sufficiently comparable to that of antidepressants, so this agent may be preferable in patients with presentations associated with poorer outcomes with antidepressants (e.g. rapid cycling, or a history of TEAS). Some instances, such as presentations with psychosis, dysphoric hypomania, or prominent insomnia or anxiety, may even favour the use of an agent such as quetiapine with more adverse effects but with more compelling evidence of utility in acute BP II depression (Calabrese et al., 2005; Thase et al., 2006), and also with a reputation for relief of symptoms of psychosis, mood elevation, insomnia and anxiety (Bowden et al., 2005; McIntyre et al., 2005; Hirschfeld et al., 2006).

Unfortunately, there are few data from randomised controlled trials to inform the making of such decisions. Nevertheless, these findings considering the utility of antidepressants as maintenance treatments in bipolar disorder are not encouraging, and suggest that tricyclic antidepressant monotherapy is no better than placebo (Prien et al., 1973; Kane et al., 1982). They also find that lithium is superior compared not only to placebo (Prien et al., 1973; Dunner et al., 1976; Fieve et al., 1976; Dunner et al., 1982; Kane et al., 1982), but also compared to tricyclic antidepressant monotherapy (Prien et al., 1973; Kane et al., 1982; Prien, 1984) and to carbamazepine monotherapy (Greil et al., 1997). Moreover, adding tricyclic antidepressants to lithium failed to provide additional efficacy compared to lithium monotherapy (Wehr and Goodwin, 1979; Quitkin et al., 1981; Prien, 1984). Some, but not all, of the above studies included patients with BP II, which limits their interpretation. For example, when considering the sub-set of patients with BP II Disorder or Bipolar Disorder NOS, limited data suggest that carbamazepine may have advantages over lithium maintenance (Greil et al., 1998; Greil and Kleindienst, 1999). In a more recent trial, lamotrigine appeared effective compared to placebo, on some outcome measures, in maintenance treatment of rapid-cycling bipolar disorder, with the benefit driven by particular efficacy in rapid-cycling BP II (Calabrese et al., 2000).

Randomised controlled studies of maintenance treatment with atypical antipsychotics in patients with BP II are lacking. In BP I patients, olanzapine (Tohen et al., 2005, 2006) and aripiprazole (Keck et al., 2006) appeared to be effective maintenance treatments, but with both agents the benefit appeared to be efficacy in preventing mood elevation, rather than depression.

This proposed schema has substantial limitations, including an inadequate evidence base to confirm the validity of such a subtyping of BP II, or the utility of these agents for either the acute treatment (with the exception of quetiapine) – or maintenance treatment (with the possible exception of lamotrigine in rapid cyclers) – of BP II. Nevertheless, this formulation may provide testable hypotheses regarding the heterogeneity of BP, and relationships to treatment responses.

Parker points to the possible value of adjunctive therapies such as fish oil (omega-3 fatty acid). Although the evidence base for such therapies is limited and benefits may be modest, the adjunctive use of 'nutriceuticals' such as fish oil or folic acid appears to entail minimal risk of adverse effects, can enhance the therapeutic alliance (particularly if these interventions are proposed by the patient), and may provide a benign way to satisfy the urge to intervene pharmaco-logically, thus permitting existing therapies sufficient time to take effect.

Bipolar depression

Syndromal and sub-syndromal depression is by far the most pervasive problem for patients with BP II (Judd *et al.*, 2003). For patients with Bipolar II B, using antidepressants as foundational agents as described by Parker may minimise adverse effects and is supported by some systematic evidence (Himmelhoch *et al.*, 1991; Amsterdam, 1998; Amsterdam *et al.*, 1998, 2004; Amsterdam and Garcia-Espana, 2000; Amsterdam and Brunswick, 2003). Parker describes the following step-based strategy:

(1) start with an SSRI, and temporarily add low-dose olanzapine if necessary;
(2) if ineffective, switch to a similar strategy with a broader spectrum antidepressant (venlafaxine);
(3) if ineffective, switch to a similar strategy with a yet broader spectrum antidepressant (tricyclic);
(4) if ineffective, switch to a similar strategy with an even broader spectrum antidepressant (monoamine oxidase inhibitor); and then add a mood stabiliser as an augmentor to the foundational antidepressant.

Such a ranking reflects a desire to avoid the increased risk of TEAS with venlafaxine (Vieta *et al.*, 2002; Post *et al.*, 2006); TEAS and somatic adverse effects with tricyclic antidepressants (Peet, 1994; Nemeroff *et al.*, 2001); and somatic adverse effects, drug interactions, and dietary restrictions with monoamine oxidase inhibitors. For such patients (Figure 16.1 – right) (based on controlled and observational longer-term studies in patients with rapid-cycling BP II), additional treatment options may include bupropion – provided insomnia and anxiety are not prominent (Haykal and Akiskal, 1990), and lamotrigine (Calabrese *et al.*, 2000). Also, limited data from controlled trials suggest lithium may have utility in acute BP II depression (Goodwin *et al.*, 1972; Baron *et al.*, 1975), and data from controlled and observational studies suggest that valproate may be of use (Sachs *et al.*, 2001; Winsberg *et al.*, 2001).

If there is treatment resistance, combinations that include lamotrigine (Nierenberg *et al.*, 2006b) or lithium or liothyronine (Nierenberg *et al.*, 2006a) could be considered. In view of evidence of efficacy in acute BP II depression, quetiapine (Calabrese *et al.*, 2005; Thase *et al.*, 2006) could be considered. With evidence of efficacy in acute BP I depression (Tohen *et al.*, 2003; Brown *et al.*, 2006), and accelerating response in treatment-resistant acute unipolar major depression (Shelton *et al.* 2005), olanzapine-fluoxetine combination therapy could also be considered. In such patients, interventions with atypical antipsychotics may be limited by the risk of adverse effects, more than with other agents.

However, for patients with Bipolar II A (Figure 16.1 – left), a different approach could prove preferable. This would be based on concerns regarding the risks of inadequate efficacy for acute depressive symptoms or mood destabilisation with antidepressants (Ghaemi *et al.*, 2003), and the evidence of the utility of quetiapine in acute BP II depression (Calabrese *et al.*, 2005; Thase *et al.*, 2006) and lamotrigine maintenance treatment in rapid-cycling BP II (Calabrese *et al.*, 2000). For patients with psychosis or dysphoric hypomania, or prominent insomnia or anxiety, the need for an agent with evidence of efficacy for such symptoms may favour quetiapine, in spite of lamotrigine's better adverse effects profile. As noted above, limited data from controlled trials suggest lithium has utility in acute BP II depression (Goodwin *et al.*, 1972; Baron *et al.*, 1975), and controlled and observational studies suggest that valproate may have value (Sachs *et al.*, 2001; Winsberg *et al.*, 2001).

If there is treatment resistance in the Bipolar II A patient, combinations that include lamotrigine (Nierenberg *et al.*, 2006b) or lithium or liothyronine (Nierenberg *et al.*, 2006a) could be considered. Evidence of efficacy in acute BP I depression (Tohen *et al.*, 2003; Brown *et al.*, 2006), and accelerating response in treatment-resistant acute unipolar major depression (Shelton *et al.*, 2005), suggests olanzapine-fluoxetine combination therapy could also be considered. Also, emerging evidence suggests that adjunctive pramipexole (Goldberg *et al.*, 2004; Zarate *et al.*, 2004) and adjunctive modafinil (Frye *et al.*, 2007) may have utility in treatment-resistant BP II depression.

Bipolar 'highs' or hypomania

As Parker notes, in comparison to BP I, there may be less acute urgency regarding the need to address symptoms of mood elevation with medication in most patients with BP II. Lifestyle interventions such as maintaining regular sleep-wake cycles and good sleep hygiene, managing interpersonal and occupational stress and avoiding illicit drugs and excessive use of alcohol can offer substantial benefits.

Some patients may see little need to address euphoric hypomanias with medication or even lifestyle changes. However, although their hypomanias are pleasant, patients should be mindful that these may potentiate subsequent depressive episodes. Life charting is a useful tool in assessing the relationship between hypomanic and depressive episodes. If such a relationship is demonstrated, and hypomanic episodes are indeed the 'parents of depressive episodes', then lifestyle and/or medication interventions ought to be considered, to attenuate symptoms of mood elevation to the extent that they do not yield subsequent depression. In some instances this may be straightforward, entailing only modest lifestyle changes (e.g. ensuring a minimum six hours of sleep per night). In other cases, considerable skill may be needed to assess and manage such problems. For example, patients with a prior hyperthymic temperament (chronic sustained sub-syndromal hypomanic but not depressive symptoms) may aspire to return to this temperament, and may even be able to return to some degree of hyperthymia without triggering depression. In contrast, patients with a prior cyclothymic temperament (chronic oscillation between sub-syndromal hypomanic and sub-syndromal depressive symptoms) may not be able to sustain even sub-syndromal hypomanic symptoms without triggering subsequent depression.

Non-drug management components

Parker emphasises the importance of education, mood charting and wellbeing plans in the integrated management of BP II. Individual and group psychoeducation and peer-support group interventions can assist newly diagnosed patients to put their illness in perspective. In addition, emphasising a collaborative interactive approach can help patients to see themselves as active participants rather than passive recipients of pharmacotherapy. Choosing a medication in a collaborative fashion, integrating evidence from clinical trials with the patient's personal history and concerns regarding adverse effects, and then objectively assessing therapeutic and adverse effects of that intervention also means that individuals can embrace a model in which the medication rather than the patient is on trial.

Education

Several useful sources of educational information are described by Parker, and the need to carefully select sources appropriate for individual patients and their families is emphasised. An additional useful publication for patients with BP II is Ronald Fieve's *Moodswing* (Fieve, 1997). Peer-support organisations such as the Depression and Bipolar Support Alliance (DBSA) (http://www.dbsalliance.org/) can also provide important information.

Mood charting

Mood charting as described by Parker is useful for patients and their families, as well as clinicians. Mood charts are a direct way for patients to become active participants in the management of their mood fluctuations. They are particularly useful for patients with frequent episodes, in order to more effectively communicate the clinical course with caregivers and to enable analysis of illness course parameters (e.g. relationship of menstrual cycle to mood symptoms), as well as responses to psychosocial stressors and to treatments. Additionally, mood charts are useful for depressed patients, where state-dependent memory minimises or forgets prior periods of euthymia and mood elevation. Mood charts in these settings are also personalised reminders of prior success, and provide hope of future improvement, as well as underlining the prior limitations and consequences of permitting mood elevation. Such charts come in various formats, one of which is available in the Wellness Toolbox section of the DBSA website.

Wellbeing plans

As Parker observes, active participation of patients and their families in efforts to prevent episodes and enhance wellness are important. Emphasising such efforts (as compared to acute interventions) should commence, arguably, as soon as acute symptoms are controlled. The Wellness Toolbox section of the DBSA website includes several useful tools for patients and their families. Mood charting is just one clinician-initiated approach.

Wellness enhancement programmes need to be patient-initiated and patient-centred to maximise patient participation in the successful management of their illness. Interested clinicians can contribute to patient attendance of support groups by periodically presenting at such meetings, covering new therapeutic developments and providing 'Ask the Doctor' sessions. Clinicians and patients can disseminate patient-devised components of successful wellbeing plans to other patients, acknowledging the importance of patient-initiated contributions to enhancing and maintaining wellness. An active mastery-oriented approach to living with bipolar disorder, compared with a passive victimised point of view, is more likely to yield better control of mood symptoms, and also permit personal growth that can increase the likelihood of better functional outcomes.

Adjunctive psychotherapy

Parker highlights the importance of adjunctive psychotherapy in the management of patients with bipolar disorder. Substantive psychological issues are commonly encountered in BP II management. For example, given the less severe intensity of mood elevation with BP II, differentiating normality and bipolar features can be more challenging than for patients with BP I. Moreover, patients can have significant conflicts regarding relationships between superior performance and mood symptoms, particularly if treatments interfere with continued superior performance. Tackling such issues directly may avoid future treatment non-adherence. Despite the psychological problems being individualised and complex, the last few years have seen remarkable advances in establishing systematic adjunctive psychotherapeutic interventions for patients with BP II.

As indicated above, psychoeducation is useful and, indeed, is a common feature of several effective psychotherapeutic approaches to bipolar disorder (Colom *et al.*, 2003; Lam *et al.*, 2003; Miklowitz *et al.*, 2003; Frank *et al.*, 2005). Thus, an adjunctive psychoeducation group was superior to a non-structured group as prophylaxis over 24 months for BP I and BP II patients (Colom *et al.*, 2003). Similarly, adjunctive family-focused therapy for relapse prevention was superior to crisis management (Miklowitz *et al.*, 2003) and to individual-focused therapy (Rea *et al.*, 2003) over 24 months in patients with BP I. In these studies the benefits extended beyond the psychotherapy interventions. However, there is evidence that booster sessions may be necessary. For example, in a 30-month study, although adjunctive cognitive behavioural therapy was superior to medication management for relapse prevention for BP I over the first 12 months, which included booster sessions (Lam *et al.*, 2003), the benefit was not evident in the last 18 months, which did not include booster sessions (Lam *et al.*, 2005).

Systematic efforts to modulate activities over time can yield benefits. For instance, in a 24-month study, adjunctive acute interpersonal and social rhythm therapy compared to acute intensive clinical management yielded better long-term episode prevention in patients with BP I Disorder (Frank *et al.*, 2005).

As with medication interventions, patient selection can affect the outcome of adjunctive psychotherapy. For instance, in an 18-month study, adjunctive cognitive behaviour therapy was no better overall than treatment-as-usual for patients with severe recurrent BP I and BP II disorder (Scott *et al.*, 2006), but had utility in those patients with fewer than a dozen prior episodes.

Conclusions

This commentary describes preliminary efforts to move towards evidence-based management of BP II, with a particular emphasis on addressing clinical hetero-geneity. Thus, some patients with BP II may benefit from an approach that uses antidepressants as foundational agents, as described by Parker. However, other patients may benefit from an alternative approach that utilises other medications as foundational agents. Further research is needed to provide clinicians with an evidence-based approach to address the clinical heterogeneity encountered in the management of BP II.

REFERENCES

American Psychiatric Association (2000). *Diagnostic and Statistical Manual of Mental Disorders, Fourth Edition, Text Revision (DSM–IV–TR)*. Washington. DC: American Psychiatric Association.

Amsterdam, J. (1998). Efficacy and safety of venlafaxine in the treatment of Bipolar II major depressive episode. *Journal of Clinical Psychopharmacology*, **18**, 414–17.

Amsterdam, J. D. and Brunswick, D. J. (2003). Antidepressant monotherapy for Bipolar Type II major depression. *Bipolar Disorders*, **5**, 388–95.

Amsterdam, J. D. and Garcia-Espana, F. (2000). Venlafaxine monotherapy in women with Bipolar II and unipolar major depression. *Journal of Affective Disorders*, **59**, 225–9.

Amsterdam, J. D., Garcia-Espana, F., Fawcett, J. *et al.* (1998). Efficacy and safety of fluoxetine in treating Bipolar II major depressive episode. *Journal of Clinical Psychopharmacology*, **18**, 435–40.

Amsterdam, J. D., Shults, J., Brunswick, D. J. and Hundert, M. (2004). Short-term fluoxetine monotherapy for Bipolar Type II or Bipolar NOS major depression – low manic switch rate. *Bipolar Disorders*, **6**, 75–81.

Baron, M., Gershon, E. S., Rudy, V., Jonas, W. Z. and Buchsbaum, M. (1975). Lithium carbonate response in depression. Prediction by unipolar/bipolar illness, average-evoked response, catechol-O-methyl transferase, and family history. *Archives of General Psychiatry*, **32**, 1107–11.

Bowden, C. L., Grunze, H., Mullen, J. *et al.* (2005). A randomized, double-blind, placebo-controlled efficacy and safety study of quetiapine or lithium as monotherapy for mania in bipolar disorder. *Journal of Clinical Psychiatry*, **66**, 111–21.

Brown, E. B., McElroy, S. L., Keck, P. E. Jr. *et al.* (2006). A 7-week, randomized, double-blind trial of olanzapine/fluoxetine combination versus lamotrigine in the treatment of Bipolar I depression. *Journal of Clinical Psychiatry*, **67**, 1025–33.

Calabrese, J. R., Keck, P. E. Jr., Macfadden, W. *et al.* (2005). A randomized, double-blind, placebo-controlled trial of quetiapine in the treatment of Bipolar I or II depression. *American Journal of Psychiatry*, **162**, 1351–60.

Calabrese, J. R., Suppes, T., Bowden, C. L. *et al.* (2000). Lamictal 614 Study Group. A double-blind, placebo-controlled, prophylaxis study of lamotrigine in rapid-cycling bipolar disorder. *Journal of Clinical Psychiatry*, **61**, 841–50.

Colom, F., Vieta, E., Martinez-Aran, A. *et al.* (2003). A randomized trial on the efficacy of group psychoeducation in the prophylaxis of recurrences in bipolar patients whose disease is in remission. *Archives of General Psychiatry*, **60**, 402–7.

Dunner, D. L., Stallone, F. and Fieve, R. R. (1976). Lithium carbonate and affective disorders. A double-blind study of prophylaxis of depression in bipolar illness. *Archives of General Psychiatry*, **33**, 117–20.

Dunner, D. L., Stallone, F. and Fieve, R. R. (1982). Prophylaxis with lithium carbonate: an update. *Archives of General Psychiatry*, **39**, 1344–5.

Fieve, R. R. (1997). *Moodswing* (2nd edn). New York: Bantam Books.

Fieve, R. R., Kumbaraci, T. and Dunner, D. L. (1976). Lithium prophylaxis of depression in Bipolar I, Bipolar II, and unipolar patients. *American Journal of Psychiatry*, **133**, 925–9.

Frank, E., Kupfer, D. J., Thase, M. E. *et al.* (2005). Two-year outcomes for interpersonal and social rhythm therapy in individuals with Bipolar I Disorder. *Archives of General Psychiatry*, **62**, 996–1004.

Frye, M. A., Grunze, H., Suppes, T. *et al.* (2007). A placebo-controlled evaluation of adjunctive modafinil in the treatment of bipolar depression. *American Journal of Psychiatry*, **164**, 1242–9.

Ghaemi, S. N., Hsu, D. J., Soldani, F. and Goodwin, F. K. (2003). Antidepressants in bipolar disorder: the case for caution. *Bipolar Disorders*, **5**, 421–33.

Goldberg, J. F., Burdick, K. E. and Endick, C. J. (2004). Preliminary randomized, double-blind, placebo-controlled trial of pramipexole added to mood stabilizers for treatment-resistant bipolar depression. *American Journal of Psychiatry*, **161**, 564–6.

Goodwin, F. K., Murphy, D. L., Dunner, D. L. and Bunney, W. E. Jr. (1972). Lithium response in unipolar versus bipolar depression. *American Journal of Psychiatry*, **129**, 44–7.

Greil, W. and Kleindienst, N. (1999). Lithium versus carbamazepine in the maintenance treatment of Bipolar II Disorder and Bipolar Disorder Not Otherwise Specified. *International Clinical Psychopharmacology*, **14**, 283–5.

Greil, W., Ludwig-Mayerhofer, W., Erazo, N. *et al.* (1997). Lithium versus carbamazepine in the maintenance treatment of bipolar disorders: a randomised study. *Journal of Affective Disorders*, **43**, 151–61.

Greil, W., Kleindienst, N., Erazo, N. and Müller-Oerlinghausen, B. (1998). Differential response to lithium and carbamazepine in the prophylaxis of bipolar disorder. *Journal of Clinical Psychopharmacology*, **18**, 455–60.

Haykal, R. F. and Akiskal, H. S. (1990). Bupropion as a promising approach to rapid-cycling Bipolar II patients. *Journal of Clinical Psychiatry*, **51**, 450–5.

Himmelhoch, J. M., Thase, M. E., Mallinger, A. G. and Houck, P. (1991). Tranylcypromine versus imipramine in anergic bipolar depression. *American Journal of Psychiatry*, **1487**, 910–16.

Hirschfeld, R. M., Williams, J. B., Spitzer, R. L. *et al.* (2000). Development and validation of a screening instrument for bipolar spectrum disorder: the Mood Disorder Questionnaire. *American Journal of Psychiatry*, **157**, 1873–5.

Hirschfeld, R. M., Weisler, R. H., Raines, S. R. and Macfadden, W. (2006). Quetiapine in the treatment of anxiety in patients with Bipolar I or II depression: a secondary analysis from a randomized, double-blind, placebo-controlled study. *Journal of Clinical Psychiatry*, **67**, 355–62.

Judd, L. L., Akiskal, H. S., Schettler, P. J. *et al.* (2003). A prospective investigation of the natural history of the long-term weekly symptomatic status of Bipolar II Disorder. *Archives of General Psychiatry*, **60**, 261–9.

Kane, J. M., Quitkin, F. M., Rifkin, A. *et al.* (1982). Lithium carbonate and imipramine in the prophylaxis of unipolar and Bipolar II illness: a prospective, placebo-controlled comparison. *Archives of General Psychiatry*, **39**, 1065–9.

Keck, P. E. Jr., Calabrese, J. R., McQuade, R. D. *et al.* for the Aripiprazole Study Group (2006). A randomized, double-blind, placebo-controlled 26-week trial of aripiprazole in recently manic patients with Bipolar I Disorder. *Journal of Clinical Psychiatry*, **67**, 626–37.

Lam, D. H., Watkins, E. R., Hayward, P. *et al.* (2003). A randomized controlled study of cognitive therapy for relapse prevention for bipolar affective disorder: outcome of the first year. *Archives of General Psychiatry*, **60**, 145–52.

Lam, D. H., Hayward, P., Watkins, E. R., Wright, K. and Sham, P. (2005). Relapse prevention in patients with bipolar disorder: cognitive therapy outcome after 2 years. *American Journal of Psychiatry*, **162**, 324–9.

McIntyre, R. S., Brecher, M., Paulsson, B., Huizar, K. and Mullen, J. (2005). Quetiapine or haloperidol as monotherapy for bipolar mania: a 12-week, double-blind randomised, parallel-group, placebo-controlled trial. *European Neuropsychopharmacology*, **15**, 573–85.

Miklowitz, D. J., George, E. L., Richards, J. A., Simoneau, T. L. and Suddath, R. L. (2003). A randomized study of family-focused psychoeducation and pharmacotherapy in the outpatient management of bipolar disorder. *Archives of General Psychiatry*, **60**, 904–12.

Nemeroff, C. B., Evans, D. L., Gyulai, L. *et al.* (2001). Double-blind, placebo-controlled comparison of imipramine and paroxetine in the treatment of bipolar depression. *American Journal of Psychiatry*, **158**, 906–12.

Nierenberg, A. A., Fava, M., Trivedi, M. H. *et al.* for the STAR*D Study Team (2006a). A comparison of lithium and T(3) augmentation following two failed medication treatments for depression: a STAR*D report. *American Journal of Psychiatry*, **163**, 1519–30; Quiz, 1665.

Nierenberg, A. A., Ostacher, M. J., Calabrese, J. R. *et al.* and STEP-BD Investigators (2006b). Treatment-resistant bipolar depression: a STEP-BD equipoise randomized effectiveness trial of antidepressant augmentation with lamotrigine, inositol, or risperidone. *American Journal of Psychiatry*, **163**, 210–16.

Peet, M. (1994). Induction of mania with selective serotonin re-uptake inhibitors and tricyclic antidepressants. *British Journal of Psychiatry*, **164**, 549–50.

Post, R. M., Altshuler, L. L., Leverich, G. S. *et al.* (2006). Mood switch in bipolar depression: comparison of adjunctive venlafaxine, bupropion and sertraline. *British Journal of Psychiatry*, **189**, 124–31.

Prien, R. F. (1984). NIMH report. Five-center study clarifies use of lithium and imipramine for recurrent affective disorders. *Hospital and Community Psychiatry*, **35**, 1097–8.

Prien, R. F., Caffey, E. M. Jr. and Klett, C. J. (1973). Prophylactic efficacy of lithium carbonate in manic-depressive illness. Report of the Veterans Administration and National Institute of Mental Health collaborative study group. *Archives of General Psychiatry*, **28**, 337–41.

Quitkin, F., Rifkin, A., Kane, J., Ramos-Lorenzi, J. R. and Klein, D. F. (1978). Prophylactic effect of lithium and imipramine in unipolar and Bipolar II patients: a preliminary report. *American Journal of Psychiatry*, **135**, 570–2.

Quitkin, F. M., Kane, J. M., Rifkin, A. *et al.* (1981). Lithium and imipramine in the prophylaxis of unipolar and Bipolar II depression: a prospective, placebo-controlled comparison. *Psychopharmacology Bulletin*, **17**, 142–4.

Rea, M. M., Tompson, M. C., Miklowitz, D. J. et al. (2003). Family-focused treatment versus individual treatment for bipolar disorder: results of a randomized clinical trial. *Journal of Consulting and Clinical Psychology*, **71**, 482–92.

Sachs, G., Altshuler, L., Ketter, T. et al. (2001). Divalproex versus placebo for the treatment of bipolar depression. 40th Annual Meeting of the American College of Neuropsychopharmacology, Waikaloa, Hawaii, December 9–13.

Scott, J., Paykel, E., Morriss, R. et al. (2006). Cognitive-behavioural therapy for severe and recurrent bipolar disorders: randomised controlled trial. *British Journal of Psychiatry*, **188**, 313–20.

Shelton, R. C., Williamson, D. J., Corya, S. A. et al. (2005). Olanzapine/fluoxetine combination for treatment-resistant depression: a controlled study of SSRI and nortriptyline resistance. *Journal of Clinical Psychiatry*, **66**, 1289–97.

Thase, M. E., Macfadden, W., Weisler, R. H. for the BOLDER II Study Group (2006). Efficacy of quetiapine monotherapy in Bipolar I and II depression: a double-blind, placebo-controlled study (the BOLDER II study). *Journal of Clinical Psychopharmacology*, **26**, 600–9.

Tohen, M., Vieta, E., Calabrese, J. et al. (2003). Efficacy of olanzapine and olanzapine-fluoxetine combination in the treatment of Bipolar I depression. *Archives of General Psychiatry*, **60**, 1079–88.

Tohen, M., Greil, W., Calabrese, J. R. et al. (2005). Olanzapine versus lithium in the maintenance treatment of bipolar disorder: a 12-month, randomized, double-blind, controlled clinical trial. *American Journal of Psychiatry*, **162**, 1281–90.

Tohen, M., Calabrese, J. R., Sachs, G. S. et al. (2006). Randomized, placebo-controlled trial of olanzapine as maintenance therapy in patients with Bipolar I Disorder responding to acute treatment with olanzapine. *American Journal of Psychiatry*, **163**, 247–56.

Tondo, L., Baldessarini, R. J., Floris, G. and Rudas, N. (1997). Effectiveness of restarting lithium treatment after its discontinuation in Bipolar I and Bipolar II disorders. *American Journal of Psychiatry*, **154**, 548–50.

Tondo, L., Baldessarini, R. J., Hennen, J. and Floris, G. (1998). Lithium maintenance treatment of depression and mania in Bipolar I and Bipolar II disorders. *American Journal of Psychiatry*, **155**, 638–45.

Vieta, E., Martinez-Aran, A., Goikolea, J. M. et al. (2002). A randomized trial comparing paroxetine and venlafaxine in the treatment of bipolar depressed patients taking mood stabilizers. *Journal of Clinical Psychiatry*, **63**, 508–12.

Wehr, T. A. and Goodwin, F. K. (1979). Rapid cycling in manic-depressives induced by tricyclic antidepressants. *Archives of General Psychiatry*, **36**, 555–9.

Winsberg, M. E., DeGolia, S. G., Strong, C. M. and Ketter, T. A. (2001). Divalproex therapy in medication-naive and mood-stabilizer-naive Bipolar II depression. *Journal of Affective Disorders*, **67**, 207–12.

Zarate, C., Payne, J., Singh, J. et al. (2004). Pramipexole for Bipolar II depression: a placebo-controlled proof of concept study. *Biological Psychiatry*, **56**, 54–60.

17

Management commentary

Franco Benazzi

I have treated thousands of bipolar patients (mainly BP II) in an outpatient private practice, which is more representative of real-world practice in northern Italy (instead of the National Health Service and University centres, which people avoid for fear of stigma and to avoid mixing with psychotic individuals). As detailed in this book, most treatments shown effective in BP I have not been tested for managing BP II, and, until trials show effectiveness also in BP II, BP I guidelines cannot necessarily be adopted for BP II.

Parker's pharmacological management of BP II is at odds with all or almost all BP I guidelines, which recommend first initiating a mood-stabilising agent. Instead, Parker first trials a narrow-action antidepressant, and, what is even more important, suggests trialling antidepressants long-term for mood stabilisation and to prevent recurrences. This approach is at variance with the widespread view (supported by little evidence!) that antidepressants induce cycling and switching.

In fact, Parker has been treating BP II in a way similar to my own practice for many years. Naturalistic studies have shown that antidepressants have a much lower risk of inducing switching in BP II compared with BP I (this corresponds to my clinical observations), and can prevent depression recurrences in a sub-group of BP I/BP II disorders (Benazzi, 1997; Altshuler et al., 2006; Leverich et al., 2006). Some controlled studies not designed to test this hypothesis (Amsterdam et al., 1998; Amsterdam and Garcia-Espana, 2000), naturalistic studies (Benazzi, 1997; Altshuler et al., 2006; Leverich et al., 2006), and a controlled study (Parker et al., 2006) have shown than some SSRIs can prevent depression recurrences in a BP II sub-group, without inducing cycling and switching.

Differences in management between Parker and myself relate more to the treatment of *mixed depression* (i.e. co-occurrence of a major depressive episode and hypomanic symptoms, albeit with the latter often below the minimum number of four required by DSM–IV for the diagnosis of hypomania) (Benazzi, 2005a) in relation to the use of mood-stabilising agents. Mixed depression is common in BP II. In my outpatient practice, if one probes for hypomanic

Bipolar II Disorder. Modelling, Measuring and Managing, ed. Gordon Parker. Published by Cambridge University Press. © Cambridge University Press 2008.

symptoms during the present episode of depression it is present in at least one-half of the patients. Dominant symptoms are usually irritability and racing/crowded thoughts (which are usually not spontaneously reported), and mild psychomotor agitation (which may be missed if a rating scale is not used). The bipolar character of mixed depression has been shown in many studies, as reviewed by Benazzi (2006), and is best supported by a bipolar (type I and II) family history. The complexity, however, is that several 'mixed state' symptoms (such as irritability and psychomotor agitation) could reflect the primary depressed state rather than be intrusive features of a high.

Nevertheless, acute hypomania is likely to respond to the same anti-manic agents effective in BP I. However, I have found some agents (e.g. gabapentin) shown not to be effective in acute mania, to be useful in acute hypomania or for the hypomanic symptoms of mixed depression.

Treatment of acute BP II depression has been little studied. As noted earlier, one problem in managing BP II depression, not taken into account by current studies (including those for BP I depression), is that bipolar depression is often a mixed state which antidepressants alone (i.e. not protected by mood stabilising agents) can worsen, including the occasional possible induction of suicidality. This is one of the reasons why those with BP II depression should be systematically assessed for concurrent hypomanic symptoms.

Such systematic assessment also respects the recent US Food and Drug Authority (FDA) warning on antidepressants and suicidality, which has listed irritability, psychomotor agitation and bipolarity as possible precursors to the suicidality related to antidepressant use. Further arguments emerge from studies showing that mixed depression is often present before a suicide attempt, while racing/crowded thoughts (as well as psychomotor agitation) have also been shown to be an independent predictor of suicidal ideation (Benazzi, 2005b; Balazs et al., 2006; Bauer et al., 2006). Analyses of naturalistic databases testing the impact of antidepressants on mixed depression have reported worsening of depression and higher risk of switching in BP I/BP II depression compared with non-mixed depression (Bottlender et al., 2004; Goldberg et al., 2004; Frye et al., 2006; McElroy et al., 2006). In my view, mixed depression should be treated first by a mood-stabilising agent to control its hypomanic symptoms, and antidepressants should be added later (if still necessary, as I have observed that the more the concurrent hypomanic symptoms the likelier it is that the depression will also disappear with such treatment). Controlled studies are needed to test these personal clinical observations.

The anti-suicidal effect reported for lithium in bipolar disorders may be related to its ability to prevent the onset of manic/hypomanic symptoms during a depression recurrence. While lithium has been shown to have stronger preventive effects for mania/hypomania than for depression in BP I, lithium preventive effects in BP II seem broader, as it appears that both depression and hypomania are prevented (Prien *et al.*, 1984; Tondo *et al.*, 1998). Further, for the prevention of recurrences in BP II, lithium is the only drug shown to be effective in controlled studies.

Lamotrigine has not shown clear antidepressant effects in BP I depression (Calabrese *et al.*, 1999), and it has been released only for the prevention of depression recurrences in BP I (because it somewhat delays the time to recurrence of depression). In rapid-cycling bipolar disorder, which is mainly a BP II depression, lamotrigine may reduce time to depression recurrence, but, again, it has not shown acute antidepressant effects (Calabrese *et al.*, 2000, 2005). Quetiapine has been shown effective for BP I depression, but not for BP II depression (Calabrese *et al.*, 2005; Hirschfeld *et al.*, 2006).

Despite the results of these studies, my management of BP II is based on my clinical observations, as now summarised. Firstly, if BP II depression is not 'mixed', I use antidepressants alone (SSRIs being the first choice). Secondly, if those with BP II depression become agitated while being treated with an antidepressant (i.e. mixed depression), I add a mood-stabilising agent (usually gabapentin, valproate, clonazepam, low-dose olanzapine or quetiapine). Thirdly, if BP II depression presents as a mixed state, I first use a mood-stabilising agent to control the concurrent hypomanic symptoms (which usually takes a few days or a week), then, if depression is still present, I add an antidepressant.

After remission, the treatment that led to remission is used during the continuation phase (for some 6–12 months). If there is a history of multiple depressive recurrences in the preceding 5 years, maintenance lasts 1–2 years – with the need to maintain the treatment tested (i.e. same drugs, same doses). The latter practice is based on Kraepelin's observation that the course of manic-depressive illness was variable, including bursts of episodes close together followed by long remissions (the progressive increase of recurrences was seen only in a sub-group of cases). My maintenance strategy is also guided by the frequency of hypomanic recurrences. If an individual has had only a few hypomanic episodes in his life, it is unlikely that the rate will increase during antidepressant therapy. If there is a hypomanic episode (usually seen during follow-up), I treat it, because it may induce a depression. The treatment of rapid cycling is much more complex (i.e. I follow a difficult two-pillar system, requiring many concurrent mood-stabilising agents, and also concurrent antidepressants).

The best evidence for maintenance treatment of BP II is for lithium, but, as we have more user-friendly mood-stabilising agents, I do not, commonly, use it.

REFERENCES

Altshuler, L. L., Suppes, T., Black, D. O. *et al.* (2006). Lower switch rate in depressed patients with Bipolar II than Bipolar I disorder treated adjunctively with second-generation antidepressants. *American Journal of Psychiatry*, **163**, 313–15.

Amsterdam, J. D., Garcia-Espana, F., Fawcett, J. *et al.* (1998). Efficacy and safety of fluoxetine in treating Bipolar II major depressive episode. *Journal of Clinical Psychopharmacology*, **18**, 435–40.

Amsterdam, J. D. and Garcia-Espana, F. (2000). Venlafaxine monotherapy in women with Bipolar II and unipolar major depression. *Journal of Affective Disorders*, **59**, 225–9.

Balazs, J., Benazzi, F., Rihmer, Z. *et al.* (2006). The close link between suicide attempts and mixed (bipolar) depression: implications for suicide prevention. *Journal of Affective Disorders*, **91**, 133–8.

Bauer, M. S., Wisniewski, S. R., Marangell, L. B. *et al.* for the STEP-BD Investigators (2006). Are antidepressants associated with new-onset suicidality in bipolar disorder? A prospective study of participants in the systematic treatment enhancement program for bipolar disorder (STEP-BD). *Journal of Clinical Psychiatry*, **67**, 48–55.

Benazzi, F. (1997). Antidepressant-associated hypomania in outpatient depression: a 203-case study in private practice. *Journal of Affective Disorders*, **46**, 73–7.

Benazzi, F. (2005a). Family history validation of a definition of mixed depression. *Comprehensive Psychiatry*, **46**, 159–66.

Benazzi, F. (2005b). Suicidal ideation and depressive mixed states. *Psychotherapy and Psychosomatics*, **74**, 61–2.

Benazzi, F. (2006). Mood patterns and classification in bipolar disorder. *Current Opinion in Psychiatry*, **19**, 1–8.

Bottlender, R., Sato, T., Kleindienst, N., Strausz, A. and Moller, H.-J. (2004). Mixed depressive features predict maniform switch during treatment of depression in Bipolar I Disorder. *Journal of Affective Disorders*, **78**, 149–52.

Calabrese, J. R., Bowden, C. L., Sachs, G. S. *et al.* (1999). A double-blind placebo-controlled study of lamotrigine monotherapy in outpatients with Bipolar I depression. Lamictal 602 Study Group. *Journal of Clinical Psychiatry*, **60**, 79–88.

Calabrese, J. R., Suppes, T., Bowden, C. L. *et al.* (2000). A double-blind, placebo-controlled, prophylaxis study of lamotrigine in rapid-cycling bipolar disorder. Lamictal 614 Study Group. *Journal of Clinical Psychiatry*, **61**, 841–50.

Calabrese, J. R., Keck, P. E. Jr., Macfadden, W. *et al.* (2005). A randomized, double-blind, placebo-controlled trial of quetiapine in the treatment of Bipolar I or II depression. *American Journal of Psychiatry*, **162**, 1351–60.

Frye, M. A., McElroy, S. L., Hellemann, G. *et al.* (2006). Clinical correlates associated with antidepressant-related mania. Toronto: Programme and abstracts of the American Psychiatric Association Annual Meeting (abstract NR215).

Goldberg, J. F., Truman, C. J., Fordis, J. *et al.* (2004). Antidepressant use during mixed states: naturalistic outcome data from the STEP-1000. *Neuropsychopharmacology*, **29**, S144 (abstract).

Hirschfeld, R. M., Weisler, R. H., Raines, S. R. and Macfadden, W. for the BOLDER Study Group. (2006). Quetiapine in the treatment of anxiety in patients with Bipolar I or II depression: a secondary analysis from a randomized, double-blind, placebo-controlled study. *Journal of Clinical Psychiatry*, **67**, 355–62.

Leverich, G. S., Altshuler, L. L., Frye, M. A. *et al.* (2006). Risk of switch in mood polarity to hypomania or mania in patients with bipolar depression during acute and continuation trials of venlafaxine, sertraline, and bupropion as adjuncts to mood stabilizers. *American Journal of Psychiatry*, **163**, 232–9.

McElroy, S. L., Kotwal, R., Kaneria, R. and Keck, P. E. Jr. (2006). Antidepressants and suicidal behavior in bipolar disorder. *Bipolar Disorders*, **8**, 596–617.

Parker, G., Tully, L., Olley, A. and Hadzi-Pavlovic, D. (2006). SSRIs as mood stabilizers for Bipolar II Disorder? A proof of concept study. *Journal of Affective Disorders*, **92**, 205–14.

Prien, R. F., Kupfer, D. J., Mansky, P. A. *et al.* (1984). Drug therapy in the prevention of recurrences in unipolar and bipolar affective disorders. Report of the NIMH Collaborative Study Group comparing lithium carbonate, imipramine, and a lithium carbonate-imipramine combination. *Archives of General Psychiatry*, **41**, 1096–104.

Tondo, L., Baldessarini, R. J., Hennen, J. and Floris, G. (1998). Lithium maintenance treatment of depression and mania in Bipolar I and Bipolar II disorders. *American Journal of Psychiatry*, **155**, 638–45.

18

Management commentary

Michael Berk

There is a marked paucity of high quality trials for both pharmacological and psychological treatments of BP II. This stands in stark contrast to the substantial prevalence data, resulting in an evidence vacuum. As depression is the dominant clinical issue, treatment of BP II is essentially the acute and maintenance treatment of depression. In the absence of adequate data, the clinician is faced with a choice of extrapolating from either the unipolar depression or bipolar depression databases, acknowledging that even the latter is threadbare at present. In practice, the pharmacological choice is the balance in the algorithm between the role of accepted mood stabilisers and antidepressants. A core component of the decision-making process is the weighting of risk and benefit. In this context, a dominant issue is the potential for antidepressant therapy to induce rapid cycling and mixed states.

Complicating the issue of the assessment of switching and cycling is the methodology of such assessment. In general, prospective designs are likely to give far higher rates of event detection than retrospective ones. The availability of tools specifically designed to detect switching and cycling is essential, as methodologies relying on spontaneous reports of adverse events are likely to report lower rates than studies using structured tools for the purpose. SSRI-induced sexual dysfunction is a good example of a situation where, based on spontaneous reports, initial assessments of prevalence were negligible, while later studies utilising specific detection tools in prospective designs consistently reported substantial rates. It therefore comes as no surprise that studies examining switching without using specific measures in a prospective manner (Peet, 1994) reported vastly lower rates than studies that employed such measures (Leverich *et al.*, 2006). In the latter trial, of a BP I and BP II cohort, a favourable response to treatment – defined as response without switch – was only observed in 17.6% of individuals at the end of the acute phase, and 12.6% at the end of the maintenance phase. Also, while there was a more rapid rate of switching in the BP I group, by 18 months the BP II cohort had almost caught up.

A further issue is the definition of 'switch', and hence 'cycling'. The convention is to define a switch as the transition of an index episode to an episode of the

Bipolar II Disorder. Modelling, Measuring and Managing, ed. Gordon Parker. Published by Cambridge University Press. © Cambridge University Press 2008.

opposite polarity as a consequence of treatment of the index polarity, and classi-cally, the induction of mania with an antidepressant treatment. There is an alternate viewpoint, conceptualising cycling as the core feature of the disorder. In this construct, a therapeutic agent should have a broad effect – reducing the vulnerability to cycling. Such agents may have a role in reducing any of the parameters (e.g. number, duration and amplitude) of the episode waveform. In contrast, agents that increase the amplitude or duration of mood swings, or that shorten the cycle length, would be deleterious to course. The standard measure in many maintenance designs – time to a mood episode – essentially defines length-ening of the inter-episode period as the outcome of appropriate therapy. Studies have shown that antidepressants shorten cycle length (Wehr and Goodwin, 1987; Ghaemi *et al.*, 2001).

Another issue is the conceptualisation of polarity vulnerability. In BP II, the dominant vulnerability is to the depressive pole, and the innate vulnerability to mood elevation is by definition lower in BP II than in BP I disorder. The implication of this concept is that the switch in BP II may be into the polarity of vulnerability. Evidence is provided by two phenomena: offset of maintenance effect, and treatment resistance to the agent in question. Aggravation of the pattern of cycling may be thus primarily into depression. A common clinical phenomenon in bipolar disorder is offset of antidepressant action in the maintenance phase, sometimes referred to as 'poop-out'. Treatment resistance in depression, frequently associated with an undiagnosed bipolar diathesis, may be a manifes-tation of this concept (Sharma *et al.*, 2005).

Given the dominant depressive polarity vulnerability, cycle aggravation may be manifest as worsening of depression, with a lesser impact on manic symp-toms. The resultant phenomenology resembles a sub-threshold mixed state, exhibiting either a worsening agitated dysphoric picture, or the conversion of an anergic to an agitated depression. The DSM–IV system, requiring concurrent full mania and depression in order to define the presence of a mixed state, does not – by definition – recognise BP II mixed states. While some authors (Benazzi, 2003) have defined alternative classifications of sub-threshold mixed states compatible with BP II, these are not officially recognised, resulting in a system that lumps mixed features in Bipolar II Disorder with the depressive pole, and fails to recognise induction of a distinct iatrogenic state. This is a major gap in existing diagnostic systems, and one which plays a role in reducing recognition of a clinically critical issue.

The role of antidepressants in bipolar disorder remains a vexed issue, and is at present not fully answered by an adequate database. There are, however, sufficient emerging data for clinicians to be increasingly cautious, and for clinical practice to take into account the increasing data on the risk:benefit ratio.

REFERENCES

Benazzi, F. (2003). Bipolar II depressive mixed state: finding a useful definition. *Comprehensive Psychiatry*, **44**, 21–7.

Ghaemi, S. N., Ko, J. Y. and Goodwin, F. K. (2001). The bipolar spectrum and the antidepressant view of the world. *Journal of Psychiatric Practice*, **7**, 287–97.

Leverich, G. S., Altshuler, L. L., Frye, M. A. *et al.* (2006). Risk of switch in mood polarity to hypomania or mania in patients with bipolar depression during acute and continuation trials of venlafaxine, sertraline, and bupropion as adjuncts to mood stabilizers. *American Journal of Psychiatry*, **163**, 232–9.

Peet, M. (1994). Induction of mania with selective serotonin re-uptake inhibitors and tricyclic antidepressants. *British Journal of Psychiatry*, **164**, 549–50.

Sharma, V., Khan, M. and Smith, A. (2005). A closer look at treatment-resistant depression: is it due to a bipolar diathesis? *Journal of Affective Disorders*, **84**, 251–7.

Wehr, T. A. and Goodwin, F. K. (1987). Can antidepressants cause mania and worsen the course of affective illness? *American Journal of Psychiatry*, **144**, 1403–11.

19

Management commentary

Eduard Vieta

Introduction

Bipolar II Disorder is a significant public health problem, and there is a dearth of studies of effective treatment modalities for this specific condition. Literally, the evidence base for most of what we use to treat BP II comes from extrapolation of what we have learned from trials on BP I, unipolar depression, schizophrenia, and even epilepsy. Among several reasons, the two principal ones for this phenomenon are the relative 'youth' of the diagnostic category and the absence of a specific regulatory indication for marketing approval. Hence, in the practical absence of solid scientific grounds (El-Mallakh et al., 2006), opinion-based articles like the one by Parker become crucial to assist routine clinical care. I now offer some personal views.

Validity and reliability of the diagnosis of BP II Disorder

There is some evidence supporting BP II as a valid diagnostic category, but its reliability is relatively low (Vieta and Suppes, 2007). This is one of the major sources of both under-diagnosis and misdiagnosis (Akiskal, 2002). Most difficulties come from the frequently egosyntonic, pleasurable and transient nature of hypomania, which makes it very difficult to diagnose retrospectively. If this was a truly mild condition, nobody would care about under-diagnosis and misdiagnosis, but unfortunately, in my view, it is not mild. It only appears so when considered or observed cross-sectionally, but, in the long run it is associated with significant suffering, impairment and suicide (Vieta et al., 1997). Our group has also demonstrated that a good proportion of BP II patients are cognitively impaired as a result of their condition (Torrent et al., 2006). Comorbidity with substance use, anxiety and personality disorders is also very high (Vieta et al., 1999, 2000). This should be kept in mind when addressing the risk: benefit ratio of any therapeutic intervention.

Bipolar II Disorder. Modelling, Measuring and Managing, ed. Gordon Parker. Published by Cambridge University Press. © Cambridge University Press 2008.

General principles in the treatment of BP II

My view on the general principles in treating BP II is closer to those for BP I Disorder than to unipolar depression (see Table 19.1). Again, in the absence of a solid evidence base, this may be an arguable statement, but it certainly comes from my own clinical experience. Hence, following the general rule of 'first do no harm', I am, in principle, reluctant to prescribe antidepressants as monotherapy in these patients, as some may 'switch' or start cycling rapidly, although my position is not as radical in this regard as others (Ghaemi *et al.*, 2003), and I advocate cautious use of antidepressants as adjuncts to mood stabilisers (Vieta, 2003), even though BP II patients may be at lower risk than those with BP I (Altshuler *et al.*, 2006). I acknowledge that there may be a sub-group of patients who may respond to such a strategy (Parker *et al.*, 2006), but to date there is no way to identify such sub-group members in advance. The argument that switches are mild is not convincing because hypomania may be mild but it often leads to severe depression and suicide risk. I also suspect that the 'official' estimate of 15% of individuals with BP II developing BP I (Coryell *et al.*, 1989) is very conservative and the figure may be actually much higher. Therefore, the foundational treatment of BP II should be, in my opinion, mood stabilisers (including lithium, lamotrigine, valproate and carbamazepine), with atypical antipsychotics and antidepressants as adjuncts when appropriate. For instance, the combination of olanzapine and fluoxetine has been proved as effective in the depressed phase of BP I (Tohen *et al.*, 2003), and risperidone combined with lithium or anticonvulsants useful in hypomania (Vieta *et al.*, 2001). The exception may be quetiapine, which, so far, provides the only robustly evidence-based monotherapy for BP II depression (Suppes *et al.*, 2007), and which may become a first-line treatment if the long-term controlled trials are

Table 19.1. General principles when treating Bipolar II Disorder.

Bipolar II Disorder is not necessarily a milder form of manic depressive illness

Rapid cycling, comorbidity and suicidal behaviour are not rare and may be even more common than in BP I

A proportion of BP II subjects, probably over 15%, may 'switch' to a BP I condition

Antidepressants may be effective for a sub-group of BP II patients, but may induce mood switches and rapid cycling in others

The evidence available so far for lithium and anticonvulsants is quite poor for managing BP II, but may still provide first options

There is some evidence that quetiapine may be effective in BP II depression

It is still unclear if the currently available psychosocial therapies for BP I may be suitable for BP II as well positive. There is also some evidence supporting the adjunctive use of a dopamine agonist, pramipexole (Zarate *et al.*, 2004). Electroconvulsive therapy may also be useful for severe BP II depressive episodes.

Psychotherapy might be useful but there is little evidence on how to implement it in this condition. The controlled trials on psychoeducation, which is the closest to what Parker calls 'wellbeing plans', enrolled BP II as well as BP I patients, but they were not powered for sub-analysis to allow us to quantify any differential impact across bipolar subtypes. However, the general principles of psychoeducation (i.e. providing information and support, promoting treatment adherence, healthy habits and early-detection skills) should obviously apply (Colom and Vieta, 2006).

Conclusions

In the absence of evidence, some general rules should apply to the management of BP II patients. My bias is that BP II is not just a milder form of bipolar illness and that it is much closer to BP I than to unipolar disorder, and therefore I would advocate an emphasis on mood-stabilising strategies (lithium, lamotrigine and others) and cautious use of antidepressant and antipsychotic drugs, perhaps with the exception of quetiapine, which may become first-line treatment for BP II depression. Psychoeducation may also be useful, and should likely be slightly tailored for this particular subtype of bipolar illness.

Acknowledgements

Supported in part by the Spanish Ministry of Health, Red de Enfermedades Mentales (REM-TAP Network) and the Stanley Medical Research Institute.

REFERENCES

Akiskal, H. S. (2002). Towards a new classification of bipolar disorders. In *Bipolar Disorders. Clinical and Therapeutic Progress*, ed. E. Vieta, pp. 185–215. Madrid: Panamericana.

Altshuler, L. L., Suppes, T., Black, D. O. *et al.* (2006). Lower switch rate in depressed patients with Bipolar II than Bipolar I Disorder treated adjunctively with second-generation antidepressants. *American Journal of Psychiatry*, **163**, 313–15.

Colom, F. and Vieta, E. (2006). *Psychoeducation Manual for Bipolar Disorder*. New York: Cambridge University Press.

Coryell, W., Keller, M., Endicott, J. *et al.* (1989). Bipolar II illness: course and outcome over a five-year period. *Psychological Medicine*, **19**, 129–41.

El-Mallakh, R., Weisler, R. H., Townsend, M. H. and Ginsberg, L. D. (2006). Bipolar II Disorder: current and future treatment options. *Annals of Clinical Psychiatry*, **18**, 259–66.

Ghaemi, S. N., Hsu, D. J., Soldani, F. and Goodwin, F. K. (2003). Antidepressants in bipolar disorder: the case for caution. *Bipolar Disorders*, **5**, 421–33.

Parker, G., Tully, L., Olley, A. and Hadzi-Pavlovic, D. (2006). SSRIs as mood stabilizers for Bipolar II Disorder? A proof of concept study. *Journal of Affective Disorders*, **92**, 205–14.

Suppes, T., Hirschfeld, R. M., Vieta, E. *et al.* (2007). Quetiapine for the treatment of Bipolar II depression: analysis of data from two randomized, double-blind, placebo-controlled studies. *World Journal of Biological Psychiatry* (in press).

Tohen, M., Vieta, E., Calabrese, J. *et al.* (2003). Efficacy of olanzapine and olanzapine-fluoxetine combination in the treatment of Bipolar I depression. *Archives of General Psychiatry*, **60**, 1079–88.

Torrent, T., Martinez-Aran, A., Daban, C. *et al.* (2006). Cognitive impairment in Bipolar II Disorder. *British Journal of Psychiatry*, **189**, 254–9.

Vieta, E. (2003). Case for caution, case for action. *Bipolar Disorders*, **5**, 434–5.

Vieta, E. and Suppes, T. (2007). International Society for Bipolar Disorders Diagnostic Task Force on Bipolar II Disorder. *Bipolar Disorders* (in press).

Vieta, E., Colom, F., Martínez-Arán, A., Benabarre, A. and Gastó, C. (1999). Personality disorders in Bipolar II patients. *Journal of Nervous and Mental Disease*, **187**, 245–8.

Vieta, E., Colom, F., Martínez-Arán, A. *et al.* (2000). Bipolar II Disorder and comorbidity. *Comprehensive Psychiatry*, **41**, 339–43.

Vieta, E., Gastó, C., Colom, F. *et al.* (2001). The role of risperidone in Bipolar II: an open six-month study. *Journal of Affective Disorders*, **67**, 213–19.

Vieta, E., Gastó, C., Otero, A., Nieto, E. and Vallejo, J. (1997). Differential features between Bipolar I and Bipolar II disorder. *Comprehensive Psychiatry*, **38**, 98–101.

Zarate, C. A. Jr., Payne, J. L., Singh, J. *et al.* (2004). Pramipexole for Bipolar II depression: a placebo-controlled proof of concept study. *Biological Psychiatry*, **56**, 54–60.

20

Management commentary

Philip B. Mitchell

It is a difficult task to comment upon an individual's clinical model for treating 'Bipolar II Disorder' (BP II) without clarity about the criteria being used to make that diagnosis. In contemporary academic and clinical practice there is a myriad of definitions for BP II, each with associated stated and unstated connotations. There is a consequent unfortunate conflation in the use of this term, with the implicit message that 'all Bipolar II Disorder is the same'. This is in fact not true, as a quick reflection on the historical origins of the use of this term would indicate. The term 'Bipolar II Disorder' was originally coined by Fieve and Dunner (1975) to describe an attenuated form of classical bipolar disorder/manic depressive illness in which the elevated component of the illness was less severe than in Bipolar I Disorder (BP I). This concept of BP II, which became enshrined in the RDC and DSM nosological systems, and incorporates minimum durations of hypomania varying from 2 to 7 days, has been validated by being demonstrated to be genetically related to BP I.

A more recent usage has stemmed from the broad concept of the 'soft bipolar spectrum' (Akiskal and Mallya, 1987), in which conceptualisation of BP II has been extended to include brief hypomanic episodes as well as cyclothymic and hyperthymic personality traits (Akiskal *et al.*, 2000). The relationship of 'bipolar spectrum disorder' to Axis II comorbidity has been contentious, with Akiskal *et al.* (2000) arguing that for 'patients with fluctuating affective symptoms, the diagnosis of a bipolar spectrum diagnoses (sic) should take precedence over that of a personality disorder within the dramatic cluster' (p. S12, 13).

My own approach to conceiving the 'soft bipolar spectrum' is that while such a broad clinical syndrome probably does exist, its obligatory relationship to bipolar disorder is contentious, unfortunate and potentially misleading. Similar to recent developments with so-called 'paediatric bipolar disorder', a more appropriate descriptor would be some term akin to that of 'severe mood dysregulation' (Rich *et al.*, 2007). This would uncouple treatment choices from those developed specifically for bipolar disorder (or even unipolar depression), and would allow for a broader management approach which could incorporate psychological, personality and temperamental factors, in addition to biological measures.

Bipolar II Disorder. Modelling, Measuring and Managing, ed. Gordon Parker. Published by Cambridge University Press. © Cambridge University Press 2008.

What treatments have been reported for BP II? First, for the strict DSM–IV-defined condition, there have been a few reports of double-blind placebo-controlled trials in recent years. These have focused upon BP II depression, with reports of the efficacy of quetiapine (Thase *et al.*, 2006) and pramipexole – a dopamine agonist developed for the treatment of Parkinson's disease (Zarate *et al.*, 2004). Second, for broadly defined BP II (including hypomanic episodes less than 2–4 days), Parker *et al.* (2006) reported, in a placebo-controlled crossover 9-month trial in a small sample, that an SSRI antidepressant reduced the frequency and severity of at least depressed and perhaps (brief) hypomanic episodes.

Most extant national clinical practice guidelines (such as our own Australian guidelines – RANZCP, 2004) have been forced to acknowledge that there is no substantial evidence base upon which to recommend management of BP II, and that it is unclear whether extrapolation of guidance for BP I is either warranted or reasonable.

What of Parker's approach to the treatment of BP II? I will not respond *seriatim* to the fine details of his management model, which incorporates many exemplary aspects of high quality clinical care.

For the narrow (RDC/DSM) concept of BP II, I believe (unlike Parker) that it is probably reasonable to extrapolate guidance on BP I management to most patients. For that reason, I would consider it necessary for most patients with such episodes of BP II depression to require concurrent mood stabilisation along with an antidepressant, though rates of switching to hypomania or mania are clearly less prevalent than for those with BP I (Altshuler *et al.*, 2006).

For the broader 'soft bipolar spectrum' approach which Parker's recent writings (e.g. Parker *et al.*, 2006) have espoused, my major point of contention would be to commend a greater emphasis upon the personality/temperamental factors, psychological issues and comorbidities (anxiety and substance abuse) which are prevalent in patients referred to me with a prior diagnosis of 'Bipolar II Disorder'. For many of these patients, I view the relationship of the presentation to bipolar disorder as specious, and consider this rather as a broader dysfunction of mood regulation. While, for some individuals, the underlying driver is 'true' bipolar disorder, for many more there are substantial personality or temperamental issues – usually at a trait, rather than disorder, level. For example, some patients manifest an exaggerated external locus of control, responding excessively strongly to positive events such as career achievements or other successes (and correspondingly over-despondently to negative events) to the extent that 'hypomania' (or conversely clinical depression) has been diagnosed. For such individuals, psychological techniques for enhancing their capacity to regulate moods and provide a sense of control over feelings that were previously considered 'out of control' appear helpful. For others, the mood fluctuations are clearly secondary to borderline or other personality vulnerabilities, and techniques such as dialectical behaviour therapy may be of benefit. Comorbid substance abuse is not uncommon in such patients, with stimulants, alcohol or marijuana being used to either generate or control fluctuations in mood. Undoubtedly, medications such as antidepressants or mood stabilisers may also be symptomatically of benefit for a number of these patients, but often need to be provided in conjunction with sophisticated modern psychological therapies.

In conclusion, Parker's description of his clinical model for managing BP II disorder is impressive as a rare example of transparency in detailing the specifics of clinical care for a contentious area. Overall, though, the conclusion of Hadjipavlou *et al.* (2004) unfortunately still holds: 'There is a paucity of sound evidence to help guide clinicians treating BP II patients.'

REFERENCES

Akiskal, H. S., Bourgeois, M. L., Angst, J. *et al.* (2000). Re-evaluating the prevalence of and diagnostic composition within the broad clinical spectrum of bipolar disorders. *Journal of Affective Disorders*, **59** (Suppl. 1), S5–30.

Akiskal, H. S. and Mallya, G. (1987). Criteria for the 'soft' bipolar spectrum: treatment implications. *Psychopharmacology Bulletin*, **23**, 68–73.

Altshuler, L. L., Suppes, T., Black, D. O. *et al.* (2006). Lower switch rate in depressed patients with Bipolar II than Bipolar I Disorder treated adjunctively with second-generation antidepressants. *American Journal of Psychiatry*, **163**, 313–15.

Fieve, R. R. and Dunner, D. L. (1975). Unipolar and bipolar affective states. In *The Nature and Treatment of Depression*, ed. F. F. Flach and S. S. Draghi, pp. 145–60. New York: John Wiley and Sons.

Hadjipavlou, G., Mok, H. and Yatham, L. N. (2004). Pharmacotherapy of Bipolar II Disorder: a critical review of current evidence. *Bipolar Disorders*, **6**, 14–25.

Parker, G., Tully, L. and Hadzi-Pavlovic, D. (2006). SSRIs as mood stabilizers for Bipolar II Disorder? A proof of concept study. *Journal of Affective Disorders*, **92**, 205–14.

RANZCP Clinical Practice Treatment Guideline on Bipolar Disorder (2004). *Australian and New Zealand Journal of Psychiatry*, **38**, 280–305.

Rich, B. A., Schmajuk, M., Perez-Edgar, K. E. *et al.* (2007). Different psychophysiological and behavioral responses elicited by frustration in pediatric bipolar disorder and severe mood dysregulation. *American Journal of Psychiatry*, **164**, 309–17.

Thase, M. E., Macfadden, W., Weisler, R. H. *et al.* (2006). Efficacy of quetiapine monotherapy in Bipolar I and II depression: A double-blind, placebo-controlled study (the BOLDER study). *Journal of Clinical Psychopharmacology*, **26**, 600–9.

Zarate, C. A. Jr., Payne, J. L., Singh, J. *et al.* (2004). Pramipexole for Bipolar II depression: a placebo-controlled proof of concept study. *Biological Psychiatry*, **56**, 54–60.

21

Management commentary

Joseph F. Goldberg

Optimal management for patients with Bipolar II Disorder involves a tailored, individualised treatment approach that is informed, but not dictated, by the clinical trials' literature. It is precisely because of controversy and uncertainty about the nosology of BP II, and its differential diagnosis, that a systematic and thorough assessment of clinical features rightfully precedes treatment, in order to avoid premature diagnostic or therapeutic conclusions. Implementing reasonable and appropriate treatments, with clear rationales, can only occur after the careful evaluation of symptoms and clinical context in light of past history.

Consider the following vignette:

A 28-year-old man with no prior psychiatric history was referred for a second opinion after having presented with complaints of diffuse worry and mood swings. His symptoms began shortly after the break-up of a long-term relationship, which exacerbated feelings of social isolation and anxious ruminations about low self-worth. He denied suicidal thoughts or changes in appetite or sleep. Because of the patient's use of the term 'mood swings', he was begun on quetiapine 25 mg/day for a 'probable diagnosis of Bipolar II Disorder'. Sedated, but without any improvement after 2 weeks, his quetiapine was increased to 50 mg/day and lamotrigine was added at 25 mg/day. Still with no relief two weeks later, the patient returned and inquired whether or not an antidepressant would be worth taking. He was warned by his psychiatrist of the probability that 'antidepressants cause rapid cycling' and, instead, oxcarbazepine was added as 'a mood stabilizer that does not require blood tests'.

During a second opinion visit, a systematic diagnostic evaluation failed to reveal evidence of any lifetime manic or hypomanic episode that met DSM–IV criteria. In fact, the patient's use of the term 'mood swings' actually referred to waxing and waning despair about the loss of his relationship, but not a frank pattern of cyclical variation. A detailed history revealed no prior affective episodes, but longstanding fear of embarrassment in social situations, with avoidance of (and distress caused by) having to meet new people in social settings. His anxious ruminations and depressed mood were explainable by the presence of an adjustment disorder with

Bipolar II Disorder. Modelling, Measuring and Managing, ed. Gordon Parker. Published by Cambridge University Press. © Cambridge University Press 2008.

mixed anxiety and depressed mood, superimposed on a probable longer-term diagnosis of social phobia.

Aware of the patient's and referring clinician's concerns about a bipolar 'spectrum' disorder, a number of pertinent dimensions were assessed, and established that there was:

- no history of prepubescent or early adolescent depression;
- no family history of bipolar disorder, recurrent unipolar disorder, or psychotic illness;
- no history of recurrent depression in the patient, although he reported similar transient periods of distress following prior romantic break-ups;
- no history of antidepressant-induced mania or hypomania (and, indeed, no prior history of antidepressant use);
- no sign of atypical depression (i.e. involving reversed neurovegetative signs).

Although the patient was conceptualised by his referring clinician as having treatment-resistant bipolar depression, it appeared that he had neither treatment resistance nor a bipolar disorder. Further history identified a moderate degree of recent excessive alcohol use, raising concern about the potential for alcohol abuse and its consequent exacerbation of mood symptoms. It was suggested to both the patient and the referring clinician that (a) none of his existing medications were likely indicated for the problem he had, (b) counselling should occur on alcohol misuse and its effects on mood, (c) a structured individual psychotherapy, such as cognitive therapy, might be useful to target issues of self-esteem and social isolation as precipitated by the recent loss of an important relationship, and (d) a trial of a serotonergic antidepressant may be worth considering for his probable social phobia.

While the use of traditional antidepressants is controversial for patients with bipolar disorder, especially in those who previously developed mania or hypomania while taking antidepressants, concern about their 'likelihood' for inducing (hypo)mania or cycle acceleration in this case seemed rather remote. As noted in Chapter 7 of this book, such risks appear considerably less in BP II than in BP I, and likely pertain only to a minority of individuals with known bipolar illness. Even if the patient described in the preceding case *did* actually have BP II depression, the referring clinician's decision to withhold a serotonergic antidepressant would be contrary to the existing evidence base that, at least initially, supports both its safety and efficacy for BP II.

Examples such as the foregoing underscore the relevance of systematic assessment before drawing assumptions about pharmacotherapy (and psychotherapy) when considering the differential diagnosis of BP II. Discriminating comorbid conditions (such as anxiety and alcohol abuse) from those which could masquerade directly as 'bipolar spectrum' phenomena require a broad-based and comprehensive application of clinical knowledge, without shortcutting such appraisal.

Once a compelling basis *is* established for the diagnosis of BP II, clinical subtyping represents a next relevant step toward formulating a logical treatment plan. Both pharmacological and psychotherapeutic strategies may differ in patients with 'pure' depression versus mixed hypomania with depression; when DSM–IV rapid cycling or recent hypomania is present versus absent; when patients have comorbid Axis I disorders, as well as comorbid personality disorders – based on longitudinal history; and in the presence or absence of medical comorbidities (including diabetes, obesity, and risk factors for metabolic syndrome).

Establishing a lifetime history of past pharmacotherapy trials can be an onerous and, nowadays, a seemingly near-impossible task, yet without at least some knowledge of previous treatments, clinicians easily incur the risk of recreating prior failures. Ideally, one seeks to establish what mood-stabilising agents (i.e. lithium, certain anticonvulsants), antidepressants, and/or second-generation anti-psychotics may previously have been taken, for what purpose (i.e. depression, hypomania, other symptoms), at what dose, for how long, and with what out-comes (either beneficial or adverse). Known past favourable responses are always welcome news, as is information about past responses with later fade-off effects. Some authors believe that loss of response to an antidepressant, for example, may be recoverable upon rechallenge after a period of time off the medication (Byrne and Rothschild, 1998). An unambiguous favourable response to a past psycho-tropic agent compels one to reassess reintroductions, and reasons for prior cessation. (For example, if adverse effects previously seemed to outweigh thera-peutic benefits, are there remediable strategies to counteract adverse effects safely, should they recur?) A history of poor responses to other agents lends particular value to the rechallenge of a discontinued treatment that may previously have been beneficial.

Mood stabilising agents with antimanic efficacy probably are preferable to antidepressants as an initial strategy to treat BP II when there is a history of recent or persistent hypomania, whether or not depressive features coexist. Some clin-icians, for example, maintain that lithium is of particular value in 'mania-driven' forms of bipolar disorder, while an agent such as lamotrigine may be most useful in 'depression-driven' forms of illness (Ketter and Calabrese, 2002). Mood-stabilising agents other than standard antidepressants probably also remain more appropriate in the presence of rapid cycling, and in this respect quetiapine (Calabrese *et al.*, 2005) and lamotrigine (Goldberg *et al.*, 2007) probably each represent the two best-studied interventions. While their specific combination has not been exam-ined in formal clinical trials, their potential for pharmacodynamic synergy can be compelling. Notably, while some clinicians are hesitant to prescribe second-generation antipsychotics for BP II, due to concerns of potential metabolic, neuro-logical or other adverse effects, quetiapine is presently the most extensively studied agent for the treatment of BP II depression, with or without rapid cycling (Calabrese *et al.*, 2005).

Antidepressants likely represent appropriate add-on therapies to mood-stabilising agents when mood-stabilising agents such as lithium, divalproex, lamotrigine or second-generation antipsychotics such as quetiapine alone are ineffective – provided that hypomanic symptoms or rapid cycling are absent. Antidepressants may also be appropriate monotherapies, as described in the review of studies presented in Chapter 7, in the absence of recent hypomanic symptoms or rapid-cycling features. Escitalopram and sertraline probably are the best-studied serotonergic agents for bipolar depression, with positive findings in randomised trials, and they may be preferable to other serotonergic agents, at least initially. The database with bupropion, though not extensive, also appears favourable. Clinically, one might favour bupropion among patients who are overweight, interested in smoking cessation, or particularly concerned about sexual dysfunction. Data in unipolar depression suggest that serotonergic antidepressants, rather than bupropion, may be of particular value in the presence of comorbid anxiety features. Tricyclics, as well as mixed agonists such as venlafaxine, may pose greater safety issues with respect to the induction of hypomania than occurs with serotonin reuptake inhibitors or bupropion, and may be more hazardous if used without anti-manic mood-stabilising agents.

It is difficult to justify the use of antidepressants that are altogether unstudied for bipolar depression (e.g. duloxetine or mirtazapine) before introducing more evidence-based treatments. Similarly, anticonvulsants with no demonstrated efficacy for hypomania or bipolar depression are probably contrary to the standard of care unless other more established treatments have proven unsuccessful, or if they are being used for concomitant symptoms (such as anxiety or pain control) for which there may exist an independent database. Among novel strategies for BP II depression, as described in Chapter 7, modafinil or pramipexole added to mood-stabilising agents have both shown better efficacy than placebo, in preliminary controlled trials.

How long should a pharmacotherapy continue once begun? Clinicians must judge the degree of response (marked, moderate or incomplete) balanced against adverse effects, before forecasting long-term outcomes. Although some guidelines rather arbitrarily advise against the long-term use of antidepressants, clinical wisdom would suggest not perturbing homeostasis without cause. That is, patients with a marked improvement on any regimen should likely stay on that regimen without change for an indefinite period of time unless and until adverse effects or mood changes occur. At that point, practitioners must reassess their clinical status. Concern about long-term antidepressant use may partly reflect automatic assumptions that clinicians fail to identify affective cycling when it occurs. Antidepressants should likely be tapered *off* at the onset of signs of hypomania, or if a pro-cycling effect is suspected (i.e. increased vacillation of symptoms).

Curiously, practitioners are often loathe to discontinue ineffective treatments (whether antidepressant or otherwise mood-stabilising) once adequate trials have occurred – perhaps on grounds of superstition. Chaotic accrual of multiple ineffective agents can produce additive pharmacokinetic and pharmacodynamic adverse effects that may cause iatrogenic problems, which, in turn, might be indistinguishable from mood symptoms (e.g. lethargy, cognitive dulling), promote treatment non-adherence and cloud an overall clinical picture. Systematic treatment monitoring again becomes a fundamental component of serial medication changes and quality clinical care.

Finally, one would be remiss to ignore the role of structured psychotherapies and adjunctive treatments for comorbid conditions (such as alcohol recovery groups for comorbid alcohol abuse or dependence) when indicated. Comprehensive and appropriate treatment for BP II involves evaluating complex forms of psychopathology in which clinical presentations often may seem obscure. Clinical expertise involves skillful interview techniques, awareness of appropriate and available pharmacological and psychotherapeutic options, and the use of critical, creative and flexible judgement to devise logical and sound management strategies.

REFERENCES

Byrne, S. E. and Rothschild, A. J. (1998). Loss of antidepressant efficacy during maintenance therapy: possible mechanisms and treatments. *Journal of Clinical Psychiatry*, **59**, 279–88.

Calabrese, J. R., Keck, P. E. Jr., Macfadden, W. *et al.* (2005). A randomized, double-blind, placebo-controlled trial of quetiapine in the treatment of Bipolar I or II depression. *American Journal of Psychiatry*, **162**, 1351–60.

Goldberg, J. F., Bowden, C. L., Calabrese, J. R. *et al.* (2007). Six-month prospective life charting of mood symptoms with lamotrigine monotherapy versus placebo in rapid-cycling bipolar disorder. *Biological Psychiatry* (in press).

Ketter, T. A. and Calabrese, J. R. (2002). Stabilisation of mood from below versus above baseline in bipolar disorder: a new nomenclature. *Journal of Clinical Psychiatry*, **63**, 146–51.

Management commentary

Robert M. Post

I will focus on several areas of differences in nuance of interpretation of the data and in emphasis regarding the general clinical treatment paradigm suggested by Parker. As he notes, the entire field of bipolar research suffers from a paucity of systematic studies in the literature, thus opening the issue of optimal treatment approaches to a great diversity of opinion.

However, one notable difference in tactics that I would employ is to emphasise that BP II depression is similar to recurrent unipolar depression, but that recurrent depressive illness – of either the unipolar or bipolar variety – carries rather grave risks to one's psychological and medical health. The risk of suicide is high in both syndromes, and in some studies, even higher for BP II than for BP I illness (Rihmer and Pestality, 1999). Recurrence and disability rates are serious and the medical risks are substantial. For example, those who are clinically depressed are two- to four-times more likely to suffer from a myocardial infarction, and if they are depressed at the time of the heart attack, they are two- to four-times more likely to die, than those who are not depressed (Jiang et al., 2002; Malach and Imperato, 2004). Such increased medical risks for illness onset and poorer prognosis when in company with depression cut across a great variety of medical illnesses, from diabetes to complex pain syndromes. Moreover, whereas those with a history of two or fewer prior unipolar or bipolar depressions have the risk of late-life dementia equalling that of the general population, those with four or more depressions, have a doubling of risk (Kessing and Nilsson, 2003; Kessing and Andersen, 2004).

Therefore, I would make every attempt to educate patients about the inherent risks of recurrent depressive illness, indicating only that BP II hypomanic interposing episodes make the risk greater and treatment more complicated. In addition to the minor indiscretions and poor judgement of BP II hypomanias, some 40% of men and more than two-thirds of the women experience these as an uncomfortable, driven, anxious, or what might be labelled dysphoric hypomania (Suppes et al., 2005). The interposing hypomanias of BP II also make it more likely for the patient to use alcohol and other substances of abuse than do patients with

Bipolar II Disorder. Modelling, Measuring and Managing, ed. Gordon Parker. Published by Cambridge University Press. © Cambridge University Press 2008.

unipolar recurrent depression. Recurrences of depression and faster cycling are also more likely with BP II than with unipolar depressions.

Together, all of these factors suggest the critical importance of not only treating the acute episode, but also of long-term prophylaxis. One of the correlates of eventual treatment-refractoriness is a greater number of prior episodes, and in those with rapid-cycling bipolar illness (>4 episodes/year) there is a somewhat uniform reduced responsivity to most psychopharmacological treatments, including naturalistic treatment in general, compared with those with non-rapid-cycling courses. New evidence suggests that each episode of major depression (unipolar or bipolar) is associated with decrements in serum brain-derived neurotrophic factor (BDNF) in proportion to the severity of the depression (Cunha *et al.*, 2006). In addition, there is increased oxidative stress evident during each episode of depression, and this, together with the decreases in BDNF, suggests an increased liability for cellular atrophy and potential cell loss by apoptosis.

Thus, not only are recurrences of depression dysfunctional and dangerous in their own right, but they may also be associated with the possibility of exacerbation and progression of the neurobiological abnormalities underlying the recurrent affective disorders. Countering this daunting possibility are the positive data that lithium, valproate, carbamazepine, quetiapine and all antidepressants increase BDNF or counter the effects of stress in lowering BDNF (Post, 2007). New evidence suggests that these drugs can protect the brain, and improve deficits, or prevent their progression. Thus, patient education focused on the goal of long-term prevention might increase the likelihood that patients will shift their appropriate risk:benefit ratios in favour of concerted attempts at illness prevention.

In terms of therapeutics, patients should be reassured that the primary goal of long-term BP II therapies is prevention of depressive episodes. In naturalistically treated patients in one large academic outpatient clinic, BP II patients experienced 3.7 times as many days depressed as days hypomanic, and remained symptomatic for about half of the days in the year (often with milder sub-syndromal depression), despite being treated with an average of more than three different classes of medications by experts (Kupka *et al.*, 2005). Kukopoulous *et al.* (2003) reported, and we have seen in our own experience in many case series, that patients treated with antidepressants – without a concomitant mood stabiliser, emerge with more treatment-refractory and rapid-cycling depressive recurrences, even after adequate mood stabiliser treatment is initiated. This experience is in accord with most guidelines and expert consensus recommendations that antidepressants should not be used without concomitant mood stabilisers or an atypical antipsychotic (Keck *et al.*, 2004).

Although these recommendations are generally directed at those with BP I illness, we are not aware of many systematic data that would suggest that they are not also appropriate for BP II patients. The one area where there are some data available is from our outpatient network which showed that BP II patients were less likely than BP I patients to switch into hypomania or mania upon adjunctive antidepressant treatment of their bipolar depression, even when concomitant mood stabilisers or atypicals were, in fact, in the regimen (Altshuler *et al.*, 2006; Leverich *et al.*, 2006). However, despite this 'coverage' of the antidepressant with a mood stabiliser, there were still a considerable number of patients 'switching' upon antidepressant augmentation.

After the acute clinical trial of 10 weeks of antidepressants, those of our outpatients who were doing relatively well were offered continuation with the antidepressant for up to one year. However, considering all the patients who were randomised either to bupropion, sertraline or venlafaxine, relatively few patients remained in the study without either experiencing a depressive recurrence or a switch into hypomania (Leverich *et al.*, 2006; Post *et al.*, 2006), suggesting that antidepressant augmentation may not be the ideal treatment for many adults with BP I or BP II illness. Interestingly, in a very small sub-group of about 15% of the patients who did show a good sustained improvement in mood that lasted for 2 months or more, several studies have suggested that these patients do better in terms of fewer depressive recurrences if antidepressant augmentation is maintained over the course of the next year (Altshuler *et al.*, 2001, 2003; Joffe *et al.*, 2005) as opposed to being discontinued, as is often recommended in many of the guidelines.

Given this somewhat disappointing long-term response to adjunctive antidepressant treatment for episodes breaking through a mood stabiliser, what are some of the other options? There is something appealing about the use of lamotrigine monotherapy because it has a profile that is most congruent with that of BP II, that is, it is a better agent for preventing depression than mania. While the original Calabrese *et al.* article (1999) has not been replicated in several multi-centre company-based trials to provide definitive evidence for acute antidepressant effects of lamotrigine, the studies of Frye *et al.* (2000) and Obrocea *et al.* (2002) in our laboratory, that of Sachs *et al.* from the STEP-BD study (Marangell *et al.*, 2004), and a recent European study of lithium augmentation (Nolen *et al.*, 2007) all show excellent acute antidepressant effects of lamotrigine. Aside from the realistic concerns about the presence of a severe rash in about one in 5000 individuals, its side-effect profile appears to be relatively ideal for BP II patients. Lamotrigine is not sedating, is weight neutral, causes no sexual dysfunction, and its slightly activating effects in some individuals may be useful in targeting the hypersomnia of bipolar depression. Moreover, as an agent that also, to a lesser extent, has the ability to prevent manic and mixed states, it would appear to have considerable advantages over the traditional unimodal antidepressants.

Although valproate has somewhat of a mixed profile for effects in either acute depression or its prophylaxis, recent data reported by Davis *et al.* (2005) suggest excellent acute antianxiety and antidepressant effects, and an open study of Winsberg and colleagues (2001) suggested excellent response in a high proportion of BP II patients treated with valproate monotherapy.

Lithium, obviously, remains a good option for many BP II patients, particularly those with a positive family history of affective disorders in first-degree relatives, and in those with problems of acute or chronic suicidality. Likewise, carbamazepine appears useful in BP II patients, particularly those with more complicated presentations of substance abuse comorbidities, anxiety disorders, mood-incongruent delusions, and a negative family history of bipolar illness in first-degree relatives (Post *et al.*, 2002).

Among the atypical antipsychotics, quetiapine is an obvious first choice, since the recent replication of the original Calabrese *et al.* study (2005) by Thase *et al.* (2006) indicates that quetiapine exhibits significant antidepressant, antianxiety and anti-insomnia effects in both BP II and BP I patients. It may have some advantages over olanzapine in the long-term treatment of BP II individuals because it is less likely to be associated with as much acute or sustained weight gain.

Although aripiprazole has not yet been systematically studied in BP II patients, recent open data by McElroy and associates (2007) in adjunctive treatment of bipolar patients, and the controlled study of Nickel *et al.* (2006) in patients with borderline personality disorder indicating highly significant antidepressant and antianxiety effects over placebo, suggest the likely utility of this agent for BP II patients. Aripiprazole also has an excellent short-term and long-term side-effect profile as well as being weight neutral in adults.

Therefore, it would appear prudent to recommend using a mood stabiliser or an atypical antipsychotic, either alone, or with an adjunctive antidepressant if necessary, in the treatment of BP II as well as in BP I. In this regard, there are several reasons to recommend bupropion over serotonin-selective antidepressants (SSRIs) or, in particular, the serotonin-norepinephrine reuptake inhibitors (SNRIs), the latter of which appear to have an increased proclivity for inducing switching in patients, perhaps related to their additional noradrenergic properties (Post *et al.*, 2006). In general, this investigator would avoid the older tricyclic antidepressants in favour of the second-generation agents, not only in light of their less favourable side-effect profile, but also their higher likelihood of lethality in overdose.

Parker's recommendation of careful mood charting and longitudinal monitoring of patients with BP II disorder has much appeal in enhancing the therapeutic alliance, detecting early break-through symptoms, and helping achieve the ideal psychotherapeutic and psychopharmacological treatments that are sufficient to attain and sustain remission. Thus, my only point of departure with his overall therapeutic approach would be the attempt to more directly educate patients as to the very considerable risks of both inadequate and interrupted treatment. The conceptual shift would involve two elements:

(1) like recurrent unipolar illness, BP II illness is a highly recurrent, potentially progressive medical illness that is associated with well-replicated alterations in brain and somatic biochemistry, physiology and even structural anatomy; and

(2) although this message is potentially frightening, it can be moderated by the new perspective that not only will long-term prophylaxis help prevent depressive recurrences, but it may help reverse or prevent some of these underlying neurobiological alterations as well.

The idea of helping to protect the brain and its functioning and restorative processes may add sufficient weight to the risk: benefit ratio to persuade patients to minimise the impact of their illness with appropriate long-term sustained treatment.

REFERENCES

Altshuler, L., Kiriakos, L., Calcagno, J. *et al.* (2001). The impact of antidepressant discontinuation versus antidepressant continuation on one-year risk for relapse of bipolar depression: a retrospective chart review. *Journal of Clinical Psychiatry*, **62**, 612–16.

Altshuler, L., Suppes, T., Black, D. *et al.* (2003). Impact of antidepressant discontinuation after acute bipolar depression remission on rates of depressive relapse at one-year follow-up. *American Journal of Psychiatry*, **160**, 1252–62.

Altshuler, L. L., Suppes, T., Black, D. O. *et al.* (2006). Lower switch rate in depressed patients with Bipolar II than Bipolar I disorder treated adjunctively with second-generation antidepressants. *American Journal of Psychiatry*, **163**, 313–15.

Calabrese, J. R., Bowden, C. L., Sachs, G. S. *et al.* (1999). A double-blind placebo-controlled study of lamotrigine monotherapy in outpatients with Bipolar I depression. Lamictal 602 Study Group. *Journal of Clinical Psychiatry*, **60**, 79–88.

Calabrese, J. R., Keck, P. E. Jr., Macfadden, W. *et al.* (2005). A randomized, double-blind, placebo-controlled trial of quetiapine in the treatment of Bipolar I or II depression. *American Journal of Psychiatry*, **162**, 1351–60.

Cunha, A. B., Frey, B. N., Andreazza, A. C. *et al.* (2006). Serum brain-derived neurotrophic factor is decreased in bipolar disorder during depressive and manic episodes. *Neuroscience Letter*, **398**, 215–19.

Davis, L. L., Bartolucci, A. and Petty, F. (2005). Divalproex in the treatment of bipolar depression: a placebo-controlled study. *Journal of Affective Disorders*, **85**, 259–66.

Frye, M. A., Ketter, T. A., Kimbrell, T. A. *et al.* (2000). A placebo-controlled study of lamotrigine and gabapentin monotherapy in refractory mood disorders. *Journal of Clinical Psychopharmacology*, **20**, 607–14.

Jiang, W., Krishnan, R. R. and O'Connor, C. M. (2002). Depression and heart disease: evidence of a link, and its therapeutic implications. *CNS Drugs*, **16**, 111–27.

Joffe, R. T., MacQueen, G. M., Marriott, M. and Young, L. T. (2005). One-year outcome with antidepressant treatment of bipolar depression. *Acta Psychiatrica Scandinavica*, **112**, 105–9.

Keck, P. E. Jr., Perlis, R. H., Otto, M. W. *et al.* (2004). The Expert Consensus Guideline Series: Treatment of Bipolar Disorder 2004. *Postgraduate Medicine*, Dec., 1–120.

Kessing, L. V. and Nilsson, F. M. (2003). Increased risk of developing dementia in patients with major affective disorders compared to patients with other medical illnesses. *Journal of Affective Disorders*, **73**, 261–9.

Kessing, L. V. and Andersen, P. K. (2004). Does the risk of developing dementia increase with the number of episodes in patients with depressive disorder and in patients with bipolar disorder? *Journal of Neurology, Neurosurgery and Psychiatry*, **75**, 1662–6.

Koukopoulos, A., Sani, G., Koukopoulos, A. E. *et al.* (2003). Duration and stability of the rapid-cycling course: a long-term personal follow-up of 109 patients. *Journal of Affective Disorders*, **73**, 75–85.

Kupka, R. W., Luckenbaugh, D. A., Post, R. M. *et al.* (2005). Comparison of rapid-cycling and non-rapid-cycling bipolar disorder based on prospective mood ratings in 539 outpatients. *American Journal of Psychiatry*, **162**, 1273–80.

Leverich, G. S., Altshuler, L. L., Frye, M. A. *et al.* (2006). Risk of switch in mood polarity to hypomania or mania in patients with bipolar depression during acute and continuation trials of venlafaxine, sertraline, and bupropion as adjuncts to mood stabilizers. *American Journal of Psychiatry*, **163**, 232–9.

Malach, M. and Imperato, P. J. (2004). Depression and acute myocardial infarction. *Preventative Cardiology*, **7**, 83–90.

Marangell, L. B., Martinez, J. M., Ketter, T. A. *et al.* (2004). Lamotrigine treatment of bipolar disorder: data from the first 500 patients in STEP-BD. *Bipolar Disorders*, **6**, 139–43.

McElroy, S. L., Suppes, T., Frye, M. A. *et al.* (2007). Open-label aripiprazole in the treatment of acute bipolar depression: a prospective pilot trial. *Journal of Affective Disorders* (in press).

Nickel, M. K., Muehlbacher, M., Nickel, C. *et al.* (2006). Aripiprazole in the treatment of patients with borderline personality disorder: a double-blind, placebo-controlled study. *American Journal of Psychiatry*, **163**, 833–8.

Nolen, W. A., Kupka, R. W., Hellemann, G. *et al.* (2007). Tranylcypromine versus lamotrigine as adjunctive treatment to a mood stabilizer in bipolar depression: an open randomized controlled study. *Acta Psychiatrica Scandinavica* (in press).

Obrocea, G. V., Dunn, R. M., Frye, M. A. *et al.* (2002). Clinical predictors of response to lamotrigine and gabapentin monotherapy in refractory affective disorders. *Biological Psychiatry*, **51**, 253–60.

Post, R. M. (2007). Role of BDNF in bipolar and unipolar disorder: Clinical and theoretical implications. *Journal of Psychiatric Research* (in press).

Post, R. M., Speer, A. M., Obrocea, G. V. and Leverich, G. S. (2002). Acute and prophylactic effects of anticonvulsants in bipolar depression. *Clinical Neuroscience Research*, **2**, 228–51.

Post, R. M., Altshuler, L. L., Leverich, G. S. *et al.* (2006). Mood switch in bipolar depression: comparison of adjunctive venlafaxine, bupropion and sertraline. *British Journal of Psychiatry*, **189**, 124–31.

Rihmer, Z. and Pestality, P. (1999). Bipolar II Disorder and suicidal behavior. *Psychiatric Clinics of North America*, **22**, 667–73.

Suppes, T., Mintz, J., McElroy, S. L. *et al.* (2005). Mixed hypomania in 908 patients with bipolar disorder evaluated prospectively in the Stanley Foundation Bipolar Treatment Network: a sex-specific phenomenon. *Archives of General Psychiatry*, **62**, 1089–96.

Thase, M. E., Macfadden, W., Weisler, R. H. *et al.* (2006). Efficacy of quetiapine monotherapy in Bipolar I and II depression: a double-blind, placebo-controlled study (the BOLDER II study). *Journal of Clinical Psychopharmacology*, **26**, 600–9.

Winsberg, M. E., Degolia, S. G., Strong, C. M. and Ketter, T. A. (2001). Divalproex therapy in medication-naive and mood-stabilizer-naive Bipolar II depression. *Journal of Affective Disorders*, **67**, 207–12.

23

Management commentary

Allan H. Young

While there is a general consensus that sub-sets of bipolar illness exist, there is in my view no definitive agreement upon the definition of Bipolar II Disorder or bipolar spectrum disorder. This is illustrated by the differences between the DSM–IV and ICD–10 classificatory systems. Bipolar I Disorder, BP II, cyclothymia and Bipolar Disorder Not Otherwise Specified (NOS) are itemised in DSM–IV (American Psychiatric Association, 1994) but ICD–10 (World Health Organization, 1992) only categorises different sub-sets of bipolar affective disorder and mania. DSM–IV criteria for BP II require the presence or history of one or more major depressive episodes and at least one hypomanic episode (past or present), while ICD–10 specifies two or more hypomanic/manic and depressive episodes as being necessary for bipolar affective disorder – raising the curious possibility that some might not consider first-episode mania to be part of bipolar affective disorder.

As earlier detailed in this volume, there is controversy as to whether BP II is distinct from unipolar depression, or if it exists on an overlapping continuum with unipolar depression. Benazzi (2006) reports that this depends on interpretation: BP II and unipolar depression are distinct if classic diagnostic validators are used (family history, age of onset, gender, clinical course of illness); BP II and unipolar depression are continuous if clinical features are used (lifetime manic/hypomanic symptoms, intra-depression hypomanic symptoms and intra-mania depressive symptoms). These issues have yet to be reconciled. A current or past hypomanic episode distinguishes BP II from unipolar depression but misdiagnosis can occur, depending on the diagnostic criteria used for hypomania and the fluctuating nature of bipolar illness (Angst and Gamma, 2002; Akiskal and Benazzi, 2006).

The limits of bipolar spectrum disorder are also unclear – as well detailed by Phelps in Chapter 2 of this volume. Angst (1998) has suggested that recurrent brief hypomania (1–3 days versus DSM–IV criteria of 4 days) belongs to the bipolar spectrum because of its longitudinal prevalence rate of 2.8% and its association with depression and suicidality. The Zurich study (Angst *et al.*, 2003) further suggests a broader concept of bipolarity that includes any relevant manic

Bipolar II Disorder. Modelling, Measuring and Managing, ed. Gordon Parker. Published by Cambridge University Press. © Cambridge University Press 2008.

symptoms; thus, hypomania below the threshold (not meeting current diagnostic criteria) associated with depression appears to be an important indicator of bipolarity. Angst and colleagues show us that this broader definition of bipolarity doubles the prevalence rate of BP II, making it comparable to that of unipolar depression, and this approach may reduce the diagnosis of pseudo-unipolar depression and provide more appropriate treatment approaches.

The lack of an ultimate definition of BP II leads, predictably, to unclear medication treatment strategies, as stated by Parker. In terms of narrowing the multiple options, I offer the following observations:

- Mood stabilisers (lithium and lamotrigine) are used as first-line treatment for BP II, and this strategy is widely adopted in clinical practice (Yatham, 2005).
- The use of antidepressant monotherapy in BP II is controversial (Ghaemi *et al.*, 2003; Amsterdam and Shults, 2005; Parker *et al.*, 2006), and the more commonly suggested option is to add an antidepressant (SSRI) to a mood stabiliser (Yatham, 2005).
- Atypical antipsychotic medications as monotherapy or as adjunctive therapy have been shown to be effective in open-label studies of bipolar illness (Vieta *et al.*, 2001; Janenawasin *et al.*, 2002; Dunner, 2005), but there have been few randomised controlled medication studies specifically for BP II or bipolar spectrum disorder. However, as detailed by several writers in this volume, the recent BOLDER study group evaluated the efficacy of quetiapine monotherapy in BP I and BP II depression in a randomised, double-blind, 8-week, placebo-controlled design (Calabrese *et al.*, 2005; Thase *et al.*, 2006). They reported that quetiapine monotherapy was well tolerated and efficacious for the core mood symptoms of bipolar depression, was effective in reducing suicidal ideation, and improved quality of life and sleep (Endicott *et al.*, 2007). Interestingly, quetiapine was not associated with treatment-emergent mania. The number of enrolled patients in the BOLDER studies was not sufficient to draw firm conclusions regarding the efficacy of quetiapine monotherapy in subpopulations of bipolar depression. However, significant improvement was observed in the BP II subpopulation of the BOLDER II study (Thase *et al.*, 2006) but not seen in the BOLDER I (Calabrese *et al.*, 2005) sample. The former result may represent a high response rate in the placebo group at week eight in BP II patients in the BOLDER I study. Regardless, the BOLDER studies have demonstrated that further systematic research is warranted in relation to the atypical antipsychotic drugs, in particular as a management strategy for BP II.

The bulk of the evidence in relation to drug-management strategies has thus far been from BP I or unipolar depression studies, and we now need treatment studies specifically involving BP II subjects rather than just extrapolating evidence from BP I or unipolar depression studies.

REFERENCES

Akiskal, H. S. and Benazzi, F. (2006). The DSM-IV and ICD-10 categories of recurrent [major] depressive and Bipolar II disorders: evidence that they lie on a dimensional spectrum. *Journal of Affective Disorders*, **92**, 45–54.

Amsterdam, J. D. and Shults, J. (2005). Fluoxetine monotherapy of Bipolar Type II and Bipolar NOS major depression: a double-blind, placebo-substitution, continuation study. *International Clinical Psychopharmacology*, **20**, 257–64.

American Psychiatric Association (1994). *Diagnostic and Statistical Manual of Mental Disorders*, 4th edn. Washington, DC: American Psychiatric Association.

Angst, J. (1998). The emerging epidemiology of hypomania and Bipolar II Disorder. *Journal of Affective Disorders*, **50**, 143–51.

Angst, J. and Gamma, A. (2002). A new bipolar spectrum concept: a brief review. *Bipolar Disorders*, **4** (Suppl. 1), S11–14.

Angst, J., Gamma, A., Benazzi, F., Ajdacic, V., Eich, D. and Rossler, W. (2003). Toward a re-definition of subthreshold bipolarity: epidemiology and proposed criteria for Bipolar II, minor bipolar disorders and hypomania. *Journal of Affective Disorders*, **73**, 133–46.

Benazzi, F. (2006). A continuity between Bipolar II depression and major depressive disorder? *Progress in Neuropsychopharmacology and Biological Psychiatry*, **30**, 1043–50.

Calabrese, J. R., Keck, P. E. Jr, Macfadden, W. *et al.* (2005). A randomized, double-blind, placebo-controlled trial of quetiapine in the treatment of Bipolar I or II depression. *American Journal of Psychiatry*, **162**, 1351–60.

Dunner, D. L. (2005). Atypical antipsychotics: efficacy across bipolar disorder subpopulations. *Journal of Clinical Psychiatry*, **66** (Suppl. 3), S20–7.

Endicott, J., Rajagopalan, K., Minkwitz, M., Macfadden, W. and the BOLDER Study Group (2007). A randomized, double-blind, placebo-controlled study of quetiapine in the treatment of Bipolar I and II depression: improvements in quality of life. *International Clinical Psychopharmacology*, **22**, 29–37.

Ghaemi, S. N., Hsu, D. J., Soldani, F. and Goodwin, F. K. (2003). Antidepressants in bipolar disorder: the case for caution. *Bipolar Disorders*, **5**, 421–33.

Janenawasin, S., Wang, P. W., Lembke, A. *et al.* (2002). Olanzapine in diverse syndromal and sub-syndromal exacerbations of bipolar disorders. *Bipolar Disorders*, **4**, 328–34.

Parker, G., Tully, L., Olley, A. and Hadzi-Pavlovic, D. (2006). SSRIs as mood stabilizers for Bipolar II Disorder? A proof of concept study. *Journal of Affective Disorders*, **92**, 205–14.

Thase, M. E., Macfadden, W., Weisler, R. H. *et al.* for the BOLDER II Study Group (2006). Efficacy of quetiapine monotherapy in Bipolar I and II depression: a double-blind, placebo-controlled study (the BOLDER II study). *Journal of Clinical Psychopharmacology*, **26**, 600–9.

Vieta, E., Gasto, C., Colom, F. *et al.* (2001). Role of risperidone in Bipolar II: an open 6-month study. *Journal of Affective Disorders*, **67**, 213–19.

Yatham, L. N. (2005). Diagnosis and management of patients with Bipolar II Disorder. *Journal of Clinical Psychiatry*, **66** (Suppl. 1), S13–17.

World Health Organization (1992). *The ICD–10 Classification of Mental and Behavioural Disorders*. Geneva: World Health Organization.

24

Management commentary

Guy M. Goodwin

To start with diagnosis, I have much sympathy with the educational component of the advice that is suggested in Parker's template. I am a little more cautious in accepting that hypomania is of unalloyed benefit to patients. While the subjective benefit of mood elevation may be obvious, the additional energy and self-confidence can lead both to a dissipation of goal-directed activity and increased conflict with others, which can produce a non-productive whirlwind of action. I am therefore rather cautious in accepting that even 'bipolar-lite' is anything better than friendly fire.

Aspects of Parker's medical management plan are delightfully unorthodox. To make SSRIs the first-line treatment both for mood stabilisation and for bipolar depression associated with mood disorder is not in any guideline! It is based very much on clinical experience and on the correct perception that the dangers of 'switch' in bipolar depression are rather overstated, particularly by American authorities.

However, in many Western countries there has been a sensitisation to the idea that SSRIs cause harm through their actions on arousal, or even 'suicidality'. While this is not the place to address this litigation-fuelled belief, there is no doubt that it has affected, in an adverse way, the environment in which SSRIs are used. Furthermore, we have all seen mood instability or hypomania occur after prescribing a SSRI, whether or not we can be sure it is caused by it. So, my own preference is usually for lamotrigine when the burden of the illness or presentation is acute depression. While I remain mindful of the risks of rash or even the Stevens–Johnson syndrome, in practice I have not had problems in this regard and, of course, always employ a slow-dose taper at the start. I am more likely to add quetiapine than olanzapine as an augmenting strategy because of quetiapine's better trial data on efficacy and lesser short-term metabolic consequences, which I think are difficult to justify to the patient group we are dealing with here.

To speak of mood stability in BP II often implies a cyclical or rapid-cycling course, which is widely acknowledged to be difficult to treat. I try not to be slow to propose either the use of lithium or divalproate. Where patients find the adverse

Bipolar II Disorder. Modelling, Measuring and Managing, ed. Gordon Parker. Published by Cambridge University Press. © Cambridge University Press 2008.

effects of either of the latter drugs difficult to tolerate (and where weight gain is a big problem), I have in recent months been using oxcarbazepine with apparent benefit (but without controlled data for efficacy). While, in theory, these drugs may be worth trying as monotherapy, the burden of illness is usually depression, against which they are often unsatisfactory. Thus, I often find myself adding lithium, divalproate or oxcarbazine to lamotrigine, since the latter often appears to reduce the depressive symptoms without full control of manic symptoms or hypomania.

To escalate treatment for a clear-cut depressive episode from lamotrigine or an SSRI to either an alternative treatment, or to a combination treatment is a pragmatic decision. I am certainly prepared to use the SSRIs, venlafaxine, or indeed the MAO inhibitors for the treatment of BP II patients. In practice, I find the order and the preference is determined in large measure by previous experience of patients, since they rarely come to me treatment-naïve. The place of quetiapine is assuming increasing interest because of its demonstrated benefits in both BP I and BP II depression and the relative ease with which it can be added to other medications. However, it is not well tolerated at the doses trialled for bipolar depression (300 and 600 mg).

Probably for arbitrary reasons of structure, the role of education, mood charting and a wellbeing plan is placed in the final section of Parker's template. These deserve the highest priority. Such proposals provide a non-optional foundation to treatment, about which there is rather less controversy than the pharmacological approaches. I wholeheartedly endorse what is said.

The role of psychotherapy as distinct from psychoeducation is more problematic. Many psychotherapies are so eclectic that it is difficult to know where psycho-education ends and therapy begins. Moreover, non-specific factors of empathy and understanding accompany all good psychiatric consultation. But, the obvious potential for reducing inter-episode mood instability and anxiety through a focused psychotherapy appears very attractive. Cognitive behaviour therapy (CBT) has the clearest claims to be a specific intervention for depression, based more or less on Beck's ideas about how cognitions shape mood. The problem has always been that mood also shapes cognition. Hence the likely benefit of a CBT intervention will depend on which side the balance lies. Most of us who see bipolar patients con-ceptualise their mood changes as largely endogenous, and the negative cognitions as usually driven rather than driving. Hence the preliminary support for the idea that CBT is effective in preventing relapse to depression (Lam *et al.*, 2003) was of great interest, if a little surprising. It has been cast into some doubt by the large Medical Research Council (MRC) trial recently reported in this country (Scott *et al.*, 2006). The latter was conducted by a group of therapists who were extremely surprised to find how ineffective their intervention proved to be, compared with treatment as usual. Thus the assumption that CBT, as usually delivered, is particularly well suited to the majority of patients with severe bipolar disorder, may be premature.

Mindfulness-based Cognitive Therapy (MBCT) combines aspects of cognitive therapy with training in meditation. MBCT teaches people skills that enable them to become more aware of their thoughts without judgement, viewing negative thoughts as passing mental events rather than as facts. MBCT has proven effective in preventing relapse in recurrent depression (Teasdale *et al.*, 2000) and is based on an approach that is known to be helpful in the treatment of anxiety disorders (Mindfulness-based Stress Reduction: Miller *et al.*, 1995). Additionally, preliminary findings suggest an important impact on between-episode anxiety in bipolar patients, a major neglected problem. Further work is needed to define MBCT's potential to prevent relapse in bipolar patients.

REFERENCES

Lam, D. H., Watkins, E. R., Hayward, P. *et al.* (2003). Randomized controlled study of cognitive therapy for relapse prevention for Bipolar Affective Disorder: outcome of the first year. *Archives of General Psychiatry*, **60**, 145–52.

Miller, J., Fletcher, K. and Kabat-Zinn, J. (1995). Three-year follow-up and clinical implications of a mindfulness meditation-based stress reduction intervention in the treatment of anxiety disorder. *General Hospital Psychiatry*, **17**, 192–200.

Scott, J., Paykel, E., Morriss, R. *et al.* (2006). Cognitive-behavioural therapy for bipolar disorder. *British Journal of Psychiatry*, **188**, 313–20.

Teasdale, J. D., Segal, Z. V., Williams, J. M. G. *et al.* (2000). The prevention of relapse/recurrence of major depression by mindfulness-based cognitive therapy. *Journal of Consulting and Clinical Psychology*, **68**, 615–23.

25

Management commentary

Sophia Frangou

Providing a diagnosis and introducing a management plan

As Parker points out, the diagnosis of Bipolar II Disorder requires detailed history-taking from more than one informant. The identification of hypomanic episodes is more difficult than for manic ones and these may have been overlooked in previous assessments. It is also crucial to engage patients and their families in explaining the diagnosis, its implication and its treatment.

However, it is questionable whether BP II can really be described as a 'milder form' or 'bipolar lite'. At best, one could argue that the prognosis and clinical course of BP II are areas of genuine clinical uncertainty because of poor availability of relevant data. It is regrettable that even large-scale studies addressing its prognosis, treatment and outcome (such as that undertaken by the Stanley Foundation Bipolar Network) have failed to substantially increase our knowledge base about BP II. Some data from this study are, nevertheless, highly relevant in suggesting that the morbidity and disability associated with BP II is at least comparable with that for BP I. For example, Nolen and colleagues (2004) examined the one-year clinical outcome for 258 bipolar disorder patients, of whom 53 had a diagnosis of BP II. They found that the mean overall severity of bipolar disorder was related to the severity of the depressive – and not the manic/hypomanic features. It is perhaps true that psychosis is not a clinical feature of BP II, but this is perhaps of limited clinical importance given the limited prognostic significance of psychosis for the course and outcome of the disorder (Keck *et al.*, 2003).

I also find it difficult to subscribe to the idea of the 'romance' of bipolar disorder. It may be helpful to patients and their families to maintain a positive view of bipolar disorder, but neither existing evidence nor my clinical experience suggest that patients are overall more creative or more productive. In fact, regardless of subtype, most patients with bipolar disorder are significantly disadvantaged by their illness and suffer from mood symptoms, mostly depressive, about a third or more of their lives (Post *et al.*, 2003; Judd *et al.*, 2005). The predicament of BP II

Bipolar II Disorder. Modelling, Measuring and Managing, ed. Gordon Parker. Published by Cambridge University Press. © Cambridge University Press 2008.

patients may be worse than faced by those with BP I in this respect. Judd and colleagues (2003) focused on BP II and obtained weekly symptomatic ratings from 86 patients over a mean period of 13.4 years. These patients were symptomatic for 53.9% of the time; depressive symptoms predominated (being present for 50.3% of follow-up weeks), while manic/hypomanic and cycling/mixed states were present for 1.3% and 2.3% of the time respectively. I am happy to accept that, for some patients, their experiences while depressed or elated may inspire their work or promote a deeper understanding of the human condition – but overall the disorder is a burden rather than a blessing. Our challenge is to minimise this burden as much as we can so that bipolar patients can enjoy as 'normal' a life as possible. Part of this difficult task is to manage patients' expectations. To a large degree, presenting a very optimistic outlook where BP II is presented as rather inconsequential in terms of its impact on patients' aspirations may not be helpful in the long term.

Medication strategies

I agree with Parker that symptom resolution and sustained mood stabilisation should be the primary objectives in the management of BP II. Bipolar disorder is perhaps one of the few psychiatric disorders where we can meaningfully apply a model of recovery and social reintegration if symptoms are sufficiently controlled (Judd *et al.*, 2005). Although response rates to psychotropic drugs are generally not ideal, and despite our current inability to provide individualised prescribing, the majority of people with bipolar disorder benefit from medication. Choosing the right medication regime is invariably complex and the pharmacological properties of the drugs are only one dimension. Despite this, it is important to consider both the pharmacological properties and the assumed efficacy of the different drugs in the management of the different phases of bipolar disorder.

Lithium and a number of antiepileptic drugs (carbamazepine, sodium valproate and lamotrigine, to mention those most commonly used) are often referred to as 'mood stabilisers'. It would be perhaps more accurate to refer to them as anti-manic as they are most efficacious in the acute treatment and prevention of manic rather than depressive features of bipolar disorder (Bauer and Mitchner, 2004), with the notable exception of lamotrigine. Although not explicitly stated, I believe that the predominantly anti-manic action of mood stabilisers may have influenced Parker's choice of antidepressant monotherapy as the first line of treatment in BP II. My only reservation here is that this strategy carries a risk of manic switch or rapid cycling which, although not a particular feature of BP II (Schneck *et al.*, 2004; Kupka *et al.*, 2005), needs to be managed carefully with regular monitoring. This requires both a responsive model of care provision and good patient engagement.

When either or both of these provisions are lacking or are questionable, it is perhaps safer to combine an antidepressant with either a classic mood stabiliser or with quetiapine, or to use quetiapine as monotherapy (Calabrese *et al.*, 2005). Emerging evidence suggests that quetiapine may prove the first true mood-stabilising drug as it has both antidepressant and anti-manic properties (Bowden *et al.*, 2005). In contrast, other atypical antipsychotic drugs, such as olanzapine advocated here, may be comparable or even superior to other anti-manic drugs such as lithium but they seem to have minimal impact on the depressive pole of bipolar disorder (Perlis *et al.*, 2006; Tohen *et al.*, 2003, 2005). Although Parker reports good results with olanzapine in combination with antidepressants, my preference is to avoid prescribing this drug as its superiority over other available agents is questionable, while it carries a higher risk of metabolic side effects (Guo *et al.*, 2006).

Other treatment strategies

Parker rightly emphasises the importance of non-pharmacological treatments in the management of BP II. It is regrettable that, despite the evidence for the beneficial effect of psychoeducation in the outcome of bipolar disorder (e.g. Colom *et al.*, 2005), such interventions are rarely available clinically in a formal and systematic fashion as provided in randomised controlled trials to patients.

References

Bauer, M. S. and Mitchner, L. (2004). What is a "mood stabilizer"? An evidence-based response. *American Journal of Psychiatry*, **161**, 3–18.

Bowden, C. L., Grunze, H., Mullen, J. *et al.* (2005). A randomized, double-blind, placebo-controlled efficacy and safety study of quetiapine or lithium as monotherapy for mania in bipolar disorder. *Journal of Clinical Psychiatry*, **66**, 111–21.

Calabrese, J. R., Keck, P. E. Jr., Macfadden, W. *et al.* (2005). A randomized, double-blind, placebo-controlled trial of quetiapine in the treatment of Bipolar I or II depression. *American Journal of Psychiatry*, **162**, 1351–60.

Colom, F., Vieta, E., Sanchez-Moreno, J. *et al.* (2005). Stabilizing the stabilizer: group psycho-education enhances the stability of serum lithium levels. *Bipolar Disorders*, **7** (Suppl. 5), S32–6.

Guo, J. J., Keck, P. E. Jr., Corey-Lisle, P. K. *et al.* (2006). Risk of diabetes mellitus associated with atypical antipsychotic use among patients with bipolar disorder: a retrospective, population-based, case-control study. *Journal of Clinical Psychiatry*, **67**, 1055–61.

Judd, L. L., Akiskal, H. S., Schettler, P. J. *et al.* (2003). A prospective investigation of the natural history of the long-term weekly symptomatic status of Bipolar II Disorder. *Archives of General Psychiatry*, **60**, 261–9.

Judd, L. L., Akiskal, H. S., Schettler, P. J. *et al.* (2005). Psychosocial disability in the course of Bipolar I and II disorders: a prospective, comparative, longitudinal study. *Archives of General Psychiatry*, **62**, 1322–30.

Keck, P. E. Jr., McElroy, S. L., Havens, J. R. *et al.* (2003). Psychosis in bipolar disorder: phenomenology and impact on morbidity and course of illness. *Comprehensive Psychiatry*, **44**, 263–9.

Kupka, R. W., Luckenbaugh, D. A., Post, R. M. *et al.* (2005). Comparison of rapid-cycling and non-rapid-cycling bipolar disorder based on prospective mood ratings in 539 outpatients. *American Journal of Psychiatry*, **162**, 1273–80.

Nolen, W. A., Luckenbaugh, D. A., Altshuler, L. L. *et al.* (2004). Correlates of one-year prospective outcome in bipolar disorder: results from the Stanley Foundation Bipolar Network. *American Journal of Psychiatry*, **161**, 1447–54.

Perlis, R. H., Baker, R. W., Zarate, C. A. Jr. *et al.* (2006). Olanzapine versus risperidone in the treatment of manic or mixed states in Bipolar I Disorder: a randomized, double-blind trial. *Journal of Clinical Psychiatry*, **67**, 1747–53.

Post, R. M., Denicoff, K. D., Leverich, G. S. *et al.* (2003). Morbidity in 258 bipolar outpatients followed for one year with daily prospective ratings on the NIMH life chart method. *Journal of Clinical Psychiatry*, **64**, 680–90.

Schneck, C. D., Miklowitz, D. J., Calabrese, J. R. *et al.* (2004). Phenomenology of rapid-cycling bipolar disorder: data from the first 500 participants in the Systematic Treatment Enhancement Program. *American Journal of Psychiatry*, **161**, 1902–8.

Tohen, M., Greil, W., Calabrese, J. R. *et al.* (2005). Olanzapine versus lithium in the maintenance treatment of bipolar disorder: a 12-month, randomized, double-blind, controlled clinical trial. *American Journal of Psychiatry*, **162**, 1281–90.

Tohen, M., Ketter, T. A., Zarate, C. A. *et al.* (2003). Olanzapine versus divalproex sodium for the treatment of acute mania and maintenance of remission: a 47-week study. *American Journal of Psychiatry*, **160**, 1263–71.

Management commentary: What would Hippocrates do?

S. Nassir Ghaemi

Recent pharmacy-based data (Baldessarini *et al.*, 2007) in the USA indicate American clinicians prescribe *antidepressant monotherapy* as the most common initial treatment for diagnosed bipolar disorder, and with the same frequency in Bipolar II Disorder (BP II) and Bipolar I Disorder (BP I) patients (i.e. in about 50%; only 25% receive mood stabiliser monotherapy). In fact, the whole controversy about using antidepressants in bipolar disorder is rather recent. Despite some early studies in the 1970s and 1980s (Goodwin and Jamison, 1990), the American Psychiatric Association practice guidelines in 1994 still recommended antidepressant plus mood stabiliser as first-line treatment of acute bipolar depression (Hirschfeld *et al.*, 1994). This recommendation did not change until 2002 (Hirschfeld *et al.*, 2002), and even then only applied to non-severe acute bipolar depression. Even this mild change led to a backlash, which continues to this day, particularly in the British Commonwealth (Parker, 2002; Goodwin and Young, 2003) and some parts of Germany (Moller and Grunze, 2000; Moller *et al.*, 2006). Yet it is important to note that this divide, particularly within the English-speaking world, is quite recent – it dates not to 1776 but to 2002. And even still, many bipolar experts in the USA (Altshuler *et al.*, 2003; Keck and McElroy, 2003), and most clinicians (Baldessarini *et al.*, 2007), do not view antidepressant use as problematic. Thus, if antidepressants are in fact ineffective or sometimes harmful (Ghaemi *et al.*, 2003), then we have a major current public health problem that needs to be fixed. If not, then we (in the USA) can rest on our laurels.

Parker's group is to be commended for bringing more attention to BP II. The good news is that such scientific controversies in the end will be able to be addressed by more data, in which case some of us will be right and some wrong and, in the scientific spirit, any of us could be wrong. We need to constantly maintain humility and openness to the reality that other views may turn out to be correct. As the American philosopher Charles Sanders Peirce put it, truth is corrected error (Peirce, 1958). Peirce also emphasised that knowledge of scientific truth is not the purview of any individual but, rather, flows from the consensus of

Bipolar II Disorder. Modelling, Measuring and Managing, ed. Gordon Parker. Published by Cambridge University Press. © Cambridge University Press 2008.

the community of investigators: we are all in this together. I provide this critique in that spirit. Firstly, with brief comments on some of the empirical literature, and, secondly, offering some clinical/conceptual perspectives.

Comments on the empirical literature

Data never speak for themselves; they always need to be interpreted. This is a basic axiom of statistics and epidemiology (Rothman, 2002). Hence, these comments are not meant to be definitive, and this analysis will certainly evolve with more data. Any analysis of the empirical research should first distinguish between acute and maintenance efficacy.

In relation to *acute efficacy*, the most commonly cited randomised antidepressant studies have been post hoc analyses of the unipolar depression literature (where, before 1994, BP II was not diagnosed, and thus such subjects were not excluded). For instance, in one such study 89 BP II subjects were identified in a cohort of 839 fluoxetine-treated patients and compared with 89 age- and gender-matched unipolar patients and with 661 unmatched unipolar subjects (Amsterdam *et al.*, 1998). The efficacy of fluoxetine was reported equal in the bipolar and unipolar groups. It is important that this analysis does not establish fluoxetine was better than placebo in BP II, but rather that fluoxetine response in BP II was similar to fluoxetine response in unipolar depression; the drug–placebo difference was not reported. Further, an analysis of the published data shows that the acute manic switch rate was actually four times higher in the BP II than in the unipolar group (4% vs 1%), though the paper itself does not report this analysis. Another report (Peet, 1994), which is often cited as evidence of minimal risk with the newer antidepressants, is a review in which manic switch occurred more frequently with TCAs (11.2%) vs SSRIs (3.7%) or placebo (4.2%) (Peet, 1994).

The main problem with both of these reports is that they consisted of post hoc analyses, which lead to inflated false positive chance findings (Oxman and Guyatt, 1992). (A classic study of this topic found that astrological signs predicted cardiac mortality in a post hoc analysis of randomised data; ISIS-2, 1988.) Further, since these analyses pooled different individual studies, they removed the effects of randomisation, due to reintroduction of clinical and demographic differences between studies that may influence the results (Blettner *et al.*, 1999). Besides such chance error and confounding bias risks, these studies also risk a misclassification bias (Sosenko and Gardner, 1987): no mania rating scales were performed in either study. As discovered with studies of other adverse outcomes (e.g. sexual dysfunction), if poor outcomes are not systematically assessed, they are often overlooked (Clayton *et al.*, 1997).

Prospective studies designed to assess antidepressant efficacy in BP II depression *are* emerging. Two recent examples exist, both with small samples (Amsterdam and Shults, 2005; Parker *et al.*, 2006) of 12 and 10 subjects respectively. The small samples are the major problem with these studies. The whole point of randomisation is to remove confounding bias, so that comparison groups are equal on all parameters except those being studied (Rothman, 2002; Soldani *et al.*, 2005). Successful equalisation of variables requires a large enough sample. Small sample sizes essentially invalidate the randomisation: flipping a coin 10 times will be unlikely to lead to 50–50 heads and tails; thus larger samples are needed to allow chance differences to be unlikely (perhaps $n \geq 50$ or more) (Soldani *et al.*, 2005). These 'randomised' studies are – in fact – not randomised, but observational.

Specific to the study by Parker and colleagues (Parker *et al.*, 2006), other important methodological limitations are the crossover design and the follow-up period. The crossover design is less valid for acutely changing conditions, such as bipolar disorder, where natural mood episode changes occur with some frequency. Such a design is most valid for chronic conditions, in which short-term changes in illness are not likely (Maclure and Mittleman, 2000), as carry-over effects will bias the crossover design in unstable conditions. Ultra-rapid-cycling bipolar disorder would not seem suitable for this kind of crossover design. Nonetheless, with these limitations, the authors report an apparent pattern of response to SSRIs in 5/10 subjects. Whether this is greater than would be expected from the natural history of illness is unclear. Secondly, the follow-up period of 3 months does not demonstrate maintenance phase benefit, as the investigators appear to claim, since the maintenance phase of treatment, even in rapid cycling, is probably in the 3–6-month period (or even longer) after the acute phase (Goodwin and Jamison, 2007). If the data are valid, they still represent acute benefit, at best.

Turning to *long-term maintenance studies*, only one placebo-controlled study of BP II exists, in which imipramine was the same as placebo and less effective than lithium in a small sample ($n = 22$) (Kane *et al.*, 1982).

We are left then with a literature that is essentially observational and limited, suggesting possible short-term benefits with antidepressants for those with BP II.

A final empirical clue regarding efficacy may be found in the treatment-resistant depression literature. Since BP II was not diagnosed before DSM–IV (American Psychiatric Association, 1994), the previous depression literature included such patients, which may be relevant to the strong randomised evidence from that era of efficacy with lithium in TRD (Bauer *et al.*, 2003). More recent studies, such as STAR-D, which exclude BP II, fail to replicate previously suggested lithium efficacy (Rush *et al.*, 2006). Further, recent studies find that up to one-half of those with TRD have been misdiagnosed and instead suffer from BP II depression (Parker *et al.*,

2005; Sharma *et al.*, 2005; Inoue *et al.*, 2006). Their failure to respond to multiple adequate antidepressant trials indirectly throws further doubt on the assumption that antidepressants are effective, at least as monotherapy, in BP II depression.

Clinical/conceptual perspectives

In the face of this limited evidence, my own perspective falls into two categories: clinical and conceptual. *Clinically*, it seems to me to make sense to divide BP II patients into those who have, or do not have, rapid cycling. In the treatment of depression with rapid cycling, BP II patients appear not to do well with anti-depressants, based on the limited data available (Altshuler *et al.*, 1995; Ghaemi *et al.*, 2000). In non-rapid-cycling BP II, patients seem to respond to whatever medications are given, even mood-stabiliser monotherapy (Winsberg *et al.*, 2001). I thus recommend low-dose mood stabilisers (such as lithium carbonate 600 mg/day or divalproex sodium 500–750 mg/day), due to limited side effects at lower doses and the fact that blood levels are based on BP I studies and may not relate to BP II. One observational study found the mean level of effective divalproex usage in BP II and cyclothymia to be 32.5 ng/dl (Jacobsen, 1993). My rationale as well is that these agents may also have long-term benefits and at least will not worsen bipolar disorder. I also will use less proven agents, like gabapentin or topiramate (which may have even fewer side effects), based on observational effectiveness of these agents in BP II illness (Ghaemi *et al.*, 1998, 2001; Ghaemi and Goodwin, 2003). These data are not much less valid than the antidepressant literature cited above, and again, here we have no question of possible worsening of the illness based on mania induction.

Hence, there is no reason that clinicians should feel forced to use antidepressants. It is an option, but not an option that is any better proven than mood stabilisers, which are safer. In fact, I prefer to encourage clinicians to avoid thinking of antidepressants as an early-choice option on grounds that Chekhov put well: If a pistol enters a story, eventually it has to be fired. This gets us to the *conceptual* perspective – Hippocratic psychopharmacology (Ghaemi, 2006).

Hippocrates is often misunderstood (Holmes, 1891; McHugh, 1996; Jouanna, 2001). His main teaching was not 'First do no harm'. Often that phrase is parroted as if it simply refers to ethical conservatism in treatment. But Hippocrates had a conceptual rationale for his ethics, one based on his beliefs regarding the nature of disease. In the Hippocratic perspective, disease, though produced by nature, was also cured by nature. Thus, nature was seen as the doctor's ally, not the doctor's enemy. Unlike the surgeon, for whom cure was achieved by the artificial means of the knife, the physician served as the handmaiden to nature, not curing, but helping nature to heal.

The Hippocratics divided diseases into three groups: those which are self-remitting, those which are treatable, and those which are not treatable. No treatment is needed for the first and third groups; the second group should be actively treated. Thus, Hippocratic psychopharmacology would generally be conservative and informed by the natural history of disease, not on abstract ethical grounds, but reflecting the nature of the disease. Hippocratic psychopharmacologists would not constantly be at war with symptoms, trying to fight against nature as the enemy, believing that our pills directly are the source of cure (or even, in the long run, reduce symptoms). Rather, Hippocratic psychopharmacology would consist of, first and foremost, seeking to know the disease, treating it only when the benefits clearly outweigh the risks (as described below), and doing so with a general humility that grows from knowing that nature effects healing, with the doctor's role being to help when possible and to get out of the way when not needed.

Contemporary psychopharmacology, I would assert, is non-Hippocratic. This is not due to ethical lapses; it is not because doctors ignore 'harm'. Rather, on conceptual grounds, most doctors do not understand, or implicitly reject, the Hippocratic philosophy of disease and treatment (Ghaemi, 2006).

Applied to BP II, the rapid cycling type is self-limited: there is no need to treat the acute episode with antidepressants, especially if the episodes are shorter than one month, since antidepressant biological effects are often slow. The key issue is prevention of episodes. Even for non-rapid-cycling BP II, the average duration of depression seems to be 3–6 months, and a reason to intervene with antidepressants acutely might be for marked suicidality or severely impaired functioning. But the main problem still is long-term prevention, and antidepressants have no evidence of efficacy here, alongside the possibility of worsening of the illness.

Many clinicians are unfazed by this lack of evidence of efficacy. They argue instead that one has to prove harm – to definitively demonstrate that antidepressants cause mania or rapid cycling – to convince them to stop prescribing these drugs. This has the matter backwards.

In thinking about this problem, I turned to the work of the nineteenth century American physician Oliver Wendell Holmes (Holmes, 1891). In that century, the *materia medica* (the equivalent of today's Physician's Desk Reference, PDR) was much larger than today's PDR. Physicians used pills and potions for everything: they were quite interventionist. Holmes argued that most of those treatments did not work, and simply caused harm. He argued legalistically. In the law, a person is innocent until proven guilty. In medicine, drugs should be seen as guilty until proven innocent. There is a presumption they are harmful; most do have side effects. Thus, we need to start on the benefit side of the risk: benefit ledger. Since we presume all drugs to be harmful, none should be used until there is some proof of benefit, and, the more valid the scientific proof, the better (Ghaemi, 2002).

Another way of putting it, as William Osler said, is that all drugs are toxic; it is only indications and dosing that make them effective. With this approach, gabapentin would not have been prescribed widely for every ailment (Mack, 2003), and antidepressants would not be prescribed extensively for bipolar disorder – as they are currently – in the absence of preventive benefit (Ghaemi *et al.*, 2003). Thus, what I call Holmes' Rule (Ghaemi, 2003), requires proof of efficacy before we prescribe medications.

Holmes' Rule: All medications are presumed harmful. Have proof of benefit before assessing risks.

Most psychiatrists practise non-Hippocratically. This is not to say that they are unethical or even wrong, but simply that they believe that Nature is the enemy and they want to intervene aggressively to cure patients. In the Hippocratic approach, if one does not have an adequate treatment, then one does not treat. It is no justification of unscientific treatments to state that we do not have scientific evidence. In such cases, one should refrain from treatment, because, on the whole, one will produce more harm than good (Ghaemi, 2006).

In the case of antidepressants, the question is not what reasons should we have to *not* use them, but what reasons should we have *to* use them. It is not that every patient should be given them until we get reasons to disprove their use, the scientific approach in Hippocratic medicine is that our default position is *not* to use medications unless we have strong reasons to do so. In the case of bipolar disorder, one can make a Hippocratic case to use antidepressants later down the line. The alternative view – the non-Hippocratic one – that antidepressants should be used extensively in BP II is difficult to distinguish from other non-Hippocratic approaches to medicine in the past, such as bleeding used extensively in the nineteenth century for all conditions, and psychoanalysis used extensively in the twentieth century for all conditions. Who is to say whether the use of 'antidepressants for all' in the twenty-first century is any different?

REFERENCES

Altshuler, L. L., Post, R. M., Leverich, G. S. *et al.* (1995). Antidepressant-induced mania and cycle acceleration: a controversy revisited. *American Journal of Psychiatry*, **152**, 1130–8.

Altshuler, L., Suppes, T., Black, D. *et al.* (2003). Impact of antidepressant discontinuation after acute bipolar depression remission on rates of depressive relapse at one-year follow-up. *American Journal of Psychiatry*, **160**, 1252–62.

American Psychiatric Association (1994). *Diagnostic and Statistical Manual of Mental Disorders*, 4th edn. Washington, DC: APA.

Amsterdam, J. D. and Shults, J. (2005). Fluoxetine monotherapy of Bipolar Type II and bipolar NOS major depression: a double-blind, placebo-substitution, continuation study. *International Clinical Psychopharmacology*, **20**, 257–64.

Amsterdam, J. D., Garcia-Espana, F., Fawcett, J. *et al.* (1998). Efficacy and safety of fluoxetine in treating Bipolar II major depressive episode. *Journal of Clinical Psychopharmacology*, **18**, 435–40.

Baldessarini, R. J., Leahy, L., Arcona, S. *et al.* (2007). Patterns of psychotropic drug prescription for U.S. patients with diagnoses of bipolar disorders. *Psychiatric Services*, **58**, 85–91.

Bauer, M., Adli, M., Baethge, C. *et al.* (2003). Lithium augmentation therapy in refractory depression: clinical evidence and neurobiological mechanisms. *Canadian Journal of Psychiatry*, **48**, 440–8.

Blettner, M., Sauerbrei, W., Schlehofer, B., Scheuchenpflug, T. and Friedenreich, C. (1999). Traditional reviews, meta-analyses and pooled analyses in epidemiology. *International Journal of Epidemiology*, **28**, 1–9.

Clayton, A. H., McGarvey, E. L., Clavet, G. J. and Piazza, L. (1997). Comparison of sexual functioning in clinical and non-clinical populations using the Changes in Sexual Functioning Questionnaire (CSFQ). *Psychopharmacology Bulletin*, **33**, 747–53.

Fox-Wasylyshyn, S. M. and El-Masri, M. M. (2005). Handling missing data in self-report measures. *Research in Nursing and Health*, **28**, 488–95.

Ghaemi, S. N. (ed.) (2002). *Polypharmacy in Psychiatry*. New York: Marcel Dekker.

Ghaemi, S. N. (2003). *Mood Disorders: A Practical Guide*. Philadelphia: Lippincott, Williams, and Wilkins.

Ghaemi, S. N. (2006). Hippocrates and prozac: the controversy about antidepressants in bipolar disorder. *Primary Psychiatry*, **13**, 52–8.

Ghaemi, S. N. and Goodwin, F. K. (2003). Gabapentin treatment of the non-refractory bipolar spectrum: an open case series. *Journal of Affective Disorders*, **65**, 167–71.

Ghaemi, S. N., Stoll, A. L. and Pope, H. G. (1995). Lack of insight in bipolar disorder: the acute manic episode. *Journal of Nervous and Mental Disease*, **183**, 464–7.

Ghaemi, S. N., Katzow, J. J., Desai, S. P. and Goodwin, F. K. (1998). Gabapentin treatment of mood disorders: a preliminary study. *Journal of Clinical Psychiatry*, **59**, 426–9.

Ghaemi, S. N., Boiman, E. E. and Goodwin, F. K. (2000). Diagnosing bipolar disorder and the effect of antidepressants: a naturalistic study. *Journal of Clinical Psychiatry*, **61**, 804–8.

Ghaemi, S. N., Manwani, S. G., Katzow, J. J., Ko, J. Y. and Goodwin, F. K. (2001). Topiramate treatment of bipolar spectrum disorders: a retrospective chart review. *Annals of Clinical Psychiatry*, **13**, 185–9.

Ghaemi, S. N., Hsu, D. J., Soldani, F. and Goodwin, F. K. (2003). Antidepressants in bipolar disorder: the case for caution. *Bipolar Disorders*, **5**, 421–33.

Goodwin, F. and Jamison, K. (1990). *Manic Depressive Illness*. New York: Oxford University Press.

Goodwin, F. and Jamison, K. (2007). *Manic Depressive Illness* (2nd edn). New York: Oxford University Press.

Goodwin, G. M. and Young, A. H. (2003). The British Association for Psychopharmacology guidelines for treatment of bipolar disorder: a summary. *Journal of Psychopharmacology*, **17** (Suppl. 4), S3–6.

Hirschfeld, R. M. A., Bowden, C. L., Gitlin, M. J. *et al.* (2002). American Psychiatric Association practice guideline for the treatment of patients with bipolar disorder (revision). *American Journal of Psychiatry*, **159**, 1–50.

Hirschfeld, R., Clayton, P. and Cohen, I. (1994). Practice guidelines for the treatment of patients with bipolar disorder. *American Journal of Psychiatry*, **151**, 1–31.

Holmes, O. W. (1891). *Medical Essays 1842–1882*. Boston: Houghton Mifflin and Company.

Inoue, T., Nakagawa, S., Kitaichi, Y. *et al.* (2006). Long-term outcome of antidepressant-refractory depression: the relevance of unrecognized bipolarity. *Journal of Affective Disorders*, **95**, 61–7.

ISIS-2 (1988). Randomised trial of intravenous streptokinase, oral aspirin, both, or neither among 17,187 cases of suspected acute myocardial infarction: ISIS-2. ISIS-2 (Second International Study of Infarct Survival) Collaborative Group. *Lancet*, **2**, 349–60.

Jacobsen, F. M. (1993). Low-dose valproate: a new treatment for cyclothymia, mild rapid-cycling disorders, and premenstrual syndrome. *Journal of Clinical Psychiatry*, **54**, 229–34.

Jouanna, J. (2001). *Hippocrates*. Baltimore, MD: Johns Hopkins University Press.

Kane, J. M., Quitkin, F. M., Rifkin, A. *et al.* (1982). Lithium carbonate and imipramine in the prophylaxis of unipolar and Bipolar II illness: a prospective, placebo-controlled comparison. *Archives of General Psychiatry*, **39**, 1065–9.

Keck, P. E. Jr. and McElroy, S. L. (2003). New approaches in managing bipolar depression. *Journal of Clinical Psychiatry*, **64** (Suppl. 1), S13–18.

McHugh, P. R. (1996). Hippocrates à la mode. *National Library of Medicine*, **2**, 507–9.

Mack, A. (2003). Examination of the evidence for off-label use of gabapentin. *Journal of Managed Care Pharmacy*, **9**, 559–68.

Maclure, M. and Mittleman, M. A. (2000). Should we use a case-crossover design? *Annual Review of Public Health*, **21**, 193–221.

Moller, H. J. and Grunze, H. (2000). Have some guidelines for the treatment of acute bipolar depression gone too far in the restriction of antidepressants? *European Archives of Psychiatry and Clinical Neurosciences*, **250**, 57–68.

Moller, H. J., Grunze, H. and Broich, K. (2006). Do recent efficacy data on the drug treatment of acute bipolar depression support the position that drugs other than antidepressants are the treatment of choice? A conceptual review. *European Archives of Psychiatry and Clinical Neurosciences*, **256**, 1–16.

Oxman, A. D. and Guyatt, G. H. (1992). A consumer's guide to sub-group analyses. *Annals of Internal Medicine*, **116**, 78–84.

Parker, G. (2002). Do the newer antidepressants have mood stabilizing properties? *Australian and New Zealand Journal of Psychiatry*, **36**, 427–8.

Parker, G. B., Malhi, G. S., Crawford, J. G. and Thase, M. E. (2005). Identifying 'paradigm failures' contributing to treatment-resistant depression. *Journal of Affective Disorders*, **87**, 185–91.

Parker, G., Tully, L., Olley, A. and Hadzi-Pavlovic, D. (2006). SSRIs as mood stabilizers for Bipolar II Disorder? A proof of concept study. *Journal of Affective Disorders*, **92**, 205–14.

Peet, M. (1994). Induction of mania with selective serotonin re-uptake inhibitors and tricyclic antidepressants. *British Journal of Psychiatry*, **164**, 549–50.

Peirce, C. (1958). *Selected Writings.* New York: Dover Publications.

Rothman, K. J. (2002). *Epidemiology: An Introduction.* Oxford: Oxford University Press.

Rush, A. J., Trivedi, M. H., Wisniewski, S. R. *et al.* (2006). Acute and longer-term outcomes in depressed outpatients requiring one or several treatment steps: a STAR*D report. *American Journal of Psychiatry*, **163**, 1905–17.

Sharma, V., Khan, M. and Smith, A. (2005). A closer look at treatment-resistant depression: is it due to a bipolar diathesis? *Journal of Affective Disorders*, **84**, 251–7.

Soldani, F., Ghaemi, S. N. and Baldessarini, R. (2005). Research methods in psychiatric treatment studies. Critique and proposals. *Acta Psychiatrica Scandinavica*, **112**, 1–3.

Sosenko, J. M. and Gardner, L. B. (1987). Attribute frequency and misclassification bias. *Journal of Chronic Diseases*, **40**, 203–7.

Winsberg, M. E., DeGolia, S. G., Strong, C. M. and Ketter, T. A. (2001). Divalproex therapy in medication-naïve and mood-stabilizer-naïve bipolar II depression. *Journal of Affective Disorders*, **67**, 207–12.

27

Management commentary

Michael E. Thase

Across the past decade there has been a rather dramatic increase in interest in Bipolar II Disorder. Once viewed as a relatively minor and unreliably diagnosed variant of the 'real' illness, BP II and other depressions grouped within the so-called 'softer' end of the bipolar spectrum are now considered by some experts as the more prevalent forms of manic depressive illness (see, for example, Angst and Cassano, 2005). Not only is BP II much more common than previously appreciated, there is good evidence that the depressive episodes – which can consume one half of an afflicted adult's lifetime (Judd *et al.*, 2003) – can have devastating effects on psychosocial vocational functioning that at least match those of the 'major' form of the illness (Judd *et al.*, 2005). Such findings underscore the more pernicious and protracted nature of the depressive episodes of bipolar disorder, as well as the need for better antidepressant therapies for people who experience hypomanic episodes.

As people with BP II almost never seek treatment for the hypomanic episodes, clinicians often do not make the diagnosis of BP II until after the patient has received some sort of antidepressant therapy for some duration. Once the diagnosis is made, he or she must answer only one fundamental question when fashioning a treatment: 'Is the risk of a treatment-emergent affective switch (TEAS) sufficiently high to warrant the use of a mood stabiliser?' If the answer to this question is 'yes', then management can proceed exactly as if the clinician was treating a BP I depressive episode, as will be discussed subsequently in more detail. If the answer is 'no', then an individualised treatment plan appropriate for a patient with so-called unipolar depression would be appropriate, with the caveat that there should be a higher than usual level of surveillance for signs and symptoms of TEAS, as well as a greater level of caution about the potential of particular medications to cause cycling. For example, although the data are sparse, venlafaxine would appear to be a more problematic choice for bipolar patients than either bupropion or an SSRI (Vieta *et al.*, 2002; Post *et al.*, 2006). Moclobemide also might be thought

Bipolar II Disorder. Modelling, Measuring and Managing, ed. Gordon Parker. Published by Cambridge University Press. © Cambridge University Press 2008.

of as an alternative to SSRIs in countries in which this reversible and selective monoamine oxidase inhibitor is available.

For the BP II patient for whom a mood stabiliser appears to be clinically indicated, the challenge is to pick the right mood stabiliser. In the era of evidence-based medicine – and following several decades of research and development by the pharmaceutical industry – one might expect that there would be a number of controlled studies to guide the selection of the most appropriate therapies for bipolar depression. However, such expectations have not been met and there are only a handful of controlled studies in Bipolar I depression and not even a single prospective adequately powered, placebo-controlled study of BP II depression in the literature. With respect to conventional mood stabilisers, lithium is probably underutilised in the modern era and, given its track record, low cost, and demonstrated suppressive effect on suicidal behaviour, it certainly warrants consideration. Moreover, there is an older literature that describes a sub-set of 'unipolar' depressed patients – who would now certainly be classified within the bipolar spectrum – who are responsive to lithium salts (see, for example, Kupfer et al., 1975). Unfortunately, lithium therapy is not a great choice for those who have developed TEAS or rapid cycling on antidepressant therapy and there are real concerns about its tolerability and safety with long-term use.

Evidence in support of valproate and carbamazapine – either alone or in combination – is even scantier for treatment of bipolar depressions (see, for example, Thase, 2006), which is generally why I reserve these medications for patients who cannot tolerate lithium, who will not take it, or who have a history of rapid cycling.

When the conventional mood stabilisers are not useful, I increasingly rely upon several newer options, including the non-GABAergic anticonvulsant lamotrigine and – when symptom severity or illness burden justify use – several of the atypical antipsychotics. Although lamotrigine is formally approved only for the preventive phase of therapy of BP I, its antidepressant effects are evident in a number of studies of bipolar disorder (Calabrese et al., 1999; Frye et al., 2000; Calabrese et al., 2005; Nierenberg et al., 2006). However, as these effects have – so far – defied the level of quantification in controlled studies that are necessary to garner regulatory approval, it is probably fair to say that the antidepressant effects of lamotrigine are neither strong nor consistent. The magnitude and rapidity of antidepressant effects are no doubt dampened by the need for initiating therapy at sub-therapeutic doses and slow upward titration in order to minimise the risk of serious dermatologic reactions, the one real tolerability issue that complicates lamotrigine therapy. The utility of higher-end doses (i.e. 300–600 mg/day), which typically require 12 to 16 weeks to orchestrate, remains to be established. Nevertheless, for those patients who do not develop rash ($\sim$95%), lamotrigine is one of the best-tolerated psychotropic medications and lack of weight gain and sexual side effects are notable relative strengths. Moreover, whether or not the antidepressant effects of lamotrigine therapy are ever established, lamotrigine monotherapy has been shown to reduce the risk of relapse following both manic and depressive episodes (see, for example, Goodwin *et al.*, 2004).

Because of their broad and rapid beneficial psychotropic effects for people with bipolar disorder, the atypical antipsychotic medications probably would figure even more prominently for treatment of BP II depression if not for the potential for metabolic side-effects and cost. That said, the antidepressant effects of olanzapine (Tohen *et al.*, 2003) and quetiapine (Calabrese *et al.*, 2005; Thase *et al.*, 2006) have been demonstrated in placebo-controlled studies of bipolar depression, with the former only receiving formal FDA approval in combination with fluoxetine, and the latter approved as a monotherapy on the basis of positive studies. The strengths of these medications include symptomatic control of insomnia and anxiety and, essentially, no risk of TEAS. The performance of quetiapine was particularly strong in the two registration studies, with significant benefits established in the sub-sets of patients with BP II and rapid-cycling syndromes. As quetiapine at 300 mg (at bedtime) was as effective and somewhat better tolerated than quetiapine 600 mg (at bedtime), in practice I favour lower doses and often begin at 25 mg (rather than 50 mg) and titrate slower than the dosing protocol used in the controlled studies.

For patients who present with anergic features (i.e. psychomotor retardation coupled with either hypersomnia or increased appetite), I typically skip over the better-studied (and more sedating) atypicals in favour of ziprasidone or aripiprazole. Not only are these medications less sedating, they even appear to be activating for some bipolar depressed patients, although without the apparent risk of TEAS. Adequately powered controlled studies of these medications are underway in bipolar depression.

A last consideration involves psychotherapy, particularly the time-limited, symptom-focused and psychoeducationally oriented therapies that have been established (at least as compared to antidepressant medications) as effective treatments of outpatients with unipolar depression. Whereas psychotherapy alone would be considered a contraindicated treatment component for a patient with BP I depression – specifically because of the lack of coverage against manic switches – an 8–12 week trial of cognitive, behavioural and interpersonally focused therapy may offer a novel non-pharmacological option for BP II depressed patients who have not benefited from antidepressants and for whom mood stabilisers or atypical antipsychotics are not acceptable.

REFERENCES

Angst, J. and Cassano, G. (2005). The mood spectrum: improving the diagnosis of bipolar disorder. *Bipolar Disorders*, **7** (Suppl. 4), S4–12.

Calabrese, J. R., Bowden, C. L., Sachs, G. S. *et al.* (1999). A double-blind placebo-controlled study of lamotrigine monotherapy in outpatients with Bipolar I depression. Lamictal 602 Study Group. *Journal of Clinical Psychiatry*, **60**, 79–88.

Calabrese, J. R., Keck, P. E. Jr., Macfadden, W. *et al.* (2005). A randomized, double-blind, placebo-controlled trial of quetiapine in the treatment of Bipolar I or II depression. *American Journal of Psychiatry*, **162**, 1351–60.

Frye, M. A., Ketter, T. A., Kimbrell, T. A. *et al.* (2000). A placebo-controlled study of lamotrigine and gabapentin monotherapy in refractory mood disorders. *Journal of Clinical Psychopharmacology*, **20**, 607–14.

Goodwin, G. M., Bowden, C. L., Calabrese, J. R. *et al.* (2004). A pooled analysis of two placebo-controlled 18-month trials of lamotrigine and lithium maintenance in Bipolar I Disorder. *Journal of Clinical Psychiatry*, **65**, 432–41.

Judd, L. L., Akiskal, H. S., Schettler, P. J. *et al.* (2003). A prospective investigation of the natural history of the long-term weekly symptomatic status of Bipolar II Disorder. *Archives of General Psychiatry*, **60**, 261–9.

Judd, L. L., Akiskal, H. S., Schettler, P. J. *et al.* (2005). Psychosocial disability in the course of Bipolar I and II disorders: a prospective, comparative, longitudinal study. *Archives of General Psychiatry*, **62**, 1322–30.

Kupfer, D. J., Pickar, D., Himmelhoch, J. M. and Detre, T. P. (1975). Are there two types of unipolar depression? *Archives of General Psychiatry*, **32**, 866–71.

Nierenberg, A. A., Ostacher, M. J., Calabrese, J. R. *et al.* (2006). Treatment-resistant bipolar depression: a STEP-BD equipoise randomized effectiveness trial of antidepressant augmentation with lamotrigine, inositol, or risperidone. *American Journal of Psychiatry*, **163**, 210–16.

Post, R. M., Altshuler, L. L., Leverich, G. S. *et al.* (2006). Mood switch in bipolar depression: comparison of adjunctive venlafaxine, bupropion and sertraline. *British Journal of Psychiatry*, **189**, 124–31.

Thase, M. E. (2006). Pharmacotherapy of bipolar depression: an update. *Current Psychiatry Reports*, **8**, 478–88.

Thase, M. E., Macfadden, W., Weisler, R. H. *et al.* for the BOLDER II Study Group (2006). Efficacy of quetiapine monotherapy in Bipolar I and II depression: a double-blind, placebo-controlled study (the BOLDER II study). *Journal of Clinical Psychopharmacology*, **26**, 600–9.

Tohen, M., Vieta, E., Calabrese, J. *et al.* (2003). Efficacy of olanzapine and olanzapine-fluoxetine combination in the treatment of Bipolar I depression. *Archives of General Psychiatry*, **60**, 1079–88.

Vieta, E., Martinez-Aran, A., Goikolea, J. M. *et al.* (2002). A randomized trial comparing paroxetine and venlafaxine in the treatment of bipolar depressed patients taking mood stabilizers. *Journal of Clinical Psychiatry*, **63**, 508–12.

28

Rounding up and tying down

Gordon Parker

The reader of this volume has been presented – following an evocative Introduction, and a rich historical overview by Shorter (Chapter 1) – with considerable technical material and some quite contrasting management views for Bipolar II Disorder (BP II). While it is commonly put that medical education should prioritise tolerance of ambiguity, this is more defensible as a principle. In practice, clinicians look for guidelines and consensus to assist their management decisions. While several chapter conclusions appear poles apart from each other (*qua* 'bipolar'), there is more consensus than dissent between authors than might have been anticipated, and it is possible to identify many commonalities, reconcile some controversies and identify key areas where research work is required.

How meaningful is the BP II category?

While many would challenge whether BP II actually exists, the majority of this book's authors view BP II as a clinically meaningful category, while the impact of BP II (in terms of disability, economic cost and risk of suicide) argues strongly for its gravity. The consequences of the substantive collateral damage that can occur during the 'highs' (affecting relationships, work, finances, reputation, use of drugs and alcohol – and in ways that differ from behaviours during depressed mood states) argues even further for appreciation of the significance of this condition. To suggest that BP II does not exist, or is a slight (or 'lite') disorder, no longer appear sustainable propositions.

Modelling?

Given that BP II exists, a central and immediate question follows – how is it best modelled? Phelps (Chapter 2) cut to the bone in questioning how it can be carved at its joints – an entity or 'a point on a continuous spectrum'. He reported several studies which fail to find points of rarity between varying expressions of bipolar and unipolar disorder – thus arguing against discrete types and more for a

Bipolar II Disorder. Modelling, Measuring and Managing, ed. Gordon Parker. Published by Cambridge University Press. © Cambridge University Press 2008.

continuum. Further, he detailed the concept of 'soft bipolarity', a continuum model where, at one end, an individual may actually have a bipolar condition in the absence of any actual hypomanic or manic features. Such debates about continuum versus categorical models have long occurred in relation to the uni-polar disorders. But, if bipolar disorder is a spectrum condition, how low do we go in defining 'highs' as we move away from Bipolar I Disorder (BP I), and how do we assign individuals along a continuum? In essence, is BP II everything that is 'not BP I' or defined by cut-off scores on relevant dimensional parameters?

In practice, evidence supporting continuum models is not difficult to accrue, for we can dimensionalise everything. Breathlessness can reflect quite differing disease (e.g. asthma, pneumonia, pulmonary embolus) and non-disease (e.g. running up a mountain) processes, but be readily modelled along a severity dimension (from severe to slight). More relevant to psychiatry, a factor analysis of every clinical symptom listed in the DSM was able to generate a three-factor dimensional model. Thus, a continuum or dimensional model is an option, but is best judged in terms of its validity and worth rather than for its parsimony.

Phelps provides us with a persuasive exposition of a spectrum model, partic-ularly as he counsels us to avoid premature closure on what might be the best model of BP II, and as he offers some very practical applications for consumer, clinical and research application. For the clinician, he demonstrates how the spectrum model may influence clinical decision-making. Immediately following his chapter, the reader is offered an alternative categorical model for the bipolar disorders and for distinguishing BP I from BP II, based simply on the presence or absence of psychotic features, respectively.

Measuring, diagnosing and sub-typing?

In terms of distinguishing bipolar from unipolar disorders, our Mood Swings Questionnaire (Appendix 1) showed excellent discrimination but requires replication. Other authors note similar self-report measures, with the Mood Disorders Questionnaire being currently the most commonly cited and recommen-ded measure. While such measures assist in clinically separating bipolar and uni-polar subjects in *clinically depressed samples*, their capacity to identify individuals with bipolar disorder (let alone BP II) in general community samples is predictably limited, and is an area for research application. In contrast to attempts designed to distinguish groups into pristine and differing categories (e.g. BP I, BP II), Phelps argued – reflecting his preference for a 'bipolar spectrum' model – the possible utility of the Bipolarity Index. Research on such a measure that goes beyond symptoms to include quite variegated data including 'soft' signs, family history, age of onset, illness course and response to treatment is therefore eagerly awaited.

As detailed in Chapters 2 and 3, the clinician has two broad options for pursuing the possibility of bipolar disorder per se – inventories, and a set of clinical questions. Phelps (Chapter 2) observed that most systems – and clinicians – would make such a diagnosis on the basis of a history of highs and a set number of their symptoms. A representative list of symptom domains is provided in Chapter 2, and screening questions in Chapter 3. Such screening questions address clinical nuances beyond symptoms (e.g. a 'trend break' or evidence of mood swings emerging at a definable time; the disappearance of anxiety during a high; distinctive or over-represented melancholic features during depressed phases) that can be useful to clinicians. In relation to diagnostic criteria, several authors pointed to limitations or anomalies within both the DSM–IV and ICD–10 criteria sets. Importantly, several authors rejected the DSM-imposed duration criteria (of 7 or more days for mania, and 4 or more days for hypomania). If strictly applied, such criteria risk many individuals with true bipolar disorder (and especially BP II) not receiving such a diagnosis. Thus, the consensus was that the duration of a high should not be regarded as having any intrinsic validity.

Just as distinctions between bipolar and unipolar conditions can be problematic, distinguishing between BP II and alternative diagnoses risks false positive and false negative decisions. The reader is exposed to three categorical approaches (i.e. DSM, ICD and an 'isomer model') and one dimensional approach. DSM–IV and ICD–10 decision rules effectively assign on a categorical basis, in that individuals either meet explicit criteria or do not. Authors pointed to anomalies and paradoxes in both systems. Our own categorical model (overviewed in Chapter 3) is a parsimonious one – if an individual meets a set of clinical criteria for 'highs', they putatively have bipolar disorder. If, during any such high they have psychotic features, they are judged to have BP I and, when experiencing depressive episodes, have some likelihood of experiencing psychotic depression. If they have never had psychotic features during a high, they have a presumptive BP II condition, and would not be expected to have episodes of psychotic depression when depressed. The detailed 'isomer model' therefore positions BP I as a psychotic condition with the propensity for psychosis oscillating across the polar extremes, and BP II as a non-psychotic condition, with the propensity for mood and energy domains to oscillate from states of hypomania (i.e. elevated mood, high energy) to depression (i.e. low mood, anergia). The latter are most frequently melancholic in type (albeit with a greater likelihood of atypical features of hypersomnia and hyperphagia). By contrast, Phelps detailed a dimensional approach and its many operational advantages.

As Hadjipavlou and Yatham (Chapter 4) observed, a missed diagnosis of BP II commonly reflects a patient's failure to report hypomanic symptoms and/or the clinician not screening for such a possibility. Goldberg (Chapter 21) drew attention to the converse concern – how a false positive diagnosis of bipolar disorder can be made. In his example, the patient was described as experiencing 'mood swings', a phrase that is used by patients almost as broadly and non-specifically as the historical 'nervous breakdown' descriptor. Other authors noted how a false diagnosis of BP II can be made for individuals who have attention deficit hyperactivity disorder (ADHD) or certain personality styles (especially borderline personality disorder). As a logical extension of his continuum model, Phelps also suggested that rather than offering a categorical judgement about whether the patient has bipolar disorder or not, the clinician can make a judgement about 'how much bipolarity might the patient have'. Again, this option will benefit from studies of its utility – and of its perceived advantages and limitations by those receiving such a quantified statement. If assessment is 'indeterminate', Ketter and Wang (Chapter 16) recommend a 'rounding up' convention as worthwhile.

Phelps also sensitively observes how a diagnosis of bipolar disorder is more stigmatising than one of depression to most patients, which begs the question – should clinicians avoid offering any such emphatic or categorical diagnostic statement? Knowledge, however, is generally empowering for individuals and, while most will experience a distressing impact phase on receiving such a diagnosis, it allows relevant additional information to be pursued from their clinician and from other sources. Ketter and Wang wisely noted the need to advise patients to avoid the risks of either trivialising or catastrophising the disorder.

If we fail to define a clear boundary between BP II and BP I – and between BP II and unipolar disorder – the risks are several. Firstly, of perpetuating the common tendency to extrapolate the management of BP II from BP I guidelines. Secondly, assuming for the moment that there are differential treatment nuances for the BP I and BP II conditions, a blurred boundary may risk some patients with true BP II being effectively 'over-treated' (e.g. via receiving combinations of atypical antipsychotic, mood stabiliser or 'innovative' drugs on the basis of those clinical guidelines), and thereby being exposed to a higher rate of adverse drug reactions.

In terms of diagnosing and sub-typing, we can conclude that both DSM and ICD decision rules for distinguishing hypomania from mania – and BP II from BP I – are less than satisfactory, and worthy of revision. In terms of categorical versus dimensional models, only one model is likely to be valid, and clarification of this issue is of the highest research priority, not only to assist clinical and research definition and communication, but to clarify treatment options. The aphorism 'What's the use of running if you're on the wrong road?' is apt. Resolution strategies include the competitive testing of each model, or an iterative 'top down' and 'bottom up' process where assumptive or putative models are tweaked by data predicting treatment responsiveness and treatment failure to, in turn, shape syndrome redefinition. While such clarification would appear mandatory and urgent, if we are to learn from history, such a process risks being mired for decades. One hope is that this book's authors have clarified issues and parameters for discourse and research focus.

Treatment of BP II versus BP I – a similar or different general management model?

Theoretically, managing BP I and BP II conditions via common or differential treatment might be shaped by identifying respectively similar or differing neurobiological perturbations. Malhi's overview of neurobiological research (Chapter 6) informs us that currently available studies provide no answer as to whether neurobiological differences exist – a conclusion largely reflecting methodological limitations. Few studies have compared neurobiological markers in sufficiently large BP I and BP II sub-sets, and, as noted above, our current models for distinguishing BP I and BP II may cloud any intrinsic neurobiological distinctions being identified. The suggestion that BP II tends to 'breed true' encouraged Malhi to argue for the need to search for a BP II endophenotype. Our own 'isomer model' (Chapter 3) would argue that neurobiological distinctions may lie in the presence or absence of psychotic features (at either mood pole) and thus in the determinants of psychosis, for separating out BP I. If that model is valid, it might then theoretically argue a lesser role for the atypical antipsychotic drugs in managing BP II compared to their role in managing BP I – and particularly during acute mood elevation states – but that suggestion is drawing a long bow when we know that many treatments have true non-specific benefits across a range of conditions. As no underpinning neurobiological differences have been identified, an alternative approach is to consider the empirical effectiveness of differing therapeutic modalities, as now overviewed.

Antidepressant drugs – to use or not to use?

A key management issue – and clearly the most controversial topic considered by our authors – is the use of antidepressant monotherapy for BP II. As detailed in Chapter 8, we have long observed that a significant percentage of those with BP II report mood stabilisation (i.e. distinct benefit for depressive episodes and some attenuation of hypomanic episodes) with a narrow-spectrum SSRI, or with the dual action antidepressant venlafaxine. In Chapter 8 we also overviewed an SSRI 'proof of concept' study which quantified findings in line with those clinical impressions. However, of those who appear to respond well, a percentage experience a 'poop out' of benefit after months or years. I also concede that a percentage of individuals treated with antidepressant monotherapy experience a mood 'switch', describe or evidence 'mixed states' and/or experience more rapid cycling over time – consequences which may require lowering or ceasing the antidepressant. Despite the risk of such adverse events in some individuals, I would still argue for such antidepressant monotherapy as an initial drug strategy – as it is often the most benign of the alternative drug options in terms of the cost:benefit ratio. Further, I suggest that observant clinician and patient management (i.e. the clinician knowing when to adjust the dose of the SSRI, or cease it; the patient being warned about cycle perturbations) provides a risk: benefit ratio little different to that operating for the management of unipolar disorder (i.e. recognition that antidepressants – as for all psychotropic drugs – have side effects and require close rather than sanguine clinical management).

Book contributors offered quite varying views about antidepressant monotherapy – in essence: (i) 'qualified yes', (ii) 'uncertain' and (iii) 'no'.

In advancing a *'qualified yes'* argument, we should note Ghaemi's statement (Chapter 26) that many bipolar experts in the USA do not view antidepressant use in BP II or (BP I) disorder as problematic. My recommendation of first trialling a narrow-spectrum antidepressant is predicated on the scenario of a patient with BP II presenting to a clinician for the first time with a significant episode of depression and never having had an antidepressant previously. In such circumstances, few present with an evident 'mixed state' – which I most commonly see when patients are already receiving an antidepressant. Thus, the key issue facing me is that when a severely depressed BP II patient presents, any response to a mood stabiliser can often take 4–8 weeks. This is intolerable for many patients. By contrast, an approach weighting an antidepressant (monotherapy, or augmented, as detailed at the beginning of this chapter) is more likely to be associated with a response – and over a shorter period. If, while being maintained on the antidepressant as monotherapy, the patient reports mood-stabilising benefits, this is a distinct second advantage.

Despite commencing the SSRI at half the recommended starting dose, the most common adverse report I observe is a serotonergic reaction – whether for those with unipolar or BP II depression – which is extremely severe in about 2% of my patients, and evident in about 20%, and usually requires cessation of such a drug. For those not experiencing significant or troubling side effects, the antidepressant is then maintained to determine (by reference to mood charting and patient reporting) if the individual is noting benefits to such a maintenance strategy, and to check for any cycle changing. If there is evidence of increased cycling, or of mixed states, I trial lowering the dose, ceasing the antidepressant and/or adding a formal mood stabiliser.

Another member of the 'qualified yes' group was Benazzi (Chapter 17), who stated that he had long managed many BP II patients with antidepressant monotherapy. His key exceptions were when mixed states were present – when he would initiate a mood stabiliser before any antidepressant (if the latter was then required). A *'perhaps'* sub-set of the 'qualified yes' group included Goldberg (Chapter 7), who noted the 'small body of evidence' supporting narrow-spectrum (SSRI and venlafaxine) monotherapy as a 'reasonable first-line' treatment, and (Chapter 21) suggested that certain SSRI antidepressants (and bupropion) may be appropriate monotherapies. In addition, Hadjipavlou and Yatham (Chapter 9) conceded the possibility of antidepressant monotherapy if hypomanic episodes were mild and infrequent, and in the absence of mixed states and rapid cycling.

The *'no' group* were rarely absolute in their rejection of antidepressant monotherapy but more emphasised a need for caution. They were well represented by Berk (Chapter 18), who judged that clinicians should be 'increasingly cautious' in light of the risk:benefit ratio, with Young (Chapter 23) viewing antidepressant monotherapy as 'controversial', a view echoed by Goodwin (Chapter 24). Vieta (Chapter 19) conceded that there may be a sub-group of BP II patients who respond to antidepressant monotherapy but, as they could not be identified in advance, he clearly favoured mood stabilisers as a first-line therapy with 'cautious use of antidepressants as adjuncts'. Post (Chapter 22) noted a small sub-set of those who improved with antidepressant augmentation, but – largely extrapolating from data for BP II – detailed the risk of treatment-refractory and rapid-cycling depressive recurrences in those receiving antidepressant monotherapy. In considering antidepressant drug augmentation, Post also respected drug class differences, favouring bupropion and avoiding the tricyclic drugs. Frangou (Chapter 25) favoured antidepressant drugs being prescribed in conjunction with a mood stabiliser or quetiapine rather than as monotherapy, while Ghaemi (Chapter 26) viewed the literature as 'essentially observational and limited', albeit conceding some possible short-term benefits but without long-term efficacy.

Moving beyond such summarised positions, we might profit from considering the views of those who conceded the possibility of benefit but who either expressed major caveats or set out to define what circumstances might be associated with improvement from narrow-spectrum antidepressant monotherapy. Phelps (Chapter 2) raised 'kindling' as a major disadvantage, and suggested that it was important to ensure that antidepressants might not lead to intrinsically more frequent and more severe episodes. Many authors considering switching risk made reference to the paper by Leverich and colleagues, published in the *American Journal of Psychiatry* in 2006, where 159 bipolar patients (44 with BP II) in receipt of a mood stabiliser (i.e. lithium, an anticonvulsant or an atypical antipsychotic) were then trialled on bupropion, sertraline or venlafaxine – during either acute treatment or a one-year continuation phase. Switch rates into hypomania or mania were 11.4% and 7.9% respectively in the acute trials, and 21.8% and 14.9% in the continuation trials. However, before concluding that the introduction of antidepressants is associated with a high rate of switching, we must remember that the patient sample had bipolar disorder (where hypomanic/manic episodes would be expected in those whose illnesses were not fully controlled), and that there was no placebo group to clarify whether hypomanic and manic switch rates were necessarily increased. That study is more definitive, however, in identifying a lower rate of highs in the BP II versus the BP I patients (18.6% and 30.8%), and in quantifying a three times higher rate of switching for those receiving venlafaxine as against bupropion – and with sertraline's rates closer to those of bupropion than to venlafaxine. Such a differential rate does suggest that the *class* of antidepressant is likely to influence the risk of switching, and this might extrapolate to a similar differential risk of mixed states, with such differential class effects weighting Goldberg's recommendations (Chapter 21) in relation to prescribing antidepressant of differing classes.

In pursuing circumstances when antidepressant monotherapy might have preferential advantages and disadvantages, we observe a number of intriguing observations. Phelps (Chapter 2) suggested that there might be a point along the 'bipolar spectrum' (i.e. closer to unipolar depression) where those with BP II might preferentially respond, as against another point (i.e. closer to BP I disorder) where a mood stabiliser might be preferentially superior. Goldberg (Chapter 7) reported studies suggesting that antidepressant switching appears confined to a minority sub-group, that it is less likely to occur in BP II than in BP I, that antidepressants have 'never been shown to improve depression symptoms' during mixed states, and he further argued against their use when there is rapid cycling. Several authors noted that the risk of switching is likely to vary across the differing antidepressant drug classes, being highest in the broad spectrum tricyclic and lowest in the narrow-spectrum SSRI class.

Ketter and Wang (Chapter 16) neatly differentiated circumstances when antidepressants might be viewed as 'foundational treatments' for mood stabilisation and when best not used. The latter circumstances include the BP II condition being 'more akin to BP I', relatively frequent episodes, mixed episodes and rapid cycling. Importantly, their model (Figure 16.1) does not position all antidepressant classes within their treatment algorithm (which is limited to SSRIs and bupropion) and again respects the likelihood that differing antidepressant classes (i.e. narrow spectrum through to broad spectrum) vary in terms of their effectiveness and risk of adverse events. Thase (Chapter 27) made very similar recommendations. Goldberg (Chapter 7) also argued for the alternative use of mood stabilisers when there was evidence of high cyclicity, proneness toward hypomania in the individual's cyclical pattern, presence of mixed states, poor response to anti-depressant monotherapy, and 'poop out' over time.

Thus, there was consensus that antidepressants can cause switching (albeit less of a risk for those with BP II than previously judged), rapid cycling, mixed states and an increase in the cycling rate – but that such adverse events were not invariable. This led to two positions: first, trialling antidepressant monotherapy with close observation to check on treatment-emerging effects. Second, anti-depressant monotherapy being contraindicated. Each position was supported by a number of experts, therefore defining a key issue for resolution.

Clarification would be assisted by deriving the right model and then under-taking the appropriate randomised controlled trials. The principal hypothesis here would be that antidepressant monotherapy confers mood-stabilising benefit to a percentage of those with BP II. If demonstrated, then one would need to determine if sub-sets of responders and non-responders could be identified. Cost:benefit analyses would certainly require extended longitudinal studies to determine risks of adverse effects.

Mood stabilisers

Turning to the use of formal mood stabilisers (i.e. lithium and anticonvulsants), we were informed (Chapter 9) that these are likely to be relied on by clinicians for treating patients with diagnosed BP II, while Young (Chapter 22) viewed them (specifying lithium and lamotrigine) as the first-line treatments for BP II. Hadjipavlou and Yatham – as did Ghaemi – essentially endorsed lithium and valproate as the first-line strategy for BP II depression, and argued their strengths across a number of parameters (i.e. unassociated with cycle acceleration or switch-ing, modest antidepressant effects and prophylactic role). Importantly, and care-fully documenting their reasoning, Hadjipavlou and Yatham favoured lithium above valproate, but did not endorse lamotrigine monotherapy – albeit conceding that it might have a greater role in maintenance therapy. Lamotrigine monother-apy was nominated (along with quetiapine) by Ketter and Wang for BP II patients with BP II illnesses 'more akin to a BP I disorder'. While supportive of all formal mood stabilisers, both Goodwin (Chapter 24) and Post (Chapter 22) offered a more positive view about lamotrigine – with the latter noting a number of encouraging studies, suggested that its effectiveness in preventing depression more than mania indicated a clinical pattern consistent with BP II disorder, and also noted the relative absence of side effects. Frangou (Chapter 25) also nomi-nated lamotrigine as a first-line option. Thase (Chapter 27) expressed concerns about lithium for those who had developed affective switches or rapid cycling on antidepressant drugs and favoured lamotrigine among the mood stabilisers.

Vieta (Chapter 19) was strongly in favour of mood stabilisers as the 'foundational treatment of BP II', with antipsychotic drugs and antidepressants as adjuncts when appropriate. Goldberg (Chapter 21) also favoured mood stabilisers as the initial strategy, and suggested that lithium might be preferred when BP II was 'mania driven', and lamotrigine when 'depression driven'. Ketter and Wang (Chapter 16) suggested lithium as superior for bipolar depression and treatment-resistant depression, while Benazzi (Chapter 17) was strongly supportive of lithium for preventing episode recurrences. Goodwin (Chapter 24) described use of the anticonvulsant oxcarbaxepine for mood stabilisation. Mitchell (Chapter 20) favoured treating BP II depression akin to BP I management recommendations (i.e. using a mood stabiliser and an antidepressant).

Thus, while most commentators supported the use of mood stabilisers, quite variable views were expressed. While not universally supported, lamotrigine was nominated by many commentators.

Atypical antipsychotic drugs

The atypical antipsychotic drugs have joined the list of candidate treatments for bipolar disorder, with Fresno and Vieta (Chapter 10) noting the reasons, including the formal demonstration of some as having mood-stabilising properties. They noted the supportive – but not definitive – BOLDER data in relation to quetiapine monotherapy for BP II depressive episodes, some indicative supportive data in relation to risperidone for hypomania, and the lack of any data in relation to other atypical antipsychotic drugs for those with BP II. As noted above, quetiapine was recommended by Ketter and Wang (Chapter 16) as a first-line therapy (along with lamotrigine) for BP II patients with illnesses 'more akin to BP I disorder' – and for patients experiencing psychotic depressive episodes. Ketter and Wang, as well as Vieta (Chapter 19), Young (Chapter 23) and Thase (Chapter 27), also noted support for quetiapine as a maintenance therapy – with Vieta noting that it may be particularly useful in rapid cycling conditions. Post (Chapter 22) viewed quetiapine as the first-choice antipsychotic (albeit noting some support also for aripiprazole). Thase (Chapter 27) also broadened the general focus on quetiapine to nominate the utility of several other atypical antipsychotic drugs (i.e. aripiprazole, olanzapine, ziprasidone).

Thus, the database is surprisingly limited in relation to the role of atypical antipsychotic drugs for managing BP II. As many of the atypicals have been tested and demonstrated as having utility in managing BP I mood states, there is, again, a risk of clinicians extrapolating such use to the management of BP II. It would be preferable to undertake studies of clearly diagnosed BP II individuals, examining the capacity of the atypical antipsychotics in managing hypomania, depression and mood stabilisation, both as monotherapy and in combination with formal mood stabilisers. Importantly, if we are to argue that BP I and BP II differ (and possibly by the respective presence and absence of psychotic features), it would be important to determine if the atypical antipsychotic drugs have differing relevance across those two conditions. It may be that antipsychotic medication is too 'heavy handed' for those with BP II and/or that the cost:benefit ratio of such medications may be less acceptable than formal mood stabilisers. If they have a role, we need to know whether management dosages vary from those used to manage BP I, with Thase (Chapter 27) documenting his use of low-dose quetiapine.

It is certainly difficult to conceive of the same dose being required to manage a hypomanic episode as might be required for a manic episode. Further, while some patients with BP I may benefit from ongoing use of an atypical antipsychotic (whether as monotherapy or in combination), it is conceivable that an atypical antipsychotic might also have use on an intermittent basis for managing hypomanic or depressive extremes. As concluded by Fresno and Vieta (Chapter 10), there is a dearth of controlled studies – so disallowing any firm conclusions in relation to the role of the atypical antipsychotic drugs.

It would be important for research studies to determine if the atypical antipsychotic drugs have differential relevance across the bipolar disorders. It might be hypothesised that atypical antipsychotic drugs will be of greater mood-stabilising benefit (either as monotherapy or combination therapy) for those with BP I (if that condition mandates psychotic features), and more have an augmentation role for those with categorical non-psychotic BP II conditions. However, to the extent that these drugs are intrinsically 'mood stabilisers', a non-specific benefit across BP I and BP II could also be hypothesised.

Other drug options

In terms of more speculative strategies, Ketter and Wang (Chapter 16) supported our recommendation (Chapter 11) of fish oil augmentation. At the practical level we generally recommend that it be trialled as an augmentation strategy for 6–8 weeks. If successful, patients tend to report attenuation of mood swings and/ or the capacity to lower doses of some of their primary medications. Again, if seemingly successful, we recommend that the patient cease such augmentation for a couple of months before reinstituting it – to determine via an 'off – on – off – on' strategy whether it is likely to be providing distinctive augmentation.

Hadjipavlou and Yatham (Chapter 9) found less support for carbamazepine, topiramate and gabapentin, but did concede that each might have 'add-on' potential. Gabapentin was also noted by Benazzi (Chapter 17) for hypomania per se or hypomania in the context of a mixed depression, while Ghaemi

(Chapter 26) also stated that he would use gabapentin and topiramate, despite being 'less proven' agents. Both Goldberg (Chapter 7) and Ketter and Wang (Chapter 16) made reference to pramipexole and modafinil for treatment-resistant BP II depression.

Non-drug management strategies

Numerous authors noted the utility of education, mood charting, peer support and wellbeing plans in the 'integrated management' (Ketter and Wang, Chapter 16) of BP II, and a number of important educational sources were referenced. Post (Chapter 22) captured many of the arguments for education as put by others but also emphasised the biological consequences of failing to reduce recurrences – the exacerbation and progression of neurobiological abnormalities, possibly countered by the neuroprotective effects of many of the relevant drug treatments.

The question of the contribution of an adjunctive psychotherapy to managing BP II generated four broad – stated or inferential – positions from book contributors. Firstly, the suggestion that psychotherapy, in conjunction with medication, was mandatory. Secondly, that many of the helpful psychotherapeutic ingredients in a formal psychotherapy were part of a non-specific repertoire often described as 'good clinical management' or were subsumed in the development of a 'wellbeing plan' with a collaborative therapist. Thirdly, that any specific psychotherapy demanded a clinical target or problem independent of – or comorbid with – the BP II condition itself. Fourthly, both Mitchell (Chapter 20) and Thase (Chapter 27) considered the utility of what might be termed 'psychotherapy monotherapy' in some patients diagnosed (or misdiagnosed) with BP II.

In terms of choosing any specific psychotherapy, Goodwin (Chapter 24) prioritised cognitive behaviour therapy, but drew attention to the potential of mindfulness-based cognitive therapy. Manicavasagar (Chapter 12) well argued the capacity of psychotherapeutic strategies to contribute to 'pluralistic' management of BP II. While psychotherapy, psychoeducation and the development of wellbeing plans clearly overlap, Manicavasagar, as well as Orum (Chapter 13), delineated the individual domains and potential strengths of differing therapeutic levers. Orum emphasised a key component to a wellbeing plan – and one that differs from the psychotherapeutic and psychoeducation models – the potential of a wellbeing plan to build the patient's sense of ownership. Managing BP II is often a lifelong task, involving self-monitoring from the explicit through to the intuitive level, medication adherence, lifestyle changes, stress-managing strategies and negotiating when to involve family members and others. In essence, outcome relates to the individual's self-control. Weighting self-management in the overall 'management package' builds to self-control and a superior outcome.

Smith (Chapter 14) evocatively took us through the journey faced by many with bipolar disorder, and the progression from feeling controlled by 'It' to bringing 'It' under the individual's control – and the survival strategies that many sufferers learn – commonly painfully – from their own experience. Both Orum and Smith, highly respected clinical psychologists, described their own battles with bipolar disorder, and what they have learned. The issue then is how we can best translate such practical wisdom to the clinical management of BP II. Education (whether prepared generically as fact sheets, on web sites or as presented here), together with individualised wellbeing plan development, would appear fundamental to an overall management plan for BP II.

Romancing hypomania?

Should hypomania always be treated? This issue also polarised our writers. Several noted the imperative of treating psychotic manic episodes, to avert the major risks to reputation, relationships, work and finances. But do all hypomanic episodes necessitate 'dampening'.

Hadjipavlou and Yatham (Chapter 9) stated that there was no 'universal answer' to the question, but suggested that it may not be necessary if symptoms were mild and patients were unwilling to have such symptoms treated – subject to close follow-up. Ketter and Wang (Chapter 16) also appeared relatively sanguine, but wisely noted that patients should be mindful that such highs 'may potentiate subsequent depressive episodes'. Both Goodwin and Frangou (Chapters 24 and 25) were a categorical '*yes*', having concerns about the collateral damage. While conceding that any hypomanic episode is likely to risk a perturbing depression, as so many patients express concerns about losing their 'highs', it does strike me that it would be a worthwhile research question to examine the practical utility of mild hypomanic episodes in individuals (and not merely in very creative people).

BP II and BP I – the same or different management approach?

A key advantage to having so many independent commentators is the capacity to determine whether there is consensus or, if not, where differences lie. My reading of the many chapters is that, while there is general acceptance of clinical differences between BP I and BP II, and agreement on the non-drug commonalities to management, there are two broad positions in relation to the drug treatment of BP II.

The first position locates treatment options for BP II as being those recommended for managing BP I, with only some minor 'tweaks'. Exemplar tweaks included the suggested greater utility of lamotrigine (seemingly reflecting clinical observation), and quetiapine (reflecting a rare event in BP II data availability – the existence of a more diagnostically specific randomised controlled trial). The second position views differing drug modalities as having differential relevance across BP I and BP II – for example, arguing that antidepressant monotherapy may have greater utility for many with BP II and obviates mood stabiliser and atypical antipsychotic drugs, as well as articulating some differential effects of mood stabiliser and atypical antipsychotic drugs across the two bipolar disorders.

This book captures the current state of clinical opinion and knowledge. Advances will occur from the scientific structuring of randomised controlled trials shaped by the observations generated by those with bipolar disorder and by clinicians. As Ghaemi observed, 'we are all in this together'. And we can conclude that 'things are looking up'.

Appendix I
Black Dog Institute Self-test for Bipolar Disorder: The Mood Swings Questionnaire

This self-assessment test comprises three initial questions followed by a checklist. Only if you answer 'yes' to the first three questions should you continue on with the checklist. At the end of the test you will be given your results.

Firstly, have you had episodes of clinical depression – involving a period *of at least 2 weeks* where you were significantly depressed and unable to work or only able to work with difficulty – and had at least 4 of the following:

- Loss of interest and pleasure in most things
- Appetite or weight change
- Sleep disturbance
- Physical slowing or agitation
- Fatigue or low energy
- Feeling hopeless and helpless
- Poor concentration
- Suicidal thoughts?

If yes, proceed.

Secondly, do you have times when your mood 'cycles', that is, do you experience 'ups' as well as depressive episodes?

If yes, proceed.

Thirdly, during the 'ups' do you feel more 'wired' and 'hyper' than you would experience during times of normal happiness?

If yes, proceed.

Please complete the checklist below, rating the extent to which each item applies to you during such 'up' times.

	Much more than usual	Somewhat more than usual	No more than usual
1. Feel very confident and capable			
2. See things in a new and exciting light			
3. Feel very creative with lots of ideas and plans			
4. Become over-involved in new plans and projects			
5. Become totally confident that everything you do will succeed			
6. Feel that things are very vivid and crystal clear			
7. Spend, or wish to spend, significant amounts of money			
8. Find that your thoughts race			
9. Notice lots of coincidences occurring			
10. Note that your senses are heightened and your emotions intensified			
11. Work harder, being much more motivated			
12. Feel one with the world and nature			
13. Believe that things possess a 'special meaning'			
14. Say quite outrageous things			
15. Feel 'high as a kite', elated, ecstatic and 'the best ever'			
16. Feel irritated			
17. Feel quite carefree, not worried about anything			
18. Have much increased interest in sex (whether thoughts and/ or actions)			
19. Feel very impatient with people			
20. Laugh and find lots more things humorous			
21. Read special significance into things			
22. Talk over people			
23. Have quite mystical experiences			
24. Do fairly outrageous things			
25. Sleep less and not feel tired			
26. Sing			
27. Feel angry			

Responses in the 'much more' cell score 2, those in the 'somewhat more' cell score 1 and those in the 'no more' cell score 0. The total score is the sum of all 27 items. A score of *22 or more*, together with episodes of clinical depression, suggests possible Bipolar I or II Disorder and would warrant detailed clinical assessment.

Note: This self-assessment test may also be undertaken online: www.blackdoginstitute.org.au/bipolar/howtotell/selftest.cfm

Black Dog Institute

Hospital Road, Prince of Wales Hospital, Randwick NSW 2031

(02) 9382 4530 / (02) 9382 4523

www.blackdoginstitute.org.au

Email: blackdog@unsw.edu.au

Index

3-Methoxy-4-hydroxyphenylglycol (MHPG) 84
AA (arachidonic acid) 142
Abrams, R. 12
acute depression, and mood stabilisers 123–6
acute efficacy 270
age differences 79
age of onset 58
alcohol dependence 95, 199
    and mood stabilisers 128
alpha-linolenic acid (ALA) 141, 146, 148
American Psychiatric Association 9, 10, 12, 218,
        259, 269
anticonvulsants 120–1
    in maintenance therapy 127–8
    see also carbamazepine; gabapentin; lamotrigine;
        topiramate; valproate
antidepressants 94, 250, 286–90
    arguments against using 272, 274
    case reports/series 40
    for depression with anxiety 96–7
    destabilisation risks 39–40
    dosing 103
    empirical literature 270–2
    evidence for efficacy 36, 99–101, 220, 271
    FDA warning 26
    impact on mixed depression 233
    increasing BDNF level 253
    as initial treatment strategy 208–10
    long-term risks 41–2, 250–1
    monotherapy concerns 107
    monotherapy controversy 260, 269, 286–90
    with mood stabilisers 101–2, 210, 253–4
    negative results 254
    novel psychotropics 101
    and olanzapine augmentation 208–9
    positive response to 254
    and relapse prevention 103–4
    relative safety of 37
    safety issues 37–40, 97–9, 104
    and suicidality 38–9, 99, 202
    switching risk 37–8, 107–8
    tolerance to 102–3
    see also depression; major depression; unipolar
        depression

anxiety
    comorbid with bipolar disorder 67, 95–6
    and depression in BP II 96–7
    disappearance of during 'highs' 59
    and mindfulness therapy 264
    and paroxetine 198
    reduced by gabapentin 126
arachidonic acid (AA) 142
Aretaeus of Cappadocia 5, 61
aripiprazole 137, 222, 255, 280
assessment methodologies, conflicting results 237
atypical antipsychotic drugs 133, 280, 291–2
    as combination therapy 134
    efficacy and safety, insufficient evidence for
        134–5, 137–8
    as mood stabilisers for BP I 207–8
    see also aripiprazole; olanzapine; quetiapine,
        risperidone
automatic thoughts 159
awareness of BP II, improving 30–1

BDNF (brain-derived neurotrophic factor)
        146–7, 253
biological circadian rhythms, maintaining 164–5
biological marker studies 143
bipolar affective disorder, ICD–10 system 48, 259
bipolar disorder
    clinical definition 58–9
    comorbidity 66–9
    diagnostic process 24–7
    and disability 65–6
    economic impact of 69–70
    first descriptions of 7–8
    guidelines for treatment 135
    origins of term 7
    prevalence of 62–5, 75, 77
    self-assessment test 296–7
    social stigma of 29
    usage of term 5
    versus unipolar disorder 12
Bipolar I Disorder (BP I)
    and BP II, approach to managing 294–5
    duration of 'highs' 52
    epidemiological studies 75–8

and psychotic features 51–2
see also unipolar depression
Bipolar II Disorder (BP II) 11
    absence of psychotic features 57
    as a meaningful category 282
    and BP I, approach to managing 294–5
    danger of romanticising 265–6
    defining criteria 244
    DSM–IV recognition of 61–2
    early descriptions of 61
    prognosis 265
    special characteristics of 133–4
Bipolarity Index 23, 27–30
Bipolar Spectrum Diagnostic Scale (BSDS) 26
bipolar spectrum disorder 19, 23, 259
    and Axis II comorbidity 244
    prevalence of 62–5, 75, 77, 143
    unclear limits of 259–60
Black Dog Institute
    epidemiological studies 78–81
    essay competition 1–4
    Mood Swings Questionnaire 49–54
    online education programme 212
    self-assessment test 296–7
BOLDER (BipOLar DEpRession) studies 135, 260
Borderline Personality Disorder (BPD) 68, 128, 255
BP I *see* Bipolar I Disorder
BP II *see* Bipolar II Disorder
brain-derived neurotrophic factor (BDNF) 146–7, 253
British Association of Psychopharmacology, guidelines 107
bupropion 104, 126, 223, 250, 255, 289

calcium, changes in intracellular concentration 85
Canadian Network for Mood and Anxiety Treatments (CANMAT) 135
carbamazepine 128, 146, 253, 255, 279, 292
categorical models of diagnosis 15, 46–7, 284
    DSM system limitations 22–4
    isomer model 55–8, 284
CBT *see* Cognitive Behaviour Therapy
Classification of the Endogenous Psychoses, The (Leonhard) 10
clinical screening 58–9
cocaine dependence
    effect of mood stabilisers 128
    and rise in psychotic episodes 200
Cognitive Behaviour Therapy (CBT) 158–9
    behavioural symptoms 161–2
    cognitive symptoms 159–61
    unsuitable for severe bipolar patients 263–4
cohort effect 77–8, 79, 81
community studies, US 75–8
comorbidity 66–9, 95–6, 169
    and personality traits 245–6
    substance abuse 128, 199, 246
contemporary psychopharmacology, non-Hippocratic 273, 274
cyclical psychoses 9, 10
cycling *see* rapid cycling

'cyclothymia' 8, 9, 16, 61
    DSM classification 9
    ICD–10 classification 48–9
    treatment of 127, 272

'D' Club, member's essay 1–4
days ill (hypomanic or depressed) and use of SSRIs 113, 116
dementia, increased risk of 252
dementia praecox 8, 9
depression
    behavioural symptoms, management of 162
    comorbid with anxiety 96–7
    decrementing BDNF level 253
    disability caused by 65–6
    distinguishing from unipolar 94
    early warning signs 186
    health risks of recurrent 252–4
    medication strategies 208–10, 223–4, 263
        impact of SSRIs 111–12, 113, 198
        mood stabilisers 123–6
    'non-antidepressant' treatments 35–6
    relapse rates 103–4
    symptoms in BP I and BP II 95
    treatment resistant 253, 271–2
    see also antidepressants; major depression; unipolar depression
Depression and Bipolar Support Alliance (DBSA) 225
destabilisation induced by antidepressants 39–40
DHA *see* docosahexaenoic acid
diagnosis 284–6
    ambiguity in 219
    benefits of family involvement 205
    categorical models 15, 55–8
    complications of 46, 62–3, 134
        see also misdiagnosis of BP II
    DIGFAST mnemonic 28
    improving public awareness 30–1
    labelling issues 29–30
    partial solutions to DSM approach 27–34
    providing prior to management plan 204–6
    reliability and validity 240
    required prior to antidepressant treatment 94–6
    rigour and precision 34
    'rounding-upwards' 219
    spectrum perspective 16–17
        problems of unclear boundaries 34
    systematic assessment prior to 247–8
    see also DSM–IV diagnostic system; ICD–10 diagnostic system; screening
Diagnostic Guidelines Task Force (ISBD) 15
dietary changes, pathological consequences of 141–2
DIGFAST mnemonic, diagnosis 28
dimensional diagnostic view *see* spectrum model of bipolar disorder
disability resulting from BP I/BP II 65–6
'disease mongering' of pharmaceutical industry 30
dissociation 197

docosahexaenoic acid (DHA)
    dietary recommendations 147–8
    and increase in arachidonic acid 142
    neurophysiological mechanisms 146–7
    reduced level in BP I subjects 143
    sources of 141
    treatment studies 144–5
'Drill Cores' model of BP II 32–4
DSM–III 12
DSM–IV diagnostic system 61–2
    BP I criteria 47, 56
    BP II criteria 47, 259
    and degree of dysfunction 218–19
    diagnosis by exclusion 24–5
    and duration of 'highs' 47, 284
    and hypomania-mania distinction 47–8
    low sensitivity 26–7
    spectrum model argument 22–4
dysfunctional thoughts, challenging and changing
    158–9

eating patterns 201
ECA *see* Epidemiologic Catchment Area study
economic impact of bipolar disorder 69–70
education
    about role of medication 168
    of family and friends 153, 212
    information sources 211–12, 225
    online resources 212
    of patient and family about diagnosis 31–4
    public awareness 30–1
    see also psychoeducation
eicosapentaenoic acid (EPA)
    dietary recommendations 147–8
    and increase in arachidonic acid 142
    neurophysiological mechanisms 146–7
    sources of 141
    treatment studies 144–5
emotive techniques 161
EPA *see* eicosapentaenoic acid
Epidemiologic Catchment Area (ECA) study 63–4,
    67, 69, 75–6, 77
epidemiology
    Black Dog Institute studies 78–81
    cohort effects 77–8
    and diagnosis of BP II 62–3
    fish consumption studies 143
    prevalence of bipolar disorders 62–4, 77
    prevalence of BP II 64, 76–7
escitalopram monotherapy 100, 102, 250
    effects of 40
    randomised control trial 109
Expressed Emotion (EE) 162

families
    aiding diagnosis 205, 218, 265
    educating about BP II 31–4
Family Focused Therapy (FFT) 162–4, 227
family history 32, 50, 59, 63, 255
    see also patient history
FDA *see* Food and Drug Administration

fish oil, role in mood disorders 141, 149, 223, 292
    history of n-3 PUFAs 141–2
    public health issues 142–3
    research studies 143
        biological marker 143
        epidemiological 143
        treatment 144–5
    treatment recommendations 147–9, 207
fluoxetine monotherapy 100, 102, 137, 270
fluoxetine-olanzapine combination (OFC) 137,
    138, 280
fMRI (functional MRI) 86, 87
Food and Drug Administration (FDA)
    approval of quetiapine 135
    and olanzapine-fluoxetine combination 137, 280
    warning against prescribing antidepressants
    26, 233
functional impairment 110, 113, 171
functional MRI (fMRI) 86, 87

gabapentin 125–6, 128, 274, 292–3
gender differences 80–1, 201–2
genetic factors 89
    gene expression and PUFAs 147
    genes implicated in mood disorders 22
glucose metabolism 87

high-risk activities and triggers 187
    identifying 185–7
'highs' *see* hypomania
Hippocratic psychopharmacology 272–3, 274
Holmes' Rule 274
hospitalisation criterion for BP I 49, 51, 56
hypomania 8
    behavioural symptoms, management of 161
    creativity experienced during 193, 205–6
    dangers of trivialising 262
    deciding whether to treat 122, 294
    and decision making 198
    diagnosis
        DSM–IV criteria 47–8, 61–2
        'hard' vs. 'soft' criteria 64
        ICD–10 criteria 48
        screening 24–7, 58–9
        see also questionnaires
    distinguishing from happiness 48, 57
    drill cores model 32–4
    duration of 47, 52, 59, 62, 65
    early warning signs 186
    features of 58
    frequency of recurrences 121, 234
    Kraepelin's description 61
    maladaptive behaviours 168–9
    management of 224–5
    medication
        antidepressant effects 97–9
        changes to 210
        impact of SSRIs 112, 113
        lithium treatment for acute 122
        managing without 121–2
        valproate treatment 122

prevalence rates 64
and risks of recurrent depression 252–4
see also mania
Hypomanic Checklist (HCL-32) 57

ICD–10 diagnostic system 48–9
identities, developing alternative 197
incidence of BP II, possible increase in younger
      patients 77–8, 81
Internet, using to improve awareness of
      BP II 31
interpersonal and social rhythm therapy (IPSRT)
      164–7
interpersonal stress in families ('Expressed
      Emotion') 162
ISIS-2 270
isomer model 55–8, 284, 286

'kindling' concept 39, 40, 41

lamotrigine 220, 262
    antidepressant effects of 279–80
    and comorbid disorders 128
    monotherapy
      negative results 125
      positive results 254
    and treatment of acute depression 124–5
lifetime prevalence *see* prevalence of bipolar
      disorders
Listening to Prozac (Kramer) 198
lithium 255, 279
    as a combined mood stabiliser 123
    and acute depression 123–4, 220
    effectiveness of 126–7
    prescription patterns 120
    reducing suicidality 126, 233–4
    with valproate for acute mania 122
    versus valproate for rapid cycling 127
long-term treatment 250–1
    and antidepressants 36, 41–2, 104
      destabilisation risks 39–40
      and relapse prevention 103–4
    concerns over 168, 172
    mood stabilisers 126–9
    and prevention 153
      recurrent depression 253–6

maintenance treatment 220, 234
    and antidepressants 103–4
    with atypical antipsychotics 222
    and hypomania 122
    and lamotrigine 222, 279–80, 290
    and mood stabilisers 126–9
    and omega-3 148
    single long-term study 271
major depression 11, 12, 217
    see also unipolar depression
maladaptive assumptions 159
management plans
    advice to patients 219–20
    involving family in 205

mania
    antidepressant effects 97–9
    diagnosis and DSM–IV criteria 16–17, 47–8
    early warning signs 186
    and melancholia, alternation of 5
    mood stabilisers for 122
    see also hypomania
manic-depression
    early cases of 6
    and family background 11
    first classification of 8, 222
    Kraepelin's work 8–9
    Leonhard's work 9–10
    usage of term 5
Manic-Depressive Illness (Goodwin and Jamison) 211
MBCT (Mindfulness-based Cognitive Therapy) 264
MDQ (Mood Disorders Questionnaire) 25, 26, 27,
      57, 219
medication 206, 220, 260, 266–7
    ambivalence about taking 205–6
    for bipolar depression 208–10, 223–4
    deciding not to take 198–9
    Hippocratic approach 272–3, 274
    Holmes' perspective 273–4
    for hypomania 210, 224–5
    inducing thirst 201
    lifetime history of 249
    mood stabilisation 206–8, 220–3
    non-compliance
      psychological strategies 172
      reasons for 168
    unorthodox 262
melancholia
    alternation with mania 5–7
    diagnosis of 12
    features of 54, 59
    see also unipolar depression
mercury poisoning from fish consumption 148
metabolites
    choline 88
    myoinositol 88
    N-acetylaspartate (NAA) 88
methodological limitations, Parker study 271
MHPG (3-Methoxy-4-hydroxyphenylglycol) 84
Mindfulness-based Cognitive Therapy (MBCT) 264
mindfulness techniques 192–3
misdiagnosis of BP II 62–3, 66, 70, 94, 218, 240, 247–8
mixed states/symptoms 20–2
    and antidepressants 38, 98
    and disability 66
    gender differences 66
    mixed depression 232–3, 234
    and suicidality 38–9, 233
    see also rapid cycling
modafinil 101, 224, 250
monoamine oxidase inhibitors (MAOIs) 99, 100
monopolar depression 10, 11
mood charting 167–8, 212–13, 226, 255–6
Mood Disorders Questionnaire (MDQ) 25, 26, 27,
      57, 219
'mood spectrum' 30, 42

mood stabilisation 262–3
  and atypical antipsychotics 207–8
  Bipolar II subtypes A and B 221–3
  choices of medication 266–7
  fish oil supplementation 207, 223
  with SSRIs 117–18, 207
mood stabilisers 129, 206–7, 290–1
  and acute depression 123–6
  anticonvulsants as 121
  antimanic action of 266
  complications of 37
  component of treatment regime 102
  definition of 121
  hypomania, management of 121–2
  as initial treatment strategy 249–50
  lack of controlled trials 120
  low doses 272
  in maintenance therapy 126–9
  prescription patterns 120
  selecting 279
  using prior to antidepressants 101–2
Moodswing (Fieve) 225
Mood Swings Questionnaire 49, 283
  outpatients study 50–4
  self-testing for 59–60
  sensitivity and specificity 57
  website study 49–50
motivational differences between BP I and BP II
    179–81
MR Spectroscopy 87–8
'multipolar disorder' 5–6

n-3 PUFAs (omega-3) 141
  biological marker studies 143
  and diet change 141–2
  epidemiological studies 143
  and hypomanic switching 145–6
  neuroscientific mechanisms 146–7
  treatment recommendations 147–9
n-6 PUFAs (omega-6)
  dietary recommendations 148
  increased levels in depressed patients 143
  increase in n-6/n-3 ratio 141–2, 143
  and rise in neurological disorders 142
National Comorbidity Survey (NCS) 18, 63–4,
    76, 77
National Comorbidity Survey Replication (NCS-R)
    69, 76, 77
National Institute for Health and Clinical Excellence
    (NICE) 121, 128
  guidelines 128
National Institute of Mental Health Systematic
    Treatment Enhancement Program for
    Bipolar Disorder (NIMH STEP-BD) 98, 99
negative thinking styles 159
neurobiology 83, 89–90
  chemistry
    3-Methoxy-4-hydroxyphenylglycol (MHPG) 84
    calcium 85
    Protein Kinase C (PKC) 84–5
  differences between BP I and BP II 286

genetic factors 89
n-3 PUFAs, effect on mood disorders 146–7
neurocognition 88–9
neuroimaging research 86
  functional neuroimaging studies 86–7
  MR Spectroscopy 87–8
  structural neuroimaging studies 86
neurocognitive deficits 88–9
NIMH STEP-BD 98, 99
non-drug management strategies 210–11, 225,
    293–4
  educational information 211–12, 225
  mood charting 226
  see also wellbeing plans
non-prescription drugs 200

olanzapine 136–7, 208–9, 222, 267
olanzapine-fluoxetine combination 137, 280
omega-3 fatty acids *see* n-3 PUFAs
omega-6 fatty acids *see* n-6 PUFAs
oxidative stress, causes of 148–9, 253

patient history 50, 68, 96
  Bipolarity Index 27–8
  and diagnosis 16–17
  and misdiagnosis 248
  prescribing information (PI) warning 26
  of prior medication 249
  see also family history
patient mood chart (PMC) 109–10, 111
personality/temperament 245–6
  SSRIs modifying 198
pharmaceutical industry, 'disease mongering' 30
phasic (periodic) psychoses 7, 9, 10, 11
PKC (Protein Kinase C) 84–5
pluralistic treatment approach 152, 215–16
PMC (patient mood chart) 109–10, 111
PMD *see* psychomotor disturbance
polarity debate 12–13
polarity vulnerability 238
polyunsaturated fats *see* PUFAs
'poop-out' phenomenon, antidepressants 103, 238
positron emission tomography (PET) 86–7
post hoc analyses 270
pramipexole 101, 224, 250
prevalence of bipolar disorders 62–5, 75
  and economic costs 70
  epidemiological studies 75–8
  and increased consumption of omega-6 142
  see also epidemiology
Protein Kinase C (PKC) 84–5
proton spectroscopy 87–8
psychoeducation 157–8, 164, 227
  randomised controlled trials 157, 242
  see also education
psychological interventions 151, 156–7, 173–4
  BP I vs. BP II 152
  Cognitive Behaviour Therapy 158–62
  engaging carers, friends and others 153
  Family Focused Therapy (FFT) 162–4, 227
  interpersonal and social rhythm therapy 164–7

for longstanding BP II 155–6
long-term aims 153
main strategies for BP II 152–3
managing specific phases
    acute symptoms 168–9
    early warning signs 167–8
    psychosocial issues 171–2
    relapse prevention 170–1
medication non-compliance 172
for newly diagnosed patient 153–5
pluralistic approach 152
psychoeducation 151–2, 157–8
psychosocial factors 152
and self-monitoring 151
and stage of illness 153
suicide prevention 173
and the therapeutic alliance 157
treatment compliance 172
see also psychotherapy
psychomotor disturbance (PMD) 54, 55, 59, 101, 280
    and anxious depression 96
    and mixed depression 233
psychosocial issues 171–2
    related to relapse 171
psychotherapy 214–15, 226–7, 263–4, 280
    see also psychological interventions
psychotic features 47, 49, 51
    distinguishing BP I from BP II 51–2, 55–6, 59
public awareness of BP II, increasing 30–1
PUFAs (polyunsaturated fatty acids)
    increase in n-6/n-3 ratio 141–2
    see also n-3 PUFAs (omega-3); n-6 PUFAs (omega-6)

quality of life, improving 192–4
questionnaires 25–6, 49–54, 59–60, 283–4
    see also Mood Disorders Questionnaire; Mood
        Swings Questionnaire
quetiapine 135–6, 255, 262, 263, 280
    for acute depression 224, 241–2, 245
    BOLDER study 260
    controlled data supporting 220
    first true mood stabiliser 267
    for rapid cycling 249

randomisation and sample size 271
RANZCP, Australian guidelines 245
rapid cycling 66, 237–8
    antidepressants
        contra-indicated 273
        effects of 98
        inducing 38, 107
    assessment methods 237
    DSM–IV definition of 116
    and lithium 127
    mood stabilisers for 127–8
    risks of 38–9, 66
    and SSRIs 118
    treatment-refractory 253
    versus non-rapid-cycling 272
recovery, meaning of 193
recreational drugs 199–200

relapse
    and antidepressants 103–4
    and CBT 263–4
    detection of early warning signs 167–8
    families reducing risk of 153
    and family-focused therapy 162, 227
    and IPSRT 165
    and lamotrigine monotherapy 280
    and Mindfulness-based Cognitive
        Therapy 264
    and medication cessation 168
    omega-3 treatment 148
    psychosocial factors 171
Research Diagnostic Criteria (RDC) 11
risperidone 136, 138

screening 283–4
    clinical screening 58–9
    questionnaires 25–6, 59–60
    see also diagnosis
seasons, effect on mood 199
selective serotonin reuptake inhibitors (SSRIs)
    advantages of 118
    for anxious depression 97
    effect on hypomanic episodes 108
    for mood stabilisation 207
        proof of concept study 108–16
            discussion 116–17
            methods 109–11
            results 111–16
    problems with 262
    subtle personality changes 198
Self-Assessment Test 59–60, 296–7
self-monitoring
    mindfulness techniques 192–3, 264
    of prodromal symptoms 167
    see also mood charting; Wellbeing plans
serotonin norepinephrine reuptake inhibitors
        (SNRIs) 103, 255
sertraline 40, 103, 250
side-effects
    lamotrigine and skin rash 254, 279
    mood stabilisers vs. SSRIs 117
    olanzapine 209
    reason for stopping medication 168
    SSRIs 114–16
single photon emission computed tomography
        (SPECT) 86–7
sleep-inducing drugs 200
sleep patterns 165
SNRIs see serotonin norepinephrine reuptake
        inhibitors
social rhythms, establishing regular/stable 165
soft bipolarity 18–20, 244–5
spectrum model of bipolar disorder 15, 282–3
    current diagnostic process 24–7
    diagnostic perspective 16–17
    evidence supporting 17–18
    inadequacy of DSM model 22–4
    and mixed states 20–2
    and soft bipolarity 18–20

spectrum model of bipolar disorder (cont.)
    solutions to DSM-based approach 27–34
    treatment implications 35–42
SSRIs *see* selective serotonin reuptake inhibitors
Stanley Bipolar Network 97, 98
structural neuroimaging studies 86
substance use, management of 199–200
sub-syndromal symptoms and improved
        functioning 66
sub-threshold bipolarity 18, 23, 42, 69–70
suicidality
    and antidepressants 38–9, 99
    and FDA warning 233
    and mixed symptoms/rapid cycling 66
    psychological intervention 173
    reduced by lithium 126, 233–4
    risk higher for BP II 65
    surviving suicidal thoughts 202–3
survival strategies 195–6
    adopting alternative identities 197
    choices about medication 198–9
    deferring major decisions 198
    developing the 'bipolar personality' 196–7
    losing weight 200–1
    stressful events, monitoring 199
    substance use, management of 199–200
    suicidal thoughts 202–3
    women and BP II 201–2
switching 237–8
    assessment methodologies 237
    and class of antidepressant 288–9
    induced by antidepressants 37–8, 107–8
    and n-3 PUFAs 145–6
    see also rapid cycling

TEAS (treatment-emergent affective switch) 217,
        223, 278–9, 280
topiramate 126, 128
treatment
    for comorbid conditions 251
    compliance with, strategies for 172
    duration of 250–1
    evidence base for 245
    extrapolation from BP I 245
    general principles 241–2
    guidelines 135
    implications of spectrum perspective 35–42
    and long-term prevention of depression 253
    medication non-compliance 172
    n-3 PUFA 144–5
    pluralistic approach 152, 215–16
    polypharmacy for mood stabilisation 128–9
    and response to previous medication 249
    for 'soft bipolar spectrum' 245–6
    stopping ineffective 251
    see also long-term treatment; medication
treatment-emergent affective switch (TEAS) 217,
        223, 278–9, 280
treatment resistant depression (TRD) 271–2
tricyclic antidepressant monotherapy, non-efficacy
        of 222

unipolar depression 10–11, 12, 17–18
    antidepressants 250
    assessment 51
    continuum controversy 259
    fluoxetine response 270
    health risks of recurrent 252
    prevalence 64–5, 76
    see also antidepressants; depression; major
        depression
Unquiet Mind, An (Jamison) 211

valproate 121, 279, 290
    and alcohol dependence 128
    and Borderline Personality Disorder 128
    compared with lithium for rapid-cycling
        BP 127
    with lithium
        reducing acute mania 122
        reducing depression 124
    monotherapy 124, 255
    see also mood stabilisers
vegetarians, sources of omega-3 for 148
venlafaxine 208, 250
    dose effects 103
    monotherapy 102
        mood stabilising benefits 108, 207
        and rapid cycling 98–9, 118
    risk of TEAS 223, 278
    and switching risk 288–9
vitamin supplements 149

weight gain 200–1
Wellbeing plans 177–9, 213–14, 226
    checklist 182
    collaboration, benefits of 191–2
    early intervention 189, 190
    early warning signs
        for depression 186
        feedback on 188–9
        for hypomania/mania 186
        identifying 185
    finding motivation for 181–3
    individual differences in 191
    involving others 183–4
    motivational differences between BP I and BP II
        179–81
    past efforts by others, debriefing 184–5
    Plans A and B 188
    quality of life commitment 190, 192–4
    recovery, aim for stages of 190–1
    relationship strengths and weaknesses
        189–90
    risk factors and triggers, identifying 185–7
    safety measures 189
    secrets of managing bipolar disorder 192
women, higher rates of BP II Disorder 201–2
World Health Organization (WHO) 133, 259

ziprasidone 280
'zones of rarity' 17–18
Zurich Cohort Study 76–7